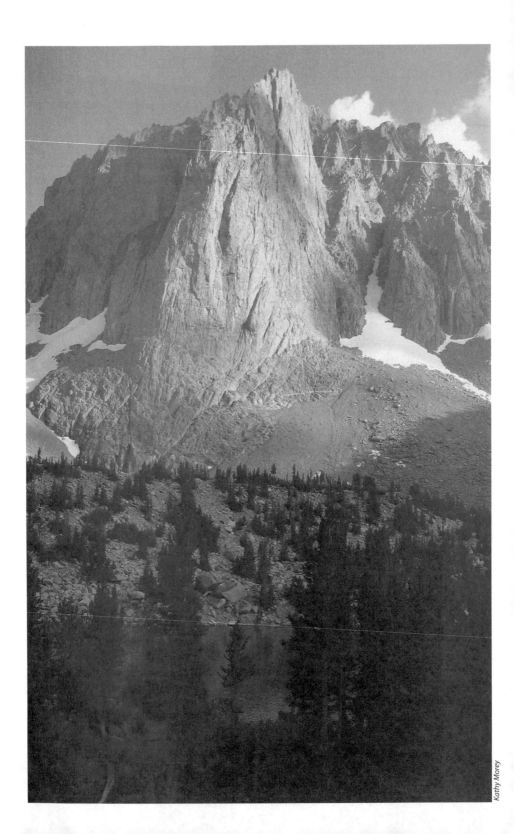

SIERRA SOUTH

BACKCOUNTRY TRIPS IN CALIFORNIA'S SIERRA NEVADA

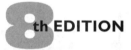 **th EDITION**

**KATHY MOREY
& MIKE WHITE**
with **STACY CORLESS, ANALISE ELLIOT,
CHRIS TIRRELL & THOMAS WINNETT**

 WILDERNESS PRESS ... *on the trail since 1967*

Sierra South: Backcountry Trips in California's Sierra Nevada

8th EDITION 2006
  6th printing 2016

Front cover photo copyright © 2006 by Dan Patitucci/PatitucciPhoto
Interior photos, except where noted, by the authors
Maps: Bart Wright/Lohnes+Wright
Book & cover design: Larry B. Van Dyke, Lisa Pletka
Book editor: Eva Dienel

ISBN: 978-0-89997-414-9

Manufactured in United States of America

Published by: **Wilderness Press**
                Keen Communications
                2204 First Avenue South, Suite 102
                Birmingham, AL 35233
                (800) 443-7227; FAX (205) 326-1012
                info@wildernesspress.com
                www.wildernesspress.com

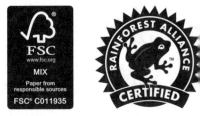

Visit our website for a complete listing of our books and for ordering information.

Distributed by Publishers Group West

Cover photo: Mt. Mendel at sunset
Frontispiece: Temple Crag above Third Lake (Trip 71)

SAFETY NOTICE: Although Wilderness Press and the author have made every attempt to ensure that the information in this book is accurate at press time, they are not responsible for any loss, damage, injury, or inconvenience that may occur to anyone while using this book. You are responsible for your own safety and health while in the wilderness. The fact that a trail is described in this book does not mean that it will be safe for you. Be aware that trail conditions can change from day to day. Always check local conditions and know your own limitations.

ACKNOWLEDGMENTS

My thanks as always to my husband, Ed Schwartz, for his support. My thanks to Tom Winnett for inspiration, opportunity, and guidance. I'm grateful to my co-authors for their enthusiasm and support during this project. Thanks also to (in alphabetical order) J. Brian Anderson, Walt Lehmann, Steven K. Schuster, and Marshalle F. Wells for the fine photos they generously submitted. I would like to also acknowledge the forbearance of the long-suffering staff at Wilderness Press, particularly Eva Dienel and Roslyn Bullas. —KM

Working with Kathy Morey on this project proved to be quite enjoyable. As usual, thanks go to Eva Dienel and the staff at Wilderness Press for their stellar efforts. I greatly appreciated the company of Keith Catlin and Jered Singleton on the trail. —MW

Many thanks to Debbie Clausen for sharing all those trail miles; my husband, Charlie Byrne; Mark Clausen for the long drive on Beasore Road; the helpful rangers at Clover Meadows for their advice and concern; and Kathy Morey for her expert guidance. —SC

Enthusiasm, support, and accompaniment from my friends and family were indispensable. Without my parents' continual belief in my capabilities, my work on this book would not be possible. My gratitude to my best friend, fellow natural-world enthusiast, and life partner John Heid. Sharing most of the trips with powerful and inspiring women, Allison Wickland and Leah Edwards, provided hours of conversation and entertainment on the trails. Many thanks to Matt Heid for his inspiration and enthusiasm for outdoor writing. To Deborah Walker for her incredible flexibility and support. I would also like to acknowledge Eva Dienel, Roslyn Bullas, Mike White, and the staff at Wilderness Press for their ability to create stellar books cover to cover. And lastly, thanks to Kathy Morey for the opportunity to fall in love with the Southern Sierra. —AE

I would like to thank Kathy Morey for all her help and encouragement. Many thanks also to my hiking partners, Dennis Kim and Elizabeth Wall. A big thank you to Eva Dienel as well for getting me involved in the book! —CT

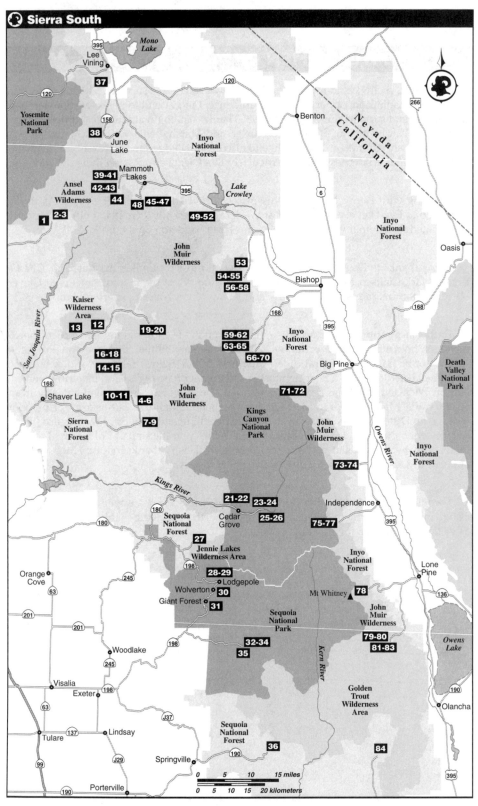

CONTENTS

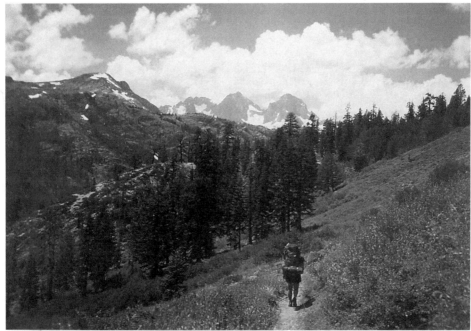

Analise Elliot

The High Trail is one of the Sierra's most scenic trails, with unforgettable views of the Ritter Range and Sierra Crest (Trip 40).

GOING HIGH TO GET HIGH
By Thomas Winnett, Wilderness Press Founder

As I write this, it is nearly 40 years since we at Wilderness Press held a celebration to promote the first edition of *Sierra North* and the upcoming *Sierra South*, one-of-a-kind books Karl Schwenke and I wrote to recommend 100 of the best backpacking trips into the northern Sierra and 100 into the southern Sierra.

It was the summer of 1967, and we celebrated in the backcountry with a high-altitude cocktail party. We invited everyone we thought would help get the word out about the book—people from the Sierra Club, outdoor writers, and friends. We held it in August, in Dusy Basin, in the eastern Sierra, 8 miles from the nearest car. The hike went over a 12,000-foot pass, so we were delighted when 15 people showed up. It was a real party. We used snow to make our martinis, ate hors d'oeuvres, and spent the night. In a mention of the event, *San Francisco Chronicle* columnist Herb Caen wondered, "How high can you get to get high?"

It was a spectacular occasion not only because we were launching the books, but because we were starting a new company. We founded Wilderness Press in 1965. Karl, a backpacking friend of mine, and I had been complaining about how hard it was to get accurate information about the out of doors. At the time, there were only one or two guidebooks to the Sierra—our favorite place—so we decided to write our own. We planned to create pre-packaged trips that specified which trails to take and where to stop each night. We would do a series of small books, each covering a 15-minute quadrangle, and they would be called the *Knapsacker/Packer Guide Series*.

In the summer of 1966, we started doing the field research. Our approach was simple: We wanted to accurately describe where the trails led and what was there. On my scouting trips, I carried more than your average backpacker. In addition to all the standard gear, I packed two cameras, two natural history books to help me indentify flowers and birds, and my Telmar tape recorder. The tape recorder ran about half the speed of the recording devices that are available today, and I'd walk along, dictating into the microphone everything I thought our customers would be interested in reading. So in addition to the basics—how to get to where you start walking, where to go, and the best campsites—we also described what we saw, the animals, flowers, birds, and trees.

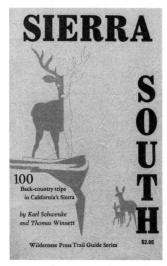

By the end of the summer, we had enough material to cover most of the trails in the northern Sierra, so we published a book of 100 trails and called it *Sierra North*. Next, we set about work on *Sierra South*, which we published in 1968.

The first edition of *Sierra South* sold like the proverbial hotcakes; we sold out our entire print run of 3000 books. Since then, this book has sold more than 140,000 copies, and it gives me great joy to see it in its eighth edition. As I think back to that high-altitude cocktail party in 1967, I wonder how many people have used this book to "go high to get high" in the Sierra. I have personally walked more than 2000 miles in this most beautiful of mountain ranges, and although I can't do that anymore, I am still hooked on the experience—the splendid isolation, the scenery that really lights up your eyeballs, the strength you feel climbing with the weight of your pack on your back, the myriad trout. I hope this guidebook hooks you, too.

TRIP CROSS-REFERENCE TABLE

TRIP NO.	OUT & BACK	SHUTTLE	LOOP	SEMILOOP	EARLY	MID	LATE	HIKING DAYS	MILEAGE	RECOMMENDED FOR BEGINNERS
		TRIP TYPE				BEST SEASON				
1				•		•	•	3	13.5	•
2				•		•	•	2	11	•
3			•			•	•	4	29	
4				•		•		4	26	
5	•					•		6	41	
6				•	•	•		4	25	
7	•					•		2	15	•
8	•					•		6	40	
9				•		•		6	34	
10	•					•		2	10	•
11				•		•		3	20	
12	•					•	•	2	9.4	•
13			•			•	•	2	21	
14	•					•	•	6	38/46	
15	•					•	•	6	43.5/51.5	
16				•		•	•	5	39	
17	•					•	•	4	33	
18		•				•	•	4	28.5/32.5	
19	•					•	•	4	16.8	•
20		•				•	•	3	19	
21	•					•	•	4	26	
22		•				•	•	6	31/33	
23	•				•		•	3	23	
24		•				•	•	7	51	
25	•					•	•	4	31	
26				•		•	•	6	41.75	
27				•	•	•		3	18.2	•
28	•					•	•	2	20	
29				•		•	•	12	110.4	
30	•					•	•	2	13	•
31		•				•	•	9	67	
32	•					•	•	2	17	
33	•					•	•	6	44	
34			•			•	•	6	40.5	
35	•					•	•	6	28	
36	•					•	•	4	19.8	
37	•					•	•	2	6.6	•
38				•	•	•		3	21	
39				•		•	•	2	17.6	
40			•			•	•	2	17.6	
41	•					•	•	2	14	•
42	•					•	•	2	16	

TRIP NO.	OUT & BACK	SHUTTLE	LOOP	SEMILOOP	EARLY	MID	LATE	HIKING DAYS	MILEAGE	RECOMMENDED FOR BEGINNERS
43			•			•	•	3	16.5	•
44				•	•	•	•	6	45	
45				•		•	•	4	25.5/26.5	
46		•			•	•	•	4	28	
47		•				•	•	3	17.4	•
48			•			•		2	15	
49	•					•	•	2	12	•
50				•			•	5	26	
51	•					•	•	2	14	•
52		•				•	•	5	30.6	
53		•				•	•	2	12/13	
54	•					•	•	2	6.6	•
55	•					•	•	4	19	
56	•					•	•	2	9.5	
57				•		•	•	4	17.75	
58				•		•	•	3	19.5	
59	•					•	•	2	14.4	
60	•					•	•	2	5.4	•
61	•					•	•	3	14	
62			•			•	•	6	39	
63		•				•	•	2	7.7	
64	•					•	•	2	13	•
65	•					•	•	2	9	
66	•					•	•	2	5	•
67				•		•	•	2	7.1	•
68	•					•	•	2	14	
69				•		•	•	6	37.5	
70		•				•	•	8	52.7	
71				•		•	•	3	15.4	
72	•					•	•	2	8.5	
73	•				•			2	16	
74	•					•	•	6	46	
75	•				•	•		2	5	•
76	•					•	•	6	27	
77	•					•	•	6	33	
78	•					•	•	5	22	
79				•		•	•	2	10.3	
80			•			•	•	4	23.3	
81		•				•	•	7	34.7	
82		•				•	•	9	54.5	
83	•					•	•	4	27	
84				•		•	•	3	20	

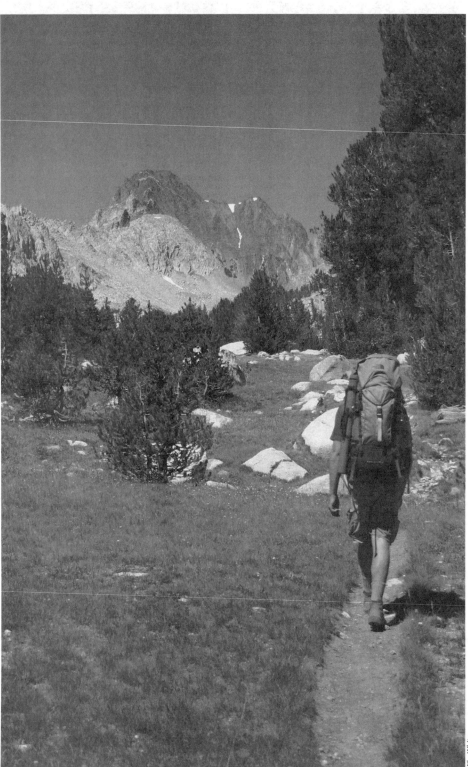

INTRODUCTION

Welcome to what we think is just about the most spectacular mountain range in the contiguous 48 states. The Sierra Nevada is a hiker's paradise filled with its hundreds of miles of wilderness uninterrupted by roads, hundreds of miles of trails, thousands of lakes, countless rugged peaks and canyons, vast forests, giant sequoias, and terrain ranging from deep, forested river valleys to sublime, treeless alpine country.

Updates for the Eighth Edition

Welcome, too, to the eighth edition of Wilderness Press's *Sierra South*. For this edition, we have some new co-authors, and we've taken a radically different approach to organizing the trips. This book is divided first into the Sierra's west and east sides and second, within the west and east sides, into road sections so you can easily locate your favorite part of the southern Sierra. Each road section includes trailheads that serve as starting points for the many individual trips in the book. Additionally, each trailhead includes a map showing every trip launching from that point, and each trip includes an elevation profile. We've also incorporated Global Positioning System (GPS) data as UTM coordinates into our trips for GPS users. We think these changes reflect the way in which you'll actually use this book better than previous editions have.

Sierra South now spans the Sierra from the southern boundary of Yosemite National Park and from Yosemite's eastern boundary south of Hwy. 120 (the Tioga Road) to the Sherman Pass area, covering a greater north-south region than previous editions. This region includes the true High Sierra, with its abundance of dramatic, above-treeline granite peaks and basins. As of its ninth edition, this book's sister, *Sierra North*, covers the Sierra from Yosemite north through the Tahoe area to I-80 and the proposed Castle Peak Wilderness just north of I-80.

Unlike the region covered by *Sierra North*, in the territory this book covers, no roads cross the range between Hwy. 120 on the north and the network of roads that cross Sherman Pass, a distance of some 140 air miles to the south. However, along those 140 air miles, many roads penetrate the range from its west and east sides, and these are the roads you'll use to get to trailheads in this book. The book's first major trip section covers the region's west side and presents roads into the west side from north to south. The second major trip section covers the Sierra's east side and, also from north to south, the roads into the range from the east.

If you have used previous editions of *Sierra South*, you'll find many of your old favorite trips here, as well as some wonderful new ones. Our coverage now includes Dinkey Lakes, Kaiser, and Jennie Lakes wildernesses, in addition to Ansel Adams, John Muir, and Golden Trout wildernesses. Most longer trips can be abbreviated to create fine, shorter ones, and many can be linked to other trips to create multiweek adventures. As before, this edition includes the must-see High Sierra Trail (now Trip 31).

It's our hope that this new edition will help you enjoy our superb southern Sierra as well as give you an incentive to work to preserve it.

We appreciate hearing from our readers. One of our goals is to keep improving these books for you. Please let us know what did and didn't work for you in this new edition and about changes you find. We're at 1200 5th St., Berkeley, CA 94710; mail@wilderness-press.com; 800-443-7227; 510-558-1666; fax 510-558-1696. Please visit us online at www.wildernesspress.com.

opposite: **Backpacker on the McGee Creek Trail (Trips 49–52)**

Care and Enjoyment of the Mountains

Be a Good Guest

The Sierra is home—the only home—to a spectacular array of plants and animals. We humans are merely guests—uninvited ones at that. Be a careful, considerate guest in this grandest of Nature's homes.

About a million people camp in the Sierra wilderness each year. The vast majority of us cares about the wilderness and tries to protect it, but it is threatened by some who still need to learn the art of living lightly on the land. The solution depends on each of us. We can minimize our impact. The saying, "Take only memories (or photos), leave only footprints," sums it up.

Learn to Go Light

John Muir, traveling along the crest of the Sierra in the 1870s with little more that his overcoat and his pockets full of biscuits was the archetype.

Muir's example may be too extreme for many, but we think he might have appreciated modern lightweight equipment and food as a great convenience. A lot of the stuff that goes into the mountains is burdensome, harmful to the wilderness, or just plain annoying to other people seeking peace and solitude. Please leave behind anything that is obtrusive or that can be used to modify the terrain: gas lanterns, radios, hatchets, gigantic tents, etc.

Carry Out Your Trash

You packed that foil and those cans and bags in when full; you can pack them out empty. Never litter or bury your trash.

Sanitation

Eliminate body wastes at least 100 feet, and preferably 200 feet, from lakes, streams, trails, and campsites. Bury feces at least 6 inches deep wherever possible. Intestinal pathogens can survive for years in feces when they're buried, but burial reduces the chances that critters will come in contact with them and carry pathogens into the water. Where burial is not possible due to lack of enough soil or gravel, leave feces where they will receive maximum exposure to heat and sunlight to hasten the destruction of pathogens. Also help reduce the waste problem in the backcountry by packing out your used toilet paper, facial tissues, tampons, sanitary napkins, and diapers. It's easy to carry them out in a heavy-duty, self-sealing plastic bag.

Protect the Water

Just because something is "biodegradable," like some soaps, doesn't mean it's okay to put it in the water. In addition, the fragile sod of meadows, lakeshores, and streamsides is rapidly disappearing from the High Sierra. Pick "hard" campsites, sandy places that can stand the use. Camp at least 200 feet from water unless that's absolutely impossible; in no case camp closer than 25 feet. Don't make campsite "improvements" like rock walls, bough beds, new fireplaces, or tent ditches.

Avoid Campfires

Use a modern, lightweight backpacking stove. (If you use a gas-cartridge stove, be sure to pack your used cartridges out.) Campfires waste a precious resource: wood that would otherwise shelter animals and, upon falling and decaying, return vital nutrients to the soil. Campfires also run the risk of starting forest fires.

Exercise special care when using an ultra-lightweight alcohol stove, as its flames tend to be uncontrollable when the pot is off the burning stove. Be sure the area is cleared for at least a cubic yard of flammable materials above, around, and below the stove.

If your stove fails and you must cook over a campfire in order to survive, here are some guidelines: If possible, camp in an established site with an existing fireplace you can use.

If you must build a fireplace, build with efficiency and restoration in mind: two to four medium-sized rocks set parallel along the sides of a narrow, shallow trench in a sandy place. Set the pot on the rocks and over the fire, which you can feed with small sticks and twigs (use only dead and downed wood). Never leave the fire unattended. Before you leave, thoroughly extinguish the fire and pour water over the ashes, and then restore the site by scattering the rocks and filling the trench.

To use a stove or have a campfire where legal, you must have a California Campfire Permit. One such permit is good for the season. Your wilderness permit can double as your California Campfire Permit. If you're taking a trip that doesn't require a wilderness permit, you still need a California Campfire Permit, available at any ranger station.

Respect the Wildlife

Avoid trampling on nests, burrows, or other homes of animals. Observe all fishing limits and keep shorelines clean and clear of litter. If angling, use biodegradable line and never leave any of it behind. If you come across an animal, just quietly observe it. Above all, don't go near any nesting animals and their young. Get "close" with binoculars or telephoto lenses.

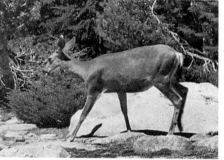
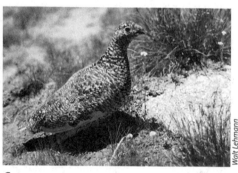

Deer

Grouse

Safety and Well Being

Hiking in the high country is far safer than driving to the mountains, and a few precautions can shield you from most of the discomforts and dangers that could threaten you.

Health Hazards

Altitude Sickness: If you normally live at sea level and come to the Sierra to hike, it may take your body several days to acclimate. Starved of your accustomed oxygen, for a few days you may experience shortness of breath even with minimal activity, severe headaches, or nausea. The best solutions are to spend time at altitude before you begin your hike and to plan a very easy first day. On your hike, light, frequent meals are best.

Giardia and Cryptosporidium: Giardiasis is a serious gastrointestinal disease caused by a waterborne protozoan, *Giardia lamblia*. Any mammal (including humans) can become infected. It will then excrete live giardia in its feces, from which the protozoan can get into even the most remote sources of water, such as a stream issuing from a glacier. Giardia can survive in snow through the winter and in cold water as a cyst resistant to the usual chemical treatments. Giardiasis can be contracted by drinking untreated water. Symptoms appear two to three weeks after exposure.

Cryptosporidium is another, smaller, very hardy pest that causes a disease similar to giardiasis. It's been found in the streams of the San Gabriel Mountains of Los Angeles, and it is spreading throughout Southern California. Probably it will eventually infest Sierra waters.

At this time, boiling and filtering are the only sure backcountry defenses against giardia and cryptosporidium. Bring water to a rolling boil; this is easy to do while you're cooking and is now judged effective at any Sierra altitude. To be effective against both giardia and the much-smaller cryptosporidium, a filter must trap particles down to 0.4 micron.

Halogen treatments (iodine, chlorine) are ineffective against cryptosporidium and hard to use properly against giardia—but they are better than no treatment at all. There

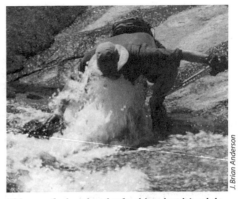

This may *feel* cool and refreshing, but it's advisable to filter or boil water before drinking it.

are chlorine-dioxide water treatments available for backpackers as well as a device that claims to zap the bugs. The chlorine-dioxide treatments reportedly take 30 minutes to kill giardia and four hours to kill cryptosporidia. Consider these treatments as back-up systems—to use only when boiling or filtering isn't possible; use only as directed.

Hypothermia: Hypothermia refers to subnormal body temperature. More hikers die from hypothermia than from any other single cause. Caused by exposure to cold, often intensified by wet, wind, and weariness, the first symptoms of hypothermia are uncontrollable shivering and imperfect motor coordination. These are rapidly followed by loss of judgment, so that you yourself cannot make the decisions to protect your own life. Death by "exposure" is death by hypothermia.

To prevent hypothermia, stay warm: Carry wind- and rain-protective clothing, and put it on as soon as you feel chilly. Stay dry: Carry or wear wool or a suitable synthetic (not cotton) against your skin, and bring raingear, even for a short hike on an apparently sunny day. If weather conditions threaten and you are inadequately prepared, flee or hunker down.

Treat shivering at once: Get the victim out of the wind and wet, replace all wet clothes with dry ones, put him or her in a sleeping bag, and give him or her warm drinks. If the shivering is severe and accompanied by other symptoms, strip him or her and yourself (and a third party if possible), and warm him or her with your own bodies, tightly wrapped in a dry sleeping bag.

Lightning: Although the odds of being struck are very small, almost everyone who goes to the mountains thinks about it. If a thunderstorm comes upon you, avoid exposed places—mountain peaks, mountain ridges, open fields, a boat on a lake—and also avoid small caves and rock overhangs. The safest place is an opening or a clump of small trees in a forest.

The best body stance is one that minimizes the area your body touches the ground. You should drop to your knees and put your hands on your knees. This is because the more area your body covers, the more chance that ground currents will pass through it. Also make sure to get all metal—such as frame packs, tent poles, etc.—away from you.

If you get struck by lightning, there isn't much you can do except pray that someone in your party is adept at CPR—or at least adept at artificial respiration if your breathing has stopped but not your heart. It may take hours for a victim to resume breathing on his or her own. If your companions are victims, attend first to those who are not moving. Those who are rolling around and moaning are at least breathing. Finally, a victim who lives should be evacuated to a hospital, because other problems often develop in lightning victims.

Wildlife Hazards

Rattlesnakes: They occur at lower elevations (they are rarely seen above 7000 feet but have been seen up to 9000 feet) in a range of habitats, but most commonly near riverbeds and streams. Their bite is rarely fatal to an adult, but a bite that carries venom may still cause extensive tissue damage.

If you are bitten, get to a hospital as soon as possible. There is no substitute for proper medical treatment.

Some people carry a snakebite kit such as Sawyer's extractor when traveling in remote areas far from help and where snake encounters are more likely: below 6000 feet along a watercourse. This kit is somewhat effective if used properly within 30 minutes after the bite—but it's still no substitute for hospital care.

Better yet, don't get bitten: Watch where you place your hands and feet; listen for the rattle. If you hear a snake rattle, stand still long enough to determine where it is, then leave in the opposite direction.

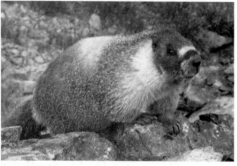

Walt Lehmann

Marmot

Rodents and Birds: Marmots live from about 6000 feet to 11,500 feet. Because they are curious, always hungry, and like to sun themselves on rocks in full view, you are likely to see them. Marmots enjoy many foods you do, including cereal and candy (especially chocolate). They may eat through a pack or tent when other entry is difficult. Marmots cannot climb trees or ropes, so you can protect your food by hanging it (though this is illegal in some areas because of bears). Smaller, climbing rodents might get into hung food. We've heard reports of jays pecking their way into bags, too. Sealed bear canisters are excellent protection against all kinds of rodents, birds, and insects. (Please see page 6 for information about bears.)

Mosquitoes: Insect repellent containing N, N diethylmeta-toluamide, known commercially as deet, will keep them off. Don't buy one without a minimum of about 30% deet. Studies show adults can use deet in moderation, but it is dangerous for children. To minimize the amount of deet on your skin, apply it to your clothes and/or hat instead—but test first to be sure that deet won't damage the garment.

A newer, time-release deet preparation works well and is much less objectionable than straight deet; however, it may be more expensive. Try this if you can't abide straight deet.

Most non-deet and low-deet repellents work much more poorly than those with 30% deet or more, and electronic repellents are useless. Clothing may also act as a bar to mosquitoes—a good reason for wearing long pants and a long-sleeved shirt. If you are a favorite target for mosquitoes (they have their preferences), you might take a head net—a hat with netting suspended all around the brim and a snug neckband.

A tent with mosquito netting makes a world of difference during mosquito season (typically, through late July). Planning your trip to avoid the height of the mosquito season is also a good preventive.

Terrain Hazards

Snow Bridges and Cornices: Stay off them.

Streams: In early season, when the snow is melting, crossing a river can be the most dangerous part of a backpack trip. Later, ordinary caution will see you across safely. If a river is running high, you should cross it only there is no safer alternative, you have found a suitable place to ford, and you use a rope—but don't tie into it; just hold onto it.

Here are some suggestions for stream-crossing:

- If a stream is dauntingly high or swift, forget it. Turn around and come back later, perhaps in late summer or early fall, when flows reach seasonal lows.
- Wear closed-toe shoes, which will protect your feet from injury and give them more secure placement.
- Cross in a stance in which you're angled upstream. If you face downstream, the water pushing against the back of your knees could cause them to buckle.
- Move one foot only when the other is firmly placed.
- Keep your legs apart for a more stable stance. You'll find a cross-footed stance unstable even in your own living room, much less in a Sierra torrent.
- One or two hiking sticks will help keep you stable while crossing. You can also use a stick to probe ahead for holes and other obstacles that may be difficult to see and judge under running water.
- One piece of advice used to be that you should unfasten your pack's hip belt in case you fell in and had to jettison the pack. However, modern quick-release buckles probably make this precaution unnecessary. Keeping the hip belt fastened will keep the pack more stable, and this will, in turn, help your stability. You may wish, however, to unfasten the sternum strap so that you have only one buckle to worry about.

The Bear Problem

The bears of the Sierra are American black bears; their coats range from black to light brown. Unless provoked, they're not usually aggressive, and their normal diet consists largely of plants. The suggestions in this section apply only to American black bears, not to the more aggressive grizzly bear, which is extinct in California.

American black bears run and climb faster than you ever will, they are immensely stronger, and they are very intelligent. Long ago, they learned to associate humans with easy sources of food. Now, keeping your food away from the local bears is a problem. Remember, though, that they aren't interested in eating you. Don't let the possibility of meeting a bear keep you out of the Sierra. Respect these magnificent creatures. Learn what you can do to keep yourself and your food safe. Some suggestions follow.

Bears—Any Time, Anywhere: You may encounter bears anywhere in the areas this book covers. If they present special problems on that trip, we mention them in the "Heads Up!" paragraph of that trip. Bears are normally daytime creatures, but they've learned that our supplies are easier to raid when we're asleep, so they're working the night shift, too. Also, it used to be that you rarely saw bears above 8000 to 9000 feet. As campers moved into the higher elevations, the bears followed.

To avoid bears while hiking, some people make noise as they go, because most American black bears are shy and will scramble off to avoid meeting you. Other people find noise-making intrusive, consider those who make noise rude, and accept the risk of meeting a bear. You will have to decide.

In camp, store your food properly and always scare bears away immediately. (See Food Storage, page 7.)

Plan Ahead: Avoid taking smelly foods and fragrant toiletries; they attract bears—bears have a superb sense of smell. Ask rangers and other backpackers where there are bear problems, and avoid those areas; also ask them what measures they take to safeguard food and chase bears away.

Carry a bear canister (see more below). If you need to counterbalance your food bags, practice the skill before you need it. After cooking, clean up food residue. Before going to sleep or leaving your camp, clean any food out of your gear and store it with the rest of your chow; otherwise, you could lose a pack to a bear that went for the granola bar you forgot in a side pocket. Don't take food into your tent or sleeping bag unless you want ursine company. Store your smelly toiletries and garbage just as carefully as you store your food. Set up and use your kitchen at a good distance from the rest of your camp. Also make sure your food, even in canisters, is stored a good distance from your campsite.

Food Storage: Backcountry management policies now hold campers responsible for keeping their food away from bears. You can even be fined for violating food-storage rules. You're also responsible for cleaning up the mess once you're sure the bear won't be back for seconds. And you have an ethical responsibility to keep bears from becoming pests, which may mean that they have to be killed.

Here are some food-storage suggestions that will help you do this:

- **Bear Canisters:** The first ones were lengths of sturdy plastic pipe fitted with a bottom and a lid only a human can open. Today there are several more choices, including lighter-weight aluminum ones and still lighter ones of exotic aerospace materials. Using these canisters is the best method for protecting your food where bear boxes (below) aren't available.

  Canisters aren't perfect, but they work very well when used properly. Using a canister is much easier and more secure than counterbalance bearbagging. They make good in-camp seats, too.

  There's also an extremely lightweight sack of bulletproof material, now available with an aluminum liner and with an odor-barrier inner sack. It is less secure than a canister, is slightly more difficult to use properly (but much easier than counterbalancing), and may not be approved for use in areas that require you to use a canister, like Sequoia and Kings Canyon national parks. You can check online or call the controlling agency(ies) to see if the areas through which you plan to pass permit use of these sacks. One of us has had good luck with them.

  The materials you receive with your permit will tell you whether canisters are required. If you don't own a canister, you can rent one from either an outdoors store or perhaps from the agency that issues your permit.

- **Counterbalance Bearbagging:** If you don't have a bear-resistant food canister or access to a bear box where you camp, counterbalance your food. Note that in areas with severe bear problems, like most of Sequoia and Kings Canyon national parks, counterbalance bearbagging is ineffective and probably against regulations.

  Assuming you're traveling in an area where bears aren't yet a severe problem, counterbalance bearbagging may protect your food not only from bears but from ground squirrels, marmots, and other creatures. It's best to get to camp early enough to get your food hung while there's light to do it. Counterbalancing is not completely secure, but it may slow the bear down. It gives you time to scare it away. When you get a permit, you may get a sheet on the counterbalance bearbagging technique. The technique is also well-covered in numerous how-to-backpack books. Practice it at home before you go.

  If a bear goes after your food, jump up and down, make a lot of noise, wave your arms—anything to make yourself seem huge, noisy, and scary. Have a stash of rocks to throw and throw them at trees and boulders to make more noise. Bang pots together. Blow whistles. The object is to scare the bear away. Never directly attack the bear itself. Note, however, that some human-habituated bears simply can't be scared off.

- **Bear Boxes (Food Storage Lockers):** Bear boxes are large steel lockers intended for storage of food only, and they will hold the food bags of several backpackers. Their latches, simple for humans, are inoperable by bears. Everyone shares the bear box; you may not put your own locks on one. Food in a properly fastened bear box is safe from bears; however, some boxes have holes in the bottom, through which, if the holes aren't plugged, mice will squeeze in to nibble on your goodies.

There are bear boxes at popular areas in Sequoia National Park and southern Kings Canyon National Park. Their locations and numbers, as well as regulations and a list of approved bear canisters, are available at or through links at www.nps.gov/seki/snrm/wildlife/food_storage.htm.

The presence of a bear box attracts campers as well as bears, and campsites around them can become overused. However, it isn't necessary for everyone to cluster right around the box. A campsite a few hundred yards away may be more secluded and desirable; the stroll to and from the bear box is a pleasant way to start and end a meal.

Bear-box don'ts: Never use a bear box as a garbage can! Rotting food is smelly and very attractive to bears. Never use a bear box as a food drop; its capacity is needed for people actually camping in its vicinity. Never leave a bear box unlatched or open, even when people are around.

- *Above timberline:* Up above the tree line, there are no trees to hang your food bags from. But there are still bears—as well as mice, marmots, and ground squirrels—anxious to share your chow. If you don't have a canister or bulletproof sack (the latter only where legal) but must hang your food, look for a tall rock with an overhanging edge, from which you can dangle your food bags high off the ground and well away from the face of the rock. Unlike bears, marmots and other critters have not learned to get your food by eating through the rope suspending it.

Another option is to bag your food and push it deep into a crack in the rocks too small and too deep for a bear to reach into—but be sure you can still retrieve it. One of us has had good luck with this technique; use it only above timberline. You may lose a little food to mice or ground squirrels, but it won't be much.

When dayhiking from a base camp where you can't put your food in a bear box or leave it in a canister, it's safer to take as much of it with you as you can.

If a Bear Gets Your Food: Never try to get your food back from a bear. It's the bear's food now, and the bear will defend it aggressively against puny you. You may hear that there are no recorded fatalities in bear-human encounters in recent Sierra history. Of course, this isn't true: Plenty of bears have been killed as a result of repeated encounters. Every time a bear gets some human food, that bear is a step closer to becoming a nuisance bear that has to be killed. And there have been very serious, though not fatal, injuries to humans in these encounters.

If, despite your best efforts, you lose your food to a bear, it may be the end of your trip but not of the world. You won't starve to death in the maximum three to four days it will take you to walk out from even the most remote Sierra spot. Your pack is now much lighter. And you can probably beg the occasional stick of jerky or handful of gorp from your fellow backpackers along the way. So cheer up, clean up the mess, get going, and plan how you can do it better on your next trip.

A Word About Cars, Theft, and Car Bears: Stealing from and vandalizing cars are becoming all too common at popular trailheads. You can't ensure that your car and its contents will be safe, but you can increase the odds. Make your car unattractive to thieves and vandals by disabling your engine (your mechanic can show you how), hiding everything you leave in the car, and closing all windows and locking all doors and compartments. Get and use a locking gas-tank cap. If you have more than one car, use the most modest one for driving to the trailhead.

Bearproof your car by not leaving any food in it and by hiding anything that looks like a picnic cooler or other food carrier—bears know what to look for. To a bear, a car with food in it is just an oversized can waiting to be opened. Some trailheads have bear boxes. Leave any food and toiletries you're not taking into the backcountry in these bear boxes rather than in your car.

The Regulations: Call, write to, or get on the website of the agency in charge of the area you plan to visit in order to learn the latest regulations, especially those concerning bears and food storage. For each trailhead in this book, you'll find the agency's name, physical address, phone number, and web address (if there is one) under Information and Permits.

Wilderness and Campfire Permits

In most places, everyone who travels overnight into a national park or national forest wilderness is required to carry a wilderness permit from the agency administering the starting trailhead. If your trip extends through more than one national forest or through both a national forest and a national park, get your permit from the forest or park where your trip starts.

A wilderness permit is issued for a single trip with a specific start date, for specific entry and exit points, and for a specified amount of time. Your permit is inflexible as to the trailhead entry point and start date. A separate permit is required for each trip. Group sizes and numbers of stock are usually restricted.

The permit system has a couple functions: The agencies responsible for the backcountry learn how many people and head of stock are using each trailhead, so they can make better decisions to prevent overuse of these areas. By giving out information with the permit on how to camp safely, avoid impact on the wilderness, and properly deal with bears, the agencies also educate wilderness users.

During the summer months, forest rangers patrol many backcountry trails, and they may ask to see your wilderness permit. If you do not have one, you may be fined and expelled from the backcountry.

There are two ways to get a permit: in person (on demand) and by advance reservation. Whether you plan to apply for your wilderness permit in advance or at the time of your trip in person, we strongly suggest you telephone the administering agency or check its website first. Rules, regulations, and procedures for issuing permits change fairly often. Further, weather, runoff conditions, and forest fires sometimes close trails in the backcountry; you can learn about this, too, in your telephone call or web research. Within each trailhead chapter, we identify the agency in charge and how to get in touch with them for more information.

HELPFUL WEBSITE

SierraNevadaWild.gov (http://sierranevadawild.gov/) is a user-friendly government source for backcountry trip planning in Sierra Nevada national parks, forests, and public lands. You'll find a wealth of wilderness information here—some via links—for all established Sierra Nevada wilderness areas, though not for proposed wilderness additions and wilderness study areas.

On-Demand Permits

You can go in person for a permit to an agency location near your entry point the day before or on the day you plan to begin your trip. The national forests and the national parks maintain a number of conveniently located facilities to serve you. Because of the severe cutbacks in funding, however, the agencies don't know from year to year which locations will be open during the summer season. Use the information provided in each trailhead section to find the visitor center, ranger station, or satellite most convenient for you.

Reserving Permits in Advance

You can also reserve a permit by mail (and sometimes by email, fax, or phone) up to six months in advance of your trip. Use the information provided in each trailhead section to discover how and when to apply.

If you apply for a permit reservation in advance:

- Know whether a fee applies; if so, include payment in the appropriate form. By mail: Include a money order or check for that amount made payable to the US Department of Agriculture—Forest Service for Forest Service wilderness areas and to the National Park Service for Sequoia and Kings Canyon national parks, or use a credit card. By fax or phone: Use a credit card. When using a credit card, supply the card type, number, and expiration date. Applications lacking the required fee will not be processed.

- If applying by mail or fax, enclose or fax a completed wilderness permit application form, one for each trip, or write a letter containing the same information. If applying by phone, be ready to supply the same information. Some agencies' websites have permit-application forms you can print out or download. If not, here is the information you need to supply: name, address, daytime phone, number of people in the party, method of travel (ski, snowshoe, foot, horse, etc.), number of stock (if applicable), start and end dates, entry and exit trailheads, principal destination, alternate dates and/or trailheads. You may also be asked for an itinerary.

- Be sure to provide a second and even a third choice of trailhead and/or entry date, in case your first choice is not available.

- If the agency will not mail your permit, find out where you should pick it up.

Quotas

For most trailheads, the agencies have set limits or quotas on the number of people who can enter a trailhead per day. Quotas are in effect mainly in the summer months; the time when they are in effect is called the quota period. Where quotas apply, only a limited number of advance reservations are accepted. The remainder of the quota is set aside for in-person applications, up to 24 hours in advance of your entry, on a first-come, first served basis.

If you plan to begin your trip from one of these trailheads, especially on the weekend, you would be wise to reserve your permit in advance. A reservation for a permit is not the same as the permit itself. Only a few agencies mail you the actual permit; most require that you pick up the permit near the trailhead entry. The purpose of the reservation is to guarantee you'll get a permit for that trailhead on the day you wish. Where no quotas apply, the only reason to reserve your permit by mail is to allow you to pick it up during off hours.

Maps and Profiles

Today's Sierra traveler is confronted by a bewildering array of maps, and it doesn't take much experience to learn that no single map fulfills all needs. There are topographic maps, base maps (US Forest Service), shaded relief maps (National Park Service), artistically drawn representational maps (California Department of Fish and Game), aerial-photograph maps, geologic maps, three-dimensional relief maps, soil-vegetation maps, and compact discs containing five levels of topographic maps already pieced together for you as well as software for drawing routes. Each map has different information to impart, and it's a good idea to use several of these maps in your planning.

For trip-planning purposes, the trailheads in this book include their own gray-scale map or maps, which show all trips and are based on the United States Geological Survey

(USGS) topographic maps or USDA Forest Service wilderness maps. (More information about these maps is on page 15.)

A useful map series for planning is the USDA Forest Service topographic series for most individual wilderness areas. The scale of most maps of this series is 1:63,360 (1 inch = 1 mile), which is very close to that of the former USGS 15′ series (1:62,500), and each conveniently covers the entire wilderness area on one map. However, you may find these maps a bit bulky for the trail.

Most backpackers prefer to use a topographic (topo) map with finer detail than the above overview/planning maps. Hikers typically prefer the USGS 7.5′ series, where the elevation is usually shown in 40-foot contour intervals (although some 7.5′ topos show 80-foot contour intervals or even 20-meter contour intervals) and the scale is 1:24,000 or about 2.625 inches per mile.

Wilderness Press still publishes and regularly updates a few 15′ topos for some areas covered by *Sierra South*. These Wilderness Press 15′ topos include indexes of the place names on them and are printed on waterproof, tear-resistant plastic. If any one or more of these maps covers all or part of a given trip, their titles appear in boldface at the beginning of the trip under the section Topo. Unlike ordinary USGS topos, these maps show details of the adjacent national forest or park for your greater convenience in trip-planning. Wilderness Press still publishes the following 15′ quads that apply to *Sierra South*: *Merced Peak, Devils Postpile, Mt. Abbott,* and *Mt. Pinchot*.

You can also use commercially available software to print out your own topographic maps at your choice of scale and detail. Protect these printouts if the ink is prone to run.

How and Where to Get Your Maps

Order Wilderness Press 15′ topos and other maps as well as books directly from Wilderness Press online at www.wildernesspress.com or by phone at 800-443-7227.

Backpacking stores and some bookstores—especially those near popular hiking areas—carry at least the topographic maps for hikes in their areas as well as the software required to print your own. USGS topographic maps and US Forest Service maps are available at many ranger stations and at stations that issue wilderness permits.

USGS's online store sells USGS maps at store.usgs.gov. Or contact the USGS Western Region office at 345 Middlefield Road, Menlo Park, CA 94025; 650-853-8300.

How to Use This Book

Terms This Book Uses

Destination/UTM Coordinates: This new edition provides UTM coordinates for GPS users. When the datum is from the field, we note this by including "(field)" after the datum. Otherwise, the datum is from mapping software. Because these data are all UTM data with the appropriate meters east (mE) and meters north (mN), we don't repeat those labels but show UTM data in this form: 11S 395115 4034251.

Trip Type: This book classifies a trip as one of four types. An **out-and-back** trip goes out to a destination and returns the way it came. A **loop** trip goes out by one route and returns by another with relatively little or no retracing of the same trail. A **semiloop** trip has an out-and-back part and a loop part; the loop part may occur anywhere along the way, and if it's in the middle, there are two out-and-back parts. A **shuttle** trip starts at one trailhead and ends at another; usually, the trailheads are too far apart for you to walk between them, so you will need to leave a car at the ending (take-out) trailhead, have someone pick you up there, or rely on California's scanty and ill-organized public transportation to get back to your starting (put-in) trailhead.

Best Season: Deciding when in the year is the best time for a particular trip is a difficult task because of yearly variations. Low early-season temperatures and mountain shadows often keep some of the higher passes closed until well into August. Early snows have been known to whiten alpine country in late July and August. Some of the trips described here are low-country ones, offered specifically for the itchy hiker who, stiff from a winter's inactivity, is searching for a warm-up excursion. These trips are labeled **early**, a period that extends roughly from late May to early July. **Mid** is from early July to the end of August, and **late** is from then to early October.

Pace: For each trip, we give the number of days you'd spend hiking at the trip's described pace—**leisurely, moderate,** or **strenuous**—as well as the number of layover days (below) you might want to take. Since this book is written for the average backpacker, we chose to describe most trips on either a leisurely or a moderate basis, depending on where the best overnight camping places were along the route. We call a few trips strenuous. A leisurely pace lets hikers absorb more of the sights, smells, and "feel" of the country they have come to see.

Layover Days: These are days when you'll want to remain camped at a particular site so you can dayhike to see other beautiful places around the area or enjoy some adventures like peakbagging. The number of layover days you take and where are purely personal choices, to be balanced with how much time you have and how much food you can carry. Our trip descriptions will help you pick where and when you want to take layover days.

Total Mileage: The trips in this book range in length between 5 and 110 miles, and many trips can be shortened or extended, based on your interest and time.

Measuring distances in the backcountry is more an art than a science. We use decimal fractions for indicating distances, but don't imagine that we measured them to the tenths and hundredths of miles. The numbers represent our best estimates of distance based on techniques like the time it took us to get from point to point. You can't represent thirds accurately as decimal fractions, so we use 0.3 for one third and 0.6 for two thirds.

Campsites: Campsites are labeled poor, fair, good, excellent, or, occasionally, Spartan, which usually means an above-timberline site with few amenities, much exposure, and breathtaking scenery. The criteria for assigning these labels were amount of use, immediate surroundings, general scenery, presence of vandalism, availability of water, kind of ground cover, and recreational potential—angling, side trips, swimming, etc. Camping is forbidden on meadows and other vegetated areas and within a certain distance of any stream or lake. You will be informed of these rules for your areas when you get your wilderness permit. "Packer campsite" indicates a semi-permanent camp (usually constructed by packers for the "comfort of their clients") characterized by things like nailed-plank table or benches, nails in the surrounding trees, and/or a large, rock fireplace.

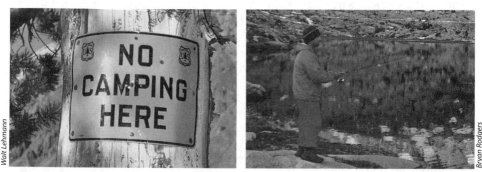

Be careful to obverve all camping and fishing regulations.

Fishing: Angling, for many, is a prime consideration when planning a trip. While we note the quality of fishing throughout the book, experienced anglers know that the size of their catch relates not only to quantity, type, and general size of the fishery, which are given, but also to water temperature, feed, angling skill, and that indefinable something known as "fisherman's luck." Generally speaking, the old "early and late" adage holds: Fishing is better early and late in the day, and early and late in the season.

Stream Crossings: Stream crossings vary greatly depending on snow-melt conditions. Often, June's raging torrent becomes September's placid creek. If a ford is described as "difficult in early season," fording that creek may be difficult because it is hard to walk through deep or fast water, and getting caught in the current would be dangerous. Whether you attempt such a crossing depends on the presence or absence of logs or other bridges, downstream rapids or waterfalls, your ability and equipment, and your judgment. We mention manmade bridges and other manmade aids for you to cross on, but we usually don't mention chance aids like logs and rocks, because they can vary from year to year. (See pages 5 and 6 for tips for crossing streams more safely.)

Trail Type and Surface: Most of the trails described here are well maintained (the exceptions are noted) and are properly signed. If the trail becomes indistinct, look for blazes (peeled bark at eye level on trees) or ducks (two or more rocks piled one atop another). Trails may fade out in wet areas like meadows, and you may have to scout around to find where they resume. Continuing in the direction you were going when the trail faded out is often, but not always, a good bet.

Two other significant trail conditions have also been described in the text: the degree of openness (type and degree of forest cover, if any, or else "meadow," "brush," or whatever) and underfooting (talus, scree, pumice, sand, "duff"—a deep humus ground cover of rotting vegetation—or other material).

A "use trail" is an unmaintained, unofficial trail that is more or less easy to follow because it is well worn by use. For example, nearly every Sierra lakeshore has a use trail worn around it by anglers in search of their prey.

Landmarks: The text contains occasional references to points, peaks, and other landmarks. These places are shown on the appropriate topographic maps cited at the beginning of the trip. For example, "Point 9426" in the text would refer to a point designated simply "9426" on the map itself.

Fire Damage: The Forest Service and the Park Service have a policy of letting fires in the backcountry burn as long as they are not a threat to people or structures. One result has been some pretty poor-looking scenery on some trips in this book. However, most of the fire-damaged areas have begun to recover soon enough that we have chosen not to delete the affected trips from the book.

How This Book Is Organized

Trips in this book are organized according to the roads and highways you must drive to get to the trailheads in this book. Unlike the region covered in *Sierra North*, no road crosses the range south of Hwy. 120 for about 140 miles to the road that goes over Sherman Pass far to the south. Rather, in this region, roads penetrate the range from the west and from the east without crossing the range. Therefore, *Sierra South* is organized first by which side of the Sierra you must start on (west or east) and then, in north to south order, by the roads you must take into the range to get to the trailheads. The trailheads appear in the order you'll find them as you drive into the range on that road.

Trailhead and Trip Organization: As previously noted, each trip is located within trailhead sections in the book. Those sections begin with a summary table, such as the fictitious one below, that uses the trailhead's name, elevation, and UTM coordinates as its title. The table briefly summarizes each trip from this trailhead:

Black Powder Trailhead   7654'; 11S 736921 4328622

DESTINATION/ UTM COORDINATES	TRIP TYPE	BEST SEASON	PACE (HIKING/ LAYOVER DAYS)	TOTAL MILEAGE
1 Bear Corral 11S 735694 4338773	Out & back	Early to mid	2/1 Moderate	18
2 Sunshine Lake 11S 733543 4347890	Out & back	Mid to late	4/1 Moderate, part cross-country	31

Following the table are details about information, permits, and driving directions to that trailhead.

Next comes the first trip from this trailhead. The trip data—UTM coordinates, total mileage, and hiking/layover days—are included with each trip entry. All trips include an elevation profile, a list of maps, and highlights. Some include **HEADS UP!**, or special considerations for that trip, and shuttle trips include directions to the take-out trailhead.

1 Bear Corral

Trip Data: 11S 735694 4338773; 18 miles; 2/1 days

Topos: *Pickle Springs*

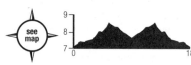

Highlights: Follow a pair of delightful streams to a secluded basin rimmed by granite cliffs on the eastern fringe of XYZ Wilderness.

DAY 1 (Black Powder Trailhead to Bear Corral, 9 miles): From the trailhead, make a short climb northeast through a canopy of lodgepole, red fir, and white fir. Birds are abundant here, especially Steller's jays, white-crowned sparrows, juncos, and chickadees. Soon the route reaches a junction with the PCT. Turn right (east) here and....

...to the good camping at forested Bear Corral (7654'; 11S 735694 4338773).

DAY 2 (Bear Corral to Black Powder Trailhead, 9 miles): Retrace your steps.

After this comes the next trip, if any, from this same trailhead. Trips in the same general area, especially multiple trips from the same trailhead, often build upon each other. For example, the first trip from a trailhead is usually the shortest—one day out to a destination, the next day back to the trailhead. The second trip will build on—extend—the first trip by following the first trip's first day and then continuing on a second and subsequent days to more distant destinations. Rather than repeat the full, detailed description for the first trip's first day, we recapitulate it as briefly as possible with the essential trail instructions to get you to that day's destination. We also identify this as a recapitulation and give you a reference to the trip and day we're recapitulating, like this: **(Recap: Trip 1, Day 1.).** If you wish, you can turn to that description to read everything we have to say about that day, which includes details about natural and human history—things that are fun to know but not essential for getting from the trailhead to the destination.

Trailhead Maps: Each trailhead section includes a map such as the one below. The legend that follows defines the symbols used in the maps in the book.

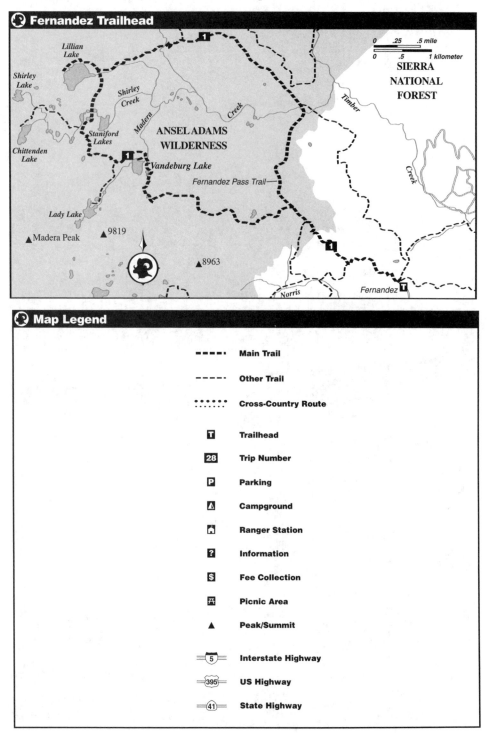

Fernandez Trailhead

0   .25   .5 mile
0   .5   1 kilometer

SIERRA
NATIONAL
FOREST

Lillian Lake

Shirley Lake

Shirley Creek

Madera

Creek

Timber

Creek

ANSEL ADAMS
WILDERNESS

Staniford Lakes

Chittenden Lake

Vandeburg Lake

Fernandez Pass Trail

Lady Lake

▲Madera Peak   ▲9819

▲8963

Norris   Fernandez

Map Legend

- - - - ∙	Main Trail
– – – – ∙	Other Trail
∙∙∙∙∙∙∙	Cross-Country Route
T	Trailhead
28	Trip Number
P	Parking
A	Campground
	Ranger Station
?	Information
$	Fee Collection
	Picnic Area
▲	Peak/Summit
5	Interstate Highway
395	US Highway
41	State Highway

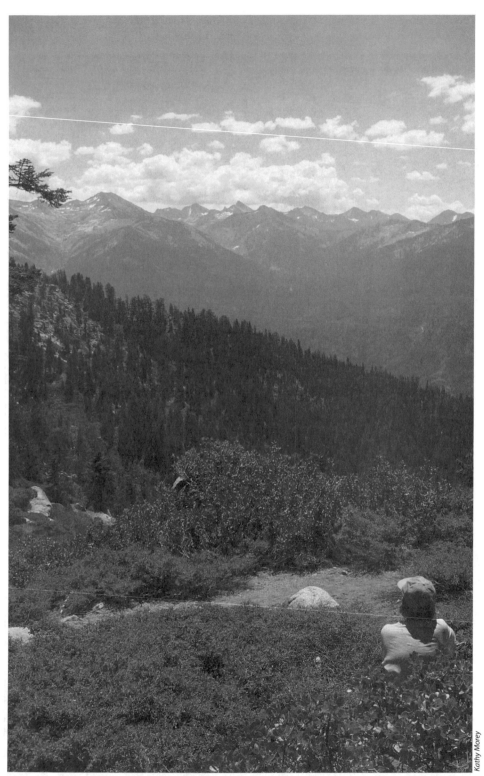

INTRODUCTION TO THE WEST SIDE

Getting to starting trailheads on the west side of the Sierra south of Yosemite means long, gradual, winding, scenic drives on mountain roads and highways from some major road in the western foothills or the Central Valley, like Hwy. 49 or Hwy. 99. Be sure to allow plenty of time to enjoy these beautiful drives. A few shuttle trips will end at roads not listed below. Along the way, small towns, tiny villages, and rustic resorts provide lodging and supplies. Especially for supplies, the larger towns nearer the roads' west ends provide better lodging and shopping choices.

On the west side, you'll enter the Sierra on these roads and highways:

State Hwy. 41 (through and then south of Yosemite)

State Hwy. 168 West Side (yes, there is an east side, too, but 168 doesn't cross the range)

Kaiser Pass Road (in some respects, a continuation of State Hwy. 168 West Side beyond Huntington Lake)

State Hwy. 180 (into Kings Canyon proper)

Generals Hwy. (links the west sides of Kings Canyon and then Sequoia national parks, passing through part of Sequoia National Forest)

State Hwy. 198 (into Mineral King)

State Hwy. 190 (into the extreme southern Sierra)

opposite: **Great Western Divide from a rest stop at Panther Gap (Trip 30)**

HWY 41

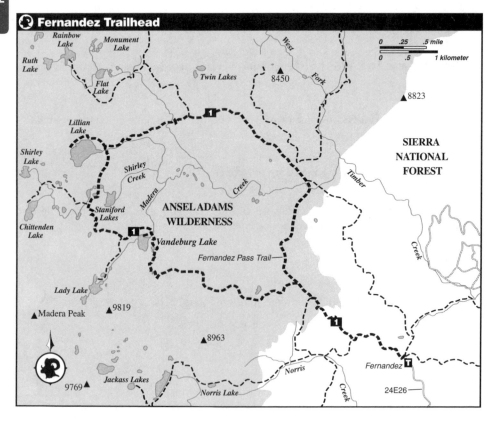

Fernandez Trailhead
9937'; 11S 395115 4034251

DESTINATION/ UTM COORDINATES	TRIP TYPE	BEST SEASON	PACE (HIKING/ LAYOVER DAYS)	TOTAL MILEAGE
I Lillian Lake 11S 291480 4159942	Semiloop	Mid to late	3/1 Moderate	13.5

Information and Permits: This trailhead is in Sierra National Forest: 1600 Tollhouse Road, Clovis, CA 93611, 559-297-0706, www.fs.fed.us/r5/sierra/. Permits are required for overnight stays, and quotas apply; reserved permits and on-demand permits are available.

Driving Directions: From Yosemite Forks on Hwy. 41, 3.5 miles north of Oakhurst and about 12 miles south of Yosemite National Park, turn east on County Road 222 toward Bass Lake. Follow this road around the lake to northeast-bound Beasore Road. Turn left onto Beasore Road (Forest Road 7), which is narrow, winding, and breathtaking—and impassable in early season due to snow.

To reach the Fernandez Trailhead, drive about 27 miles past Globe Rock, the Jackass Trailhead, and, on the right, Bowler Group Campground. Continue a little under 0.6 more mile on Beasore Road to a signed junction with a dirt road north (left) to the Norris Creek and Fernandez trailheads. Turn left onto this road and go about 2 miles, crossing Norris Creek, to a junction. Here, take the right fork northeast for another mile to reach the Fernandez parking area. Find the trail at the west side of the parking area.

Note: If you are traveling from the south, you may wish to call or go online for directions to the trailhead via Minarets Road.

I Lillian Lake

Trip Data: 11S 291480 4159942; 13.5 miles; 3/1 days

Topos: *Timber Knob*

Highlights: Nestled beneath Madera, Gale, and Sing peaks, just southwest of Yosemite National Park, the many lakes and easy mileage on this trip provide ample opportunity for exploring, fishing, and dayhiking in Ansel Adams Wilderness.

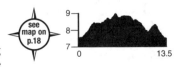

see map on p.18

HEADS UP! *For extended itineraries from Yosemite into the Granite Creek area via Isberg and Fernandez passes, see Wilderness Press's Sierra North, edition nine, trips 72 and 73.*

DAY 1 (Fernandez Trailhead to Vandeburg Lake, 4.5 miles): The Fernandez Trail begins a gentle northwestward ascent through a forest of white fir, Jeffrey pine, and lodgepole pine. Stay on this trail as it bypasses two lateral trails heading left (west) to the Norris Trailhead, eventually climbing high to gain an open ridgetop. Here, find a signed junction with the Lillian Lake loop: The right (east) fork goes directly to Lillian Lake; the left (west) fork goes to Vandeburg, Staniford, and the many other lakes in the Madera Creek drainage.

For this trip, turn left onto the loop and enter Ansel Adams Wilderness, admiring the grand views to the east. In a mixed forest of red fir, mountain hemlock, and lodgepole and western white pine, pass two meadows on the left, and then swing north to climb steeply up a rocky ridge. From the ridgetop, descend a short distance through hemlock forest to ford the outlet of Vandeburg Lake (8674´; 11S 292284 4158434). A little uphill to the west are the well-used campsites on the north side of this attractive lake. The farthest campsite to the northwest is within earshot of a lovely waterfall.

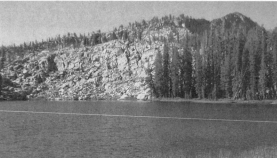

DAY 2 (Vandeburg Lake to Lillian Lake, 2.5 miles): This short but sweet hiking day gives you a chance to admire the views, discover the lakes, fish, and maybe even bag a peak from a basecamp on the trip's namesake lake.

Lillian Lake

Stacy Corless

> ### OTHER CAMPING NEAR VANDEBURG LAKE
>
> If the campsites at Vandeburg are occupied, or if you feel like hiking farther, continue on the trail at the northwest side of Vandeburg Lake. Ascend west up slabs to a signed junction with a trail going left (southwest) to Lady Lake. Take this trail; a moderate ascent of less than 0.75 mile brings you to shady campsites on the northeast side of Lady Lake, just below Madera Peak. For Day 2, return to the junction and pick up the trail directions from that junction.

From Vandeburg Lake, continue on the trail at the northwest side of Vandeburg Lake. Ascend west up slabs to a signed junction with a trail going left (southwest) to Lady Lake. Go right (north-northwest) on the main trail as it continues up more slabs dotted with lodgepole pines. Where the trail tops a low ridge, pause to take in the expansive views of the Ritter Range to the northeast.

After a short descent to the north, arrive at the first of the Staniford Lakes. Pass a signed junction with a trail west to Chittenden and Shirley lakes. Keep going ahead (north) on the main trail, pass above the largest Staniford Lake, and ford Shirley Creek. There is excellent camping at the lakes below and above the trail near the shores of these lakes.

Continuing north across granite slabs, the trail crosses several seasonal creeks before swinging west to ford the shaded outlet of Lillian Lake. Soon, the Fernandez Trail intersects a spur to Lillian Lake; turn left (west) here and shortly reach the lake. There is no camping within 400 feet of the shoreline from the outlet for approximately a quarter mile along this spur. However, several nice campsites can be found north and west of the restricted area; there also are two additional sites across the outlet on the lake's southern shore.

> ### DAYHIKES AROUND LILLIAN LAKE
>
> On a layover day, retrace your steps to the junction with the side trail to Chittenden and Shirley lakes, or go west (and uphill) on the Fernandez Pass Trail to the Fernandez Lakes, including popular Rainbow Lake (no camping). Or venture up the Post Peak Pass Trail.

DAY 3 (Lillian Lake to Fernandez Trailhead, 6.5 miles): Return to the Fernandez Trail. At the junction, turn right (south) toward the Fernandez Trailhead. At a trail junction just before the ford of Madera Creek, take the right fork eastward. During the remaining 1.5-mile walk on the loop part of this trip, curve southeast and then south, staying on the Fernandez Trail at any junctions to close the loop.

Retrace your steps southeastward to the Fernandez Trailhead from here.

Granite Creek Campground Trailhead

6978'; 11S 29955 4157469

DESTINATION/ UTM COORDINATES	TRIP TYPE	BEST SEASON	PACE (HIKING/ LAYOVER DAYS)	TOTAL MILEAGE
2 Cora Lakes 11S 299357 4163236	Semiloop	Mid to late	2/1 Leisurely	11
3 Hemlock Crossing 11S 303763 4167984	Loop	Mid to late	4/1 Strenuous	29

Information and Permits: This trailhead is in Sierra National Forest: 1600 Tollhouse Road, Clovis, CA 93611, 559-297-0706, www.fs.fed.us/r5/sierra/. Permits are required for overnight stays, and quotas apply; reserved permits and on-demand permits are available.

Driving Directions: From Yosemite Forks on Hwy. 41, 3.5 miles north of Oakhurst and about 12 miles south of Yosemite National Park, turn east on County Road 222 toward Bass Lake. Follow this road around the lake to northeast-bound Beasore Road. Turn left (north) onto Beasore Road (Forest Road 7), which is narrow, winding, and breathtaking—and impassable in early season due to snow.

To reach the Granite Creek Trailhead, drive about 27 miles past Globe Rock, the Jackass Trailhead, and, on the right, Bowler Group Campground. Continue about 6.5 more miles on Beasore Road, avoiding any turnoffs, including the turnoff to the Fernandez Trailhead, to the Clover Meadow Ranger Station.

From the Clover Meadow Ranger Station, go another 0.5 mile on Beasore Road to a junction with Forest Road 4S57. Turn right (northeast) on this road and follow it for a little more than a mile to a hikers' parking area in Granite Creek Campground.

Note: If you are traveling from the south, you may wish to call or go online for directions to the trailhead via Minarets Road.

2 Cora Lakes

Trip Data: 11S 299357 4163236; 11 miles; 2/1

Topos: *Timber Knob*

Highlights: Enjoy an easy semiloop trip that pauses in this lightly used region at a trio of charming lakes, the three little Cora Lakes.

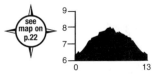

DAY 1 (Granite Creek Campground Trailhead to Middle Cora Lake, 4.5 miles): From the east end of Granite Creek Campground, take the Isberg Pass Trail north to cross a bridge and begin a dusty ascent under red fir, lodgepole, and Jeffrey pine cover. The trail steepens as it climbs a ravine, crossing and re-crossing the ravine's tiny creek. Enter Ansel Adams Wilderness and pass through the Niche, a notch west of Green Mountain and close to Granite Creek.

After fording Granite Creek (wet in early season), reach an intersection at 3 miles: right (northeast) toward Cora Creek, Chetwood Creek, and Hemlock Crossing; left (north) to Cora Lakes. Begin the loop part of this trip: Take the left fork and continue north to a ford

> **DAYHIKE FROM THE CORA LAKES**
> Spend a layover day hiking to Joe Crane Lake (9600'; 11S 295877 4166651), about 4 miles one way from the Cora Lakes north-northwest along the Isberg Pass Trail and then steeply west up a lateral that branches away from the Isberg Pass Trail. The hike affords nice views of surrounding peaks. Joe Crane Lake, tucked in the granite beneath Post Peak, also has good camping on its northeast shore.

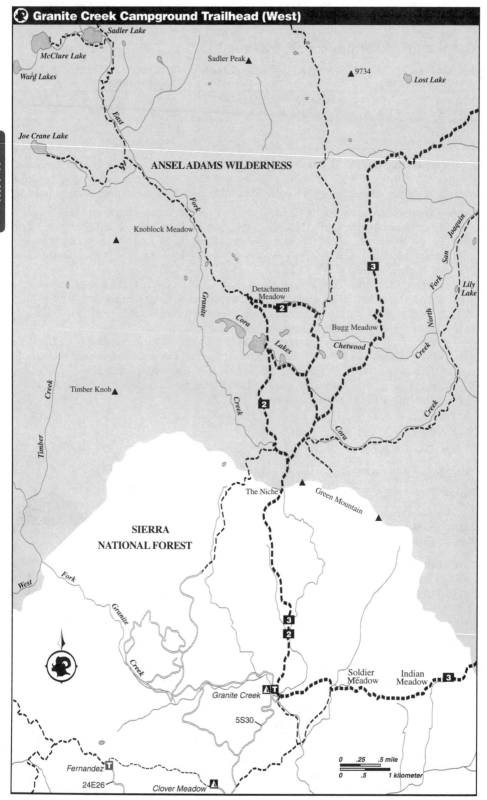

Granite Creek Campground Trailhead (West)

HWY 41

Sadler Lake

McClure Lake

Ward Lakes

Joe Crane Lake

Sadler Peak ▲

▲ 9734

Lost Lake

East

Fork

ANSEL ADAMS WILDERNESS

Knoblock Meadow

▲

Granite

Cora

Lakes

Detachment Meadow

2

Bugg Meadow

Chetwood

Lily Lake

North

Fork

San Joaquin

Creek

Creek

3

Timber Knob ▲

Timber

Creek

Creek

Creek

2

Cora

2

The Niche

Green Mountain

▲

▲

SIERRA NATIONAL FOREST

West

Fork

Granite

Creek

3

2

Soldier Meadow

Indian Meadow

3

Granite Creek

5S30

Fernandez

24E26

Clover Meadow

0   .25   .5 mile

0   .5   1 kilometer

22

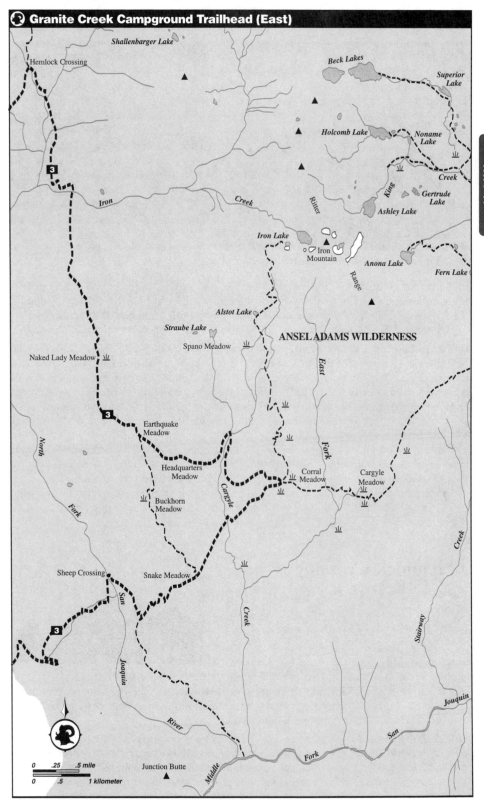

HWY 41

Shallenbarger Lake

Hemlock Crossing

Beck Lakes

Superior
Lake

Holcomb Lake

Noname
Lake

Creek

3

Iron

Creek

Ritter

King

Gertrude
Lake

Ashley Lake

Iron Lake

Iron
Mountain

Anona Lake

Fern Lake

Range

Alstot Lake

Straube Lake

ANSEL ADAMS WILDERNESS

Spano Meadow

East

Naked Lady Meadow

3

Earthquake
Meadow

Fork

North

Headquarters
Meadow

Corral
Meadow

Cargyle
Meadow

Buckhorn
Meadow

Cargyle

Fork

Creek

Sheep Crossing

Snake Meadow

San

3

Joaquin

Creek

Stairway

Jouquin

San

0   .25   .5 mile

0   .5   1 kilometer

Junction Butte

River

Middle

Fork

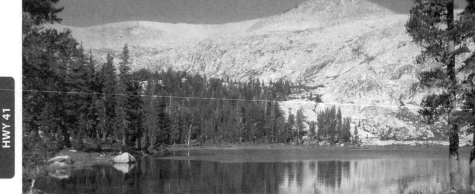

Stacy Corless

Joe Crane Lake is just a dayhike away from the Cora Lakes.

of the stream connecting Middle and Lower Cora lakes. Obeying posted camping restrictions, follow Middle Cora Lake's shoreline northward to find lovely and legal camping (8348'; 11S 299357 4163236) on the north shore or the south shore near the stream connecting Upper and Middle Cora lakes. Fishing is good, with the exception of a mid-season lull.

DAY 2 (Middle Cora Lake to Granite Creek Campground Trailhead, 6.5 miles): Today's hike continues the loop part of this trip. Leaving your campsite at Middle Cora Lake, return to the Isberg Pass Trail and turn left (north) onto it. Travel about a half mile to a junction with a lateral trail to Chetwood Creek. Turn right (southeast) onto the lateral and pass through Detachment Meadow before arriving at the remains of Chetwood Cabin. (Some maps show a junction here with a trail going north to Sadler Peak, but it isn't an obvious intersection.)

Follow the established trail as it curves right (south) away from Chetwood Cabin and goes 1.4 more miles through flower-filled meadows, passing reedy ponds before crossing the Cora Lakes' outlet stream, Cora Creek, and meeting the Hemlock Crossing Trail.

At this junction, turn right (south) and continue a half mile to the junction with the main Isberg Pass Trail. Turn left (south), closing the loop, and retrace the final 3 miles to the trailhead.

3 Hemlock Crossing

Trip Data: 11S 303763 4167984; 4/1;
29 miles

Topos: *Timber Knob, Cattle Mountain, Mount Ritter*

Highlights: This trip starts in the forested Granite Creek basin and moves into the spec-

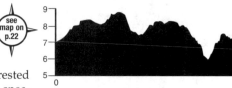

tacular North Fork San Joaquin drainage. On the way back, take the historic Mammoth Trail, once a toll route between Oakhurst and Mammoth mining district (who knew the real "gold" was in skiing?) in the 1870s and '80s.

HEADS UP! Strong and sturdy hikers could skip Day 1's leg to Cora Lakes and instead tackle the 13 miles to Hemlock Crossing in one day. But what's the hurry? Middle Cora Lake is a pretty spot; don't miss it. To avoid the dusty, 3-mile hike along a dirt road on this trip's final day, arrange a car shuttle at the Mammoth Trailhead, at the extreme east end of Road 4S60. The last day's hike also involves extreme elevation gain and loss (about 3500 feet total) to cross the North Fork San Joaquin River. You can bypass the vertical and the car shuttle altogether by making this trip an out-and-back to Hemlock Crossing from Granite Creek Campground.

DAY 1 (Granite Creek Campground Trailhead to Middle Cora Lake, 4.5 miles): *(Recap: Trip 2, Day 1.)* Ascend the Isberg Pass Trail under forest cover to the Niche. Ford Granite Creek just before a junction; from the junction, head left (north) to the stream connecting Middle and Lower Cora lakes. Ford it and, following regulations here, head for legal campsites on Middle Cora Lake (8348'; 11S 299357 4163236).

DAY 2 (Middle Cora Lake to Hemlock Crossing, 8.5 miles): Fill your hydration system at the Cora Lakes; the trail ahead can be dry in late season and has more uphill than you might expect.

Retrace your steps, crossing the stream between Middle and Lower Cora lakes, back to the trail junction south of Cora Lakes. Here, turn hard left (northeast) onto the Hemlock Crossing Trail, quickly bypassing a lateral trail right (east) to a snow-survey cabin and Lily Lake. Go ahead (north) on the Hemlock Crossing Trail here.

The dry, dusty trail rolls along steadily before a slight descent to Chetwood Creek. After crossing the creek, the trail ascends through an aspen grove and comes to the edge of the North Fork's canyon. Enjoy the dramatic views before the trail heads back into forest cover and climbs a bit to reach an unnamed creek with a poor but usable campsite, just over halfway to Hemlock Crossing.

Soon after that creek, the steep descent to Hemlock Crossing begins, and the trail (one that sees more stock traffic than foot traffic) becomes loose and rocky. Breathe a sigh of relief when the trail levels off and winds through granite outcrops, reaching a wet, meadowy area and then dropping down to two large campsites at Hemlock Crossing (7500'; 11S 303763 4167984). Here, the San Joaquin pours over a granite lip into two large, inviting, chilly pools. If the two main sites are occupied, cross the bridge and turn right (south), going a short distance to a campsite (probably illegal but tolerated, according to rangers) at a large waterfall on the river.

AT HEMLOCK CROSSING

Spend a layover day fishing or exploring the terrain to the north by taking the left fork north after crossing the bridge here. This trail gradually rises up and away from the river before passing through Yosemite-esque Stevenson Meadow (where, if you're sharing this area with a pack station group, you'll find the stock). Approximately 4 miles from Hemlock Crossing, the maintained trail ends where it meets the river again, and so does this description. Note that adventurous hikers rave about the scenic, untracked high country beyond this point: Bench Canyon to the northwest and Twin Island Lakes to the northeast, hard by the west side of the Ritter Range.

DAY 3 (Hemlock Crossing to Corral Meadow, 7 miles): Cross the bridge and turn right (south) on the descending trail that will soon rise dramatically above the river's east bank. In less than 2 miles, switchback to meet cascading Iron Creek (campsite). The trail leaves the canyon's edge to begin a gradual, forested ascent to Naked Lady Meadow, a marshy aspen grove that got its name from the bawdy images that lonely shepherds carved into tree trunks before the area's 1964 wilderness designation.

The trail skirts a hillside and drops into Earthquake Meadow, where there is a nice, spring-fed stream but very poor camping. The trail meets an unmaintained lateral route to Snake Meadow; stay on the main trail (southeast) to Corral Meadow (originally known as 77 Corral after a drought in 1877 forced shepherds to seek higher, wilder grazing lands).

In just over a mile, reach the west fork of Cargyle Creek (campsites); once past its drainage, there is evidence of a 2003 fire. The trail can be hard to follow here, but continue east-southeast to stay on track to a signed junction at Corral Meadow: left (north) to Iron Lake; right (southwest) to Clover Meadow and the trailhead; ahead (east) on the eastbound Mammoth Trail, crossing small streams to reach well-established campsites on the southeast side of the meadow (7982'; 11S 308225 4160840).

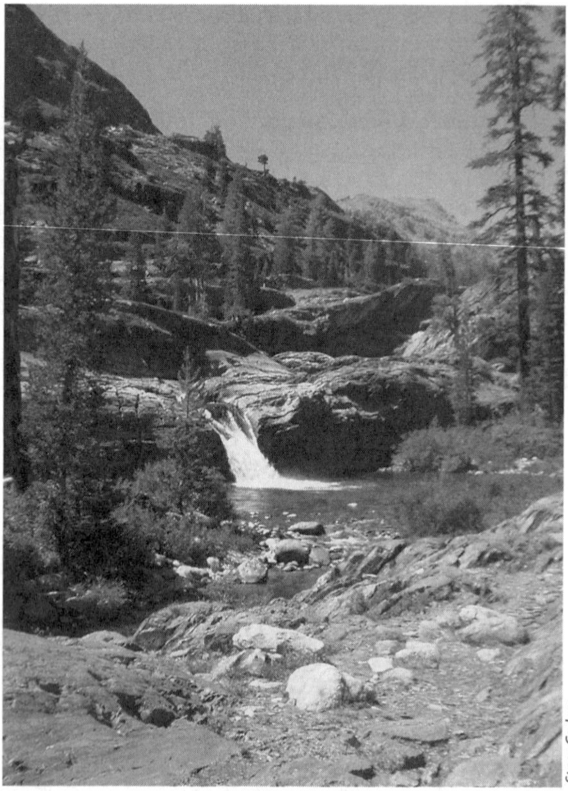

DAY 4 (Corral Meadow to Granite Creek Campground Trailhead, 9 miles): Plan to get an early start: Today's hike involves a grueling descent to a bridge over North Fork San Joaquin and then a hot climb back up to the road, which you follow back to Granite Creek Campground Trailhead.

Retrace your steps to the last junction and turn left (southwest) onto the westbound historic Mammoth Trail, a toll route that

Hemlock Crossing on the North Fork San Joaquin River

Stacy Corless

brought supplies from Fresno Flats (Oakhurst) to the eastside mining camps around Mammoth Lakes back in the 1870s and '80s.

From here, it's down, down, down. Cross Cargyle Creek before meeting the Earthquake Meadow lateral at Snake Meadow; go ahead (southwest) here toward Sheep Crossing. The trail switchbacks steeply westward down toward the river, bypassing a faint spur trail left (south). Continue the westward (toward the river) descent; as the switchbacks end, the trail swings north toward the steel bridge at Sheep Crossing. Rest and get water at Sheep Crossing before tackling the short but steep, mile-plus climb to Indian Meadow.

SHUTTLE OPTION FOR TRIP 3

Notice that there's a road east from Granite Creek Campground 3 miles to the Mammoth Trailhead, at Indian Meadow. You could cut those 3 dusty miles off Trip 3's last, tough day by staging a shuttle car there.

On the west side of the river, the trail turns south, climbing above the river a short distance before curving southwest and then switchbacking steeply up the river canyon's west wall to a roadend, the Mammoth Trailhead, at Indian Meadow. If you've dropped a car at this roadend (see sidebar above to learn how to make this trip a shuttle), your trip is over. Otherwise, follow this dusty road generally west for 3 more miles back to Granite Creek Campground Trailhead (6978'; 11S 29955 4157469); stay on the road at all junctions.

TRANS-SIERRA HIKE

For an easy trans-Sierra hike, from Corral Meadow, go east on the eastbound Mammoth Trail over East Fork Cargyle Creek and a tributary and then through beautiful Cargyle Meadow (once a popular meeting and trading place for Native American tribes from the east and west sides of the Sierra). Climb to Stairway Meadow and the Granite Stairway (neither granite, nor a stairway, oddly) to enter Inyo National Forest. Pass by Summit Meadow (not a meadow, and not at a summit) as the trail descends into Snow Canyon. At a junction with the trail to Fern and Beck lakes (good camping at Fern Lake), go ahead (northeast) to begin a pumice-y, rocky descent with great views over the Middle Fork San Joaquin River drainage.

At the bottom of the descent, ford King Creek (campsite) and curve northeast around a low ridge to reach a junction with the north-south PCT/JMT and with a spur trail ahead (north-northeast) to a junction on the riverbank. Go ahead to the riverbank junction. Turn right (briefly south and then east) over the river on a footbridge toward the Devils Postpile Trailhead. Across the river, find another junction: left (north) a quarter mile to the trailhead; right (south) to see the Postpile itself in just a few yards (why not?). See the Devils Postpile section (trips 42 and 43) for driving directions for setting up the shuttle and for more information about the area.

Wishon Reservoir—Woodchuck Trailhead

6670'; 11S 325266 4096222

DESTINATION/ UTM COORDINATES	TRIP TYPE	BEST SEASON	PACE (HIKING/ LAYOVER DAYS)	TOTAL MILEAGE
4 Halfmoon Lake 11S 335355 4102079	Semiloop	Mid	4/1 Leisurely	26
5 Blackcap Basin 11S 343726 4101161	Out & back	Mid	6/1 Moderate	41
6 Crown Lake 11S 33567 4100360	Semiloop	Early to mid	4/1 Leisurely	25

Information and Permits: This trailhead is in Sierra National Forest: 1600 Tollhouse Road, Clovis, CA 93611, 559-297-0706, www.fs.fed.us/r5/sierra/. Permits are required for overnight stays, and quotas apply; reserved permits and on-demand permits are available.

Driving Directions: From Clovis (near Fresno), take Hwy. 168 42 miles northeast to the resort town of Shaver Lake. Turn right (generally east) onto Dinkey Creek Road and follow it 26 miles to the Courtright/Wishon Y. Take the right fork south to Wishon Reservoir, 4 more miles south. Wishon Reservoir's Woodchuck Trailhead is located immediately across the dam on the left side (east) of the road.

4 Halfmoon Lake

Trip Data: 11S 335355 4102079; 26 miles; 4/1 days

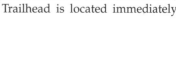

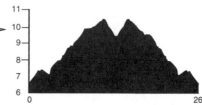

Topos: *Rough Spur, Courtright Reservoir, Blackcap Mtn.*

Highlights: Halfmoon Lake is set in an amphitheater of granite walls sculpted by vanished rivers of ice. Its shallow basin and lower elevation create relatively warm water temperatures. Head for Halfmoon Lake via Woodchuck Lake and then make a semiloop on the return via Chimney Lake.

DAY 1 (Woodchuck Trailhead to Woodchuck Lake, 8 miles): From the Woodchuck Trailhead, the trail climbs nearly 400 feet before curving east and briefly joining a dirt road. Step onto the dirt road and turn south (right) to follow the road 30 feet to a signed junction. At this junction, take the trail branching left (southeast) and continue climbing.

From the junction, the trail climbs steeply 500 feet before it swings north and begins a scenic traverse high on the forested ridge east of Wishon Reservoir. The trail undulates under dense stands of incense-cedar, white fir, and sugar pine (the latter easily identified by its large cones and its five needles per bundle), and past shallow gullies where the vegetation dramatically changes to a lush understory of bracken fern, lupine, gooseberry, columbine, and mugwort.

After nearly 2 miles, the trail turns east, swapping views of Wishon Reservoir for views north toward Lost Peak (8476') and other granitic domes. The trail tops a moraine, a mass of rock debris left behind by vanished glaciers, before it descends into Woodchuck Creek's canyon. At this point, you may hear the Helms Project Powerhouse, across the North Fork Kings River's canyon to the north.

Beyond an aspen-studded meadow, the trail curves north and descends to ford Woodchuck Creek (may be difficult in early season). From the ford, the trail ascends north under higher elevation species of red fir and lodgepole pine and then bears east to switchback 500 feet over a minor ridge hosting a campsite. From the ridge, enjoy views west toward Woodchuck Creek's canyon. Very quickly, the trail meets a signed junction (8510') with a trail to Chuck Pass (right; south-southeast).

Today's route turns left (northeast) toward Crown Pass and crosses several branches of an unnamed creek via three log bridges. Curving north again, the trail makes a short but steep ascent over another moraine to the south end of a lush meadow. Follow the track across the meadow to Moore Boys Camp (8710'), 6 miles from the trailhead and on the far side of the meadow. Fishing is poor for brook trout, and mosquitoes are voracious until late summer.

Just beyond Moore Boys Camp is a signed junction (8720') with trails right (east-northeast) to Chimney Lake and Crown Pass and left (north-northeast) toward Woodchuck Lake. Note this junction; you'll return here on Day 3.

Turn left (north-northeast) toward Woodchuck Lake, cross a couple braids of Woodchuck Creek, and meander past lodgepole pines interspersed with large boulders. As the route ascends moderately along pure lodgepole pine stands, views north reveal the sheer granite ledges that enclose Woodchuck Country. Easterners mistook the Sierra's marmots for the East's woodchucks and gave the area this erroneous name, which has stuck.

After topping out at 9840 feet, the trail descends 0.1 mile into Woodchuck Lake's basin (9812'; 11S 332701 4101144). At the lake's northwest bank, a small spur trail leads 100 yards south to large campsites. The main trail skirts the lake's sandy north shore, passing more campsites.

DAY 2 (Woodchuck Lake to Halfmoon Lake, 6 miles): En route to the south end of Woodchuck Lake, the trail crosses the eastern inlet and enters the gentle, lush terrain of the southern inlet's meadow. The trail gradually ascends out of Woodchuck Lake's basin and climbs 200 feet southward over the next mile before reaching a signed junction (9960'). The right fork goes southwest back toward Wishon Reservoir by way of a spur to Chimney Lake; note this junction, because you'll also come back here on Day 3.

For now, take the left fork (northeast) past a seasonal creek to a minor saddle where the trail briefly descends past a shallow pond. Your route then continues along barren granite slopes, climbing the south shoulder of an unnamed peak. This climb tops out 250 feet higher than upcoming Crown Pass. Descending the unnamed peak's eastern flanks, the trail reaches a junction (10,180') immediately before Crown Pass, where the right fork turns southeast toward Crown Lake (Trip 6's destination).

This day's route continues straight ahead (north-northeast) at this junction. Just beyond the signed junction, pine-filtered views lead to Scepter Peak, which separates Crown and Halfmoon lakes and their drainages (Crown to Middle Fork Kings River, and Halfmoon to North Fork Kings River).

Crown Pass (10,189') is nestled in the saddle between Crown Peak to the northeast and that unnamed higher peak (10,520') whose eastern slopes you've just descended. (For an exhilarating view, head west cross-country to the unnamed higher peak's summit for a panorama from the LeConte Divide and Kettle Ridge down the forested slopes west of Wishon Reservoir, and north-south from the Minarets near Mammoth Mountain to the high peaks of the Great Western Divide and the Kings-Kern Divide. Return to Crown Pass.)

Continuing, the rocky path descends toward Halfmoon Lake, moderately at first and then on steep switchbacks under western white and lodgepole pines. Heavily used campsites are located on the north and west banks with larger, more attractive sites situated

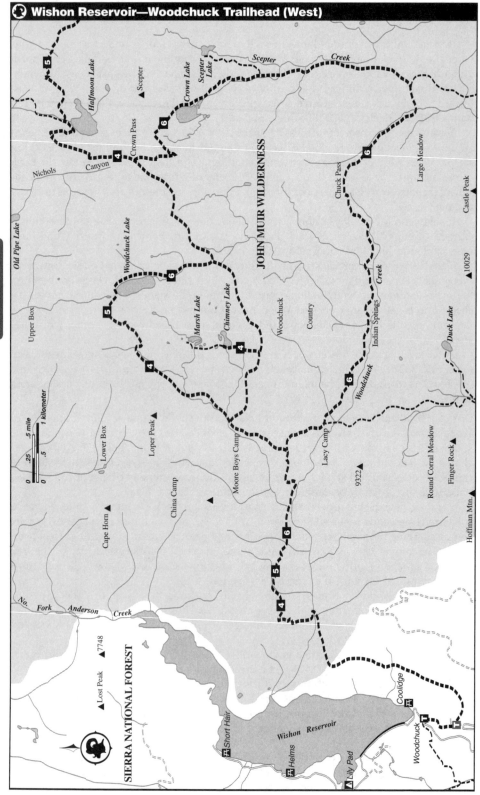

Scepter Creek

Halfmoon Lake

Scepter

Crown Lake

Scepter Lake

5

6

Crown Pass

4

Nichols

Canyon

Large Meadow

6

Chuck Pass

Castle Peak

JOHN MUIR WILDERNESS

Old Pipe Lake

Woodchuck Lake

6

▲10029

Upper Box

5

Marsh Lake

Chimney Lake

4

Woodchuck

Country

Indian Springs Creek

Duck Lake

4

Woodchuck Creek

6

1 kilometer

.5 mile

Lower Box

Loper Peak ▲

Moore Boys Camp

Lacy Camp

Round Corral Meadow

Finger Rock ▲

.25   .5

0   0

China Camp

▲

9322 ▲

Hoffman Mtn. ▲

6

Cape Horn ▲

5

No. Fork Anderson Creek

4

▲7748

Coolidge

SIERRA NATIONAL FOREST

▲Lost Peak

Short Hair

Helms

Wishon Reservoir

Lily Pad

Woodchuck

30

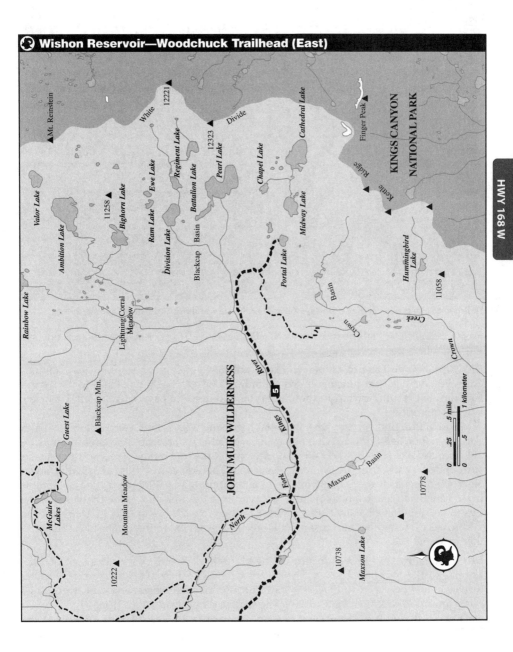

Wishon Reservoir—Woodchuck Trailhead (East)

KINGS CANYON NATIONAL PARK

JOHN MUIR WILDERNESS

Mt. Reinstein

12221

White

Divide

Cathedral Lake

Finger Peak

Regiment Lake

12323

Pearl Lake

Chapel Lake

Valor Lake

Ambition Lake

11258

Bighorn Lake

Ram Lake

Ewe Lake

Battalion Lake

Division Lake

Blackcap Basin

Midway Lake

Kettle Ridge

Hummingbird Lake

11058

Rainbow Lake

Lightning Corral Meadow

Portal Lake

Basin

Crown

Creek

Crown

Blackcap Mtn.

Guest Lake

Kings Fork River

North Fork

Maxson Basin

10778

10222

Mountain Meadow

Maxson Lake

10738

McGuire Lakes

0 .25 .5 mile

0 .5 1 kilometer

HWY 168 W

HWY 168 W

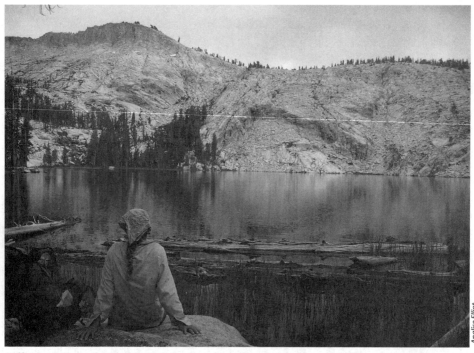

Analise Elliot

Halfmoon Lake is a jewel of the Sierra, offering excellent swimming and fishing opportunities.

across the outflow. Halfmoon Lake (9430'; 11S 354494 4016101) is a jewel in a granite setting and offers good swimming and fishing for brook and rainbow trout.

DAY 3 (Halfmoon Lake to Chimney Lake, 5 miles): Retrace your steps to the Chimney
Lake/Woodchuck Lake junction described in Day 2 (9960'). Beginning the loop part of this
trip, turn left (south) toward Wishon Reservoir and descend past outcrops left by ancient
volcanic mudflows.

In 1.5 miles, find another junction (9460'), this one with a spur trail to Chimney Lake.
Turn right (northeast) toward Chimney Lake, which the trail reaches in 0.4 mile. Campsites
at Chimney Lake (9484'; 331717 4099549) are just off the trail on the lake's northwest side,
surrounded by towering trees and lichen-covered boulders. Its shallow basin and lower
elevation mean its water is relatively warm and supports a healthy population of rainbow
trout. Chimney Lake is not as popular an overnight destination as the other lakes along
this route, due to its marshy banks, which host thick clouds of mosquitoes in the early to
mid-season. During the late season, with breeding grounds drying up, head 0.3 mile farther to Marsh Lake.

DAY 4 (Chimney Lake to Woodchuck Trailhead, 7 miles): Retrace your steps south on the
Chimney Lake spur trail, back to the junction with the main trail (9460'). At this junction,
turn right and head generally west toward the next junction where, on Day 1, you turned
north toward Woodchuck Lake (8720'). The loop part of this trip ends here.

Today, turn left (southwest) and reverse the first part of Day 1's steps through Moore
Boys Camp, past the Chuck Pass junction, and on to Wishon Reservoir and the Woodchuck
Trailhead.

5 Blackcap Basin

Trip Data: 11S 343726
4101161; 41 miles;
6/1 days

see map on p.30

Topos: *Rough Spur,
Courtright Reservoir, Blackcap Mtn.*

Highlights: One of a dozen High
Sierra lakes within Blackcap Basin,
Portal Lake occupies the top steps of a glacial staircase. Although official trails end at
Portal Lake, exploration into the vast Blackcap Basin and beyond through this "portal"
leads to exquisite scenic beauty at the west edge of the LeConte Divide and Kettle Ridge,
deep in the heart of John Muir Wilderness.

DAY 1 (Woodchuck Trailhead to Woodchuck Lake, 8 miles): *(Recap: Trip 4, Day 1.)* From the
Woodchuck Trailhead, the trail climbs nearly 400 feet, curves east, and joins a dirt road for
30 feet to a signed junction. Go left (southeast) and continue climbing steeply 500 feet,
swing north, and begin a scenic traverse. After nearly 2 miles, the path turns east, tops a
moraine, and then descends into Woodchuck Creek's canyon. The trail curves north and
descends to ford the creek (may be difficult in early season). From the ford, the path
ascends north and then bears east to switchback 500 feet over a minor ridge. The trail
meets a signed junction (8510') with a trail to Chuck Pass. Turn left (northeast) toward
Crown Pass, ford multiple branches of a creek, and, curving north again, make a short but
steep ascent over another moraine to the south end of a meadow. Follow the track across
the meadow to Moore Boys Camp (8710') and then a signed junction (8720') with trails
right (east-northeast) to Chimney Lake and Crown Pass and left (north-northeast) toward
Woodchuck Lake. Turn left (northeast) toward Woodchuck Lake and cross a couple braids
of Woodchuck Creek. After topping out at 9840 feet, the trail descends 0.1 mile into
Woodchuck Lake's basin (9812'; 11S 332701 4101144), where Day 1 ends.

DAY 2 (Woodchuck Lake to Halfmoon Lake, 6 miles): *(Recap: Trip 4, Day 2.)* Head for the
lake's south end, cross the eastern inlet, and enter the southern inlet's meadow. The gradual ascent out of Woodchuck Lake's basin climbs 200 feet southward over the next mile
before reaching a signed junction; take the left fork (northeast) to a minor saddle and
descend past a shallow pond. The track then climbs 250 feet over the south shoulder of an
unnamed peak above Crown Pass. As it descends, the trail reaches a junction (10,180') a little before Crown Pass proper; continue straight ahead (north-northeast) here to find
Crown Pass (10,189') between Crown Peak to the northeast and the unnamed higher peak
(10,520') whose eastern flanks you've just descended. Continuing, the rocky path descends
toward Halfmoon Lake (9430'; 11S 354494 4016101) to end Day 2.

DAY 3 (Halfmoon Lake to Blackcap Basin, 6.5 miles): At the lake's north side, the route
reaches a signed junction with a trail that leads straight ahead (north) toward Maxson
Meadow. Take the right fork eastward, ford the creek, and head through lodgepole and
western white pine stands.

The path climbs around a rocky ridge and then curves southeast, winding gently along
a forested bench and skirting a number of shallow gullies that have produced lush meadows, a mosquito haven during the wetter months. After a short descent and a ford of
Maxson Lake's outlet, the path meets the southeast-bound North Fork Kings River Trail
(9140') coming up on the left from Courtright Reservoir (a more heavily used trail into the
headwaters of North Fork Kings River).

From this signed junction, continue east (straight ahead), leaving the open flats of
the meadow. The hike climbs steadily up the southern slopes of the glacially polished,

HWY 168 W

narrowing walls of the Kings River's canyon, offering increasingly expansive views east-southeast toward Blackcap Basin. As the canyon narrows, the sounds of flowing water become more audible, and the path returns to the riverside. The gentle but steady ascent under the shade of a lodgepole pine forest traverses areas swept by avalanches, where vigorous willow thickets outcompete conifers. North Fork Kings River on your left (north)—sometimes near and sometimes far, sometimes meandering slowly through meadows and sometimes cascading past large granite slabs—contains a healthy population of golden, brook, and brown trout. Brisk and incredibly refreshing swimming holes scoured smooth by the crystalline river will rejuvenate weary hikers.

The trail briefly leaves the North Fork and climbs south toward Portal Lake to join its outlet stream. As the grade levels, the path leads to a picturesque and expansive meadow where a campsite marks the junction with the Crown Basin Trail (10,170'). Go left (southeast) toward Portal Lake; just beyond this campsite is the easy-to-miss ford (difficult during high water) of Portal Lake's outlet. (Hikers have missed the ford and simply followed the granite slabs southeast toward Portal Lake.) Beyond the ford, the trail climbs via short switchbacks to the small, scenic campsites on the north shore of Portal Lake (10,340'; 11S 343726 4101161). If Portal Lake's sites are full, continue northeast cross-country 0.2 mile to the banks of the neighboring unnamed lake (10,390').

EXPLORING BLACKCAP AND CROWN BASINS

From Portal Lake, you can take several easily traversed cross-country routes into Blackcap Basin and Crown Basin:

To journey deeper into Blackcap Basin: Leave Portal Lake along the barren granite slabs northeast and follow gentle terrain before briefly ascending 200 feet south of the headwaters of North Fork Kings River as it cascades below Pearl Lake (10,631'). From Pearl Lake's northwest finger, the easiest route climbs due north past a minor knoll and into the Division Lake Basin. From there, Regiment Lake (10,960') and Battalion Lake (11,050') can be reached by ascending the inlet cross-country upstream.

For Crown Basin: Follow the gentle, sloping ridge southwest above Portal Lake and continue along the open granite slabs south to several shallow unnamed lakes. From there, follow Crown Creek downstream to a small tributary that is fed by Hummingbird Lake (10,365').

DAYS 4–6 (Blackcap Basin to Woodchuck Trailhead, 20.5 miles): Retrace your steps.

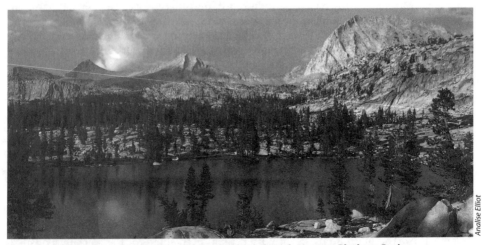

From Portal Lake, you can explore cross-country routes into the remote Blackcap Basin.

6 Crown Lake

Trip Data: 11S 33567 4100360; 25 miles;
4/1 days

Topos: *Rough Spur, Courtright Reservoir,
Blackcap Mtn.*

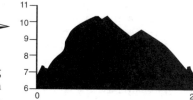

see map on p.30

Highlights: The broad, gentle terrain surrounding
Crown Lake allows excursions off the beaten path
in search of solitude. This trek provides the oppor-
tunity to commune peacefully along one of the finest series of meadows in the southern
Sierra.

DAY 1 (Woodchuck Trailhead to Woodchuck Lake, 8 miles): *(Recap: Trip 4, Day 1.)* From the
trailhead, the trail climbs nearly 400 feet, curves east, and joins a dirt road for 30 feet to a
signed junction. Go left (southeast) and continue climbing steeply 500 feet, swing north,
and begin a scenic traverse. After nearly 2 miles, the path turns east, tops a moraine, and
then descends into Woodchuck Creek's canyon. The trail curves north and descends to
ford the creek (may be difficult in early season). From the ford, the path ascends north and
then bears east to switchback 500 feet over a minor ridge. The route meets a signed junction (8510') with a trail to Chuck Pass; note this junction for your return on Day 4.

Turn left (northeast) toward Crown Pass, ford multiple branches of a creek, and, curving north again, make a short but steep ascent over another moraine to the south end of a
meadow. Follow the track across the meadow to Moore Boys Camp (8710') and then a
signed junction (8720') with trails right (east-northeast) to Chimney Lake and Crown Pass
and left (north-northeast) toward Woodchuck Lake. Turn left (northeast) toward
Woodchuck Lake and cross a couple braids of Woodchuck Creek. After topping out at 9840
feet, the trail descends 0.1 mile into Woodchuck Lake's basin (9812'; 11S 332701 4101144),
where Day 1 ends.

DAY 2 (Woodchuck Lake to Crown Lake, 3.5 miles): Head for the lake's south end, cross the
eastern inlet, and enter the southern inlet's meadow. The trail gradually ascends out of
Woodchuck Lake's basin and climbs 200 feet southward over the next mile before reaching
a signed junction; take the left fork (northeast) to a minor saddle and descend past a shallow pond. The track then climbs 250 feet over the south shoulder of an unnamed peak
above Crown Pass. As it descends, the trail reaches a junction (10,180') a little before Crown
Pass proper; turn right (south) toward Crown Lake.

From the junction, the trail descends steeply south 400 feet to the large, lodgepole-
rimmed meadow of Crown Lake (9730'; 11S 33567 4100360). Viewed from the pass, the lake
does have a crown-like shape, but its west side, containing several small pools, can be
marshy and a haven for mosquitoes. Campsites are best on the east side of the lake, where
the trail skirts along the southern slopes of the ridge above Crown Pass.

Surprise, Crown Lake is miles west of Crown Basin, and the lake's outlet flows into
Scepter Creek, which finally joins Crown Creek many miles southeast of here.

DAY 3 (Crown Lake to Indian Springs, 6 miles): The trail becomes somewhat indistinct as it
crosses the southern marshlands below Crown Lake, but it is easy to locate along the east
side of the unnamed outlet creek. Descend easily in moderate forest, at first lodgepole but
later mixed with western white pine. Intermittent marshy patches interrupt the trail's loose
duff surface as the path descends gently south on the east side of this creek.

At a junction with the Scepter Lake Trail (9420'), go ahead (south) and then cross the
creek. The trail's faint tread swings west of Scepter Creek, so that it is out of sight and
sound, but it returns to creekside at another meadow. Beyond this meadow, the route leads
to another meadow and then continues south to a junction with the Chuck Pass Trail
(9255').

HWY 168 W

Turn right (west) on this level trail and soon ford the sandy-bottomed, unnamed stream that drains Chuck Pass. Climb moderately up the southwest side of the little creek. The string of forest-bordered meadows along the creek's headwaters are, in the mountain springtime, narrow emerald ribbons interspersed with lush gardens—one of the finest series of meadows in the Sierra. After topping out at Chuck Pass (9540'), the rocky trail leads down through a park-like, spacious pine forest on a set of steep, dusty switchbacks. Soon, the route passes above a rocky, snag-strewn meadow, and then it descends to pass a series of sweeping green meadows, where the wildflower population boasts a tapestry of colors and aromas. Descending gently, the trail crosses a creek and skirts a large meadow. Soon you arrive at the attractive campsites at the west end of the meadow beside Indian Springs (8890'), between the trail and Woodchuck Creek.

DAY 4 (Indian Springs to Woodchuck Trailhead, 7.5 miles): The trail heads west down the valley of Woodchuck Creek, its tread often soft and muddy from the seepage of springs. It penetrates a dense forest of lodgepole pine and reaches a junction with the Hoffman Mountain Trail (8610').

Turn right (north) and immediately pass the ruins of an old cabin at abandoned Lacy Camp. The sandy forest path then dips west to meet the Wishon/Halfmoon Lake Trail at the Chuck Pass/Crown Pass junction, where you turned toward Crown Pass on Day 1.

From here, turn left (ahead, west) and retrace your steps to the trailhead.

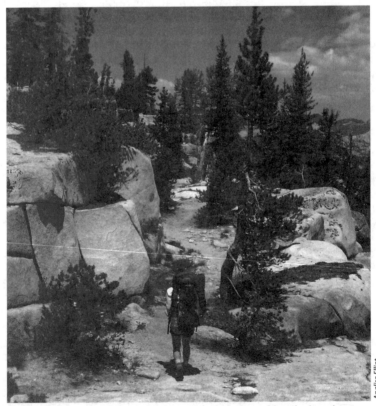

Analise Elliot

The trail tops out 250 feet above Crown Pass before reaching the junction to Crown Lake.

Courtright Reservoir—Maxson Trailhead   8040'; 11S 325593 4106033

DESTINATION/ UTM COORDINATES	TRIP TYPE	BEST SEASON	PACE (HIKING/ LAYOVER DAYS)	TOTAL MILEAGE
7 Post Corral Meadows 11S 331535 4110014	Out & back	Mid	2/0 Leisurely	15
8 Bench Valley Lakes 11S 340056 4105107	Out & back	Mid	6/1 Moderate, part cross-country	40
9 Red Mountain Basin 11S 337471 4110684	Semiloop	Mid	6/2 Moderate	34

Information and Permits: This trailhead is in Sierra National Forest: 1600 Tollhouse Road, Clovis, CA 93611, 559-297-0706, www.fs.fed.us/r5/sierra/. Permits are required for overnight stays, and quotas apply; reserved permits and on-demand permits are available.

Driving Directions: From Clovis (near Fresno), take Hwy. 168 42 miles northeast to the town of Shaver Lake. Turn right (generally east) onto Dinkey Creek Road and follow it 26 miles to the Wishon/Courtright Reservoir junction. The road to Courtright Reservoir takes the left fork, turning uphill toward the north. Follow this road another 7.5 miles to arrive at the south end of the dam. Continue to the right and cross the dam at the spillway. In another 0.6 mile, the road ends at a paved parking lot signed MAXSON TRAILHEAD.

7 Post Corral Meadows

Trip Data: 11S 331535 4110014; 15 miles; 2/0 days

Topos: *Courtright Reservoir, Ward Mountain*

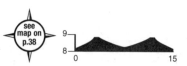

Highlights: This trip is an excellent choice for a weekend excursion. The route winds past the granite domes surrounding Courtright Reservoir, traverses sunny subalpine meadows, and climbs through open forests of pine. With moderate elevation gain, easy terrain, and an abundance of campsites, this is a fine selection for beginners.

DAY 1 (Maxson Trailhead to Post Corral Meadows, 7.5 miles): Leaving the trailhead from the west side, head north along the marked trail for 300 yards until it joins the Dusy Jeep Trail. This wide, dusty road descends briefly and then levels out over dirt and open granite slabs. After about 1 mile, an obvious log signed NO MOTOR VEHICLES bars such vehicles. The jeep trail heads left, while your route crosses the log and turns right (northeast).

The trail continues north next to a small creek for a half mile before fording it at the entrance to Maxson Meadows. Here, the trail turns into a raised path of wood and sand designed to help minimize impact on the area. Please take care to stay on the path to protect the surrounding picturesque meadows. After passing Chamberlain's Camp, the trail climbs about a mile of rocky switchbacks. While never steep, the elevation gain is steady for this mile. Beyond, the trail quickly levels off in a dense stand of lodgepole pine and comes to the signed Hobler Lake/Post Corral Meadows junction (8872'; 11S 327623 4110278). Take the right fork eastward.

The trail is briefly wide and flat and then begins to descend moderately through more pine and short switchbacks. Where the sandy trail leaves the forest, cross a seasonal creek and enter Long Meadow. The picturesque meadow is appropriately named and makes an excellent lunch and water stop. The small stream draining Long Meadow may be low during late season but will still provide water. If you got a late start, there are several campsites (8544'; 11S 329085 4110671) on the small, short rise to the north of the meadow that offer good wind protection.

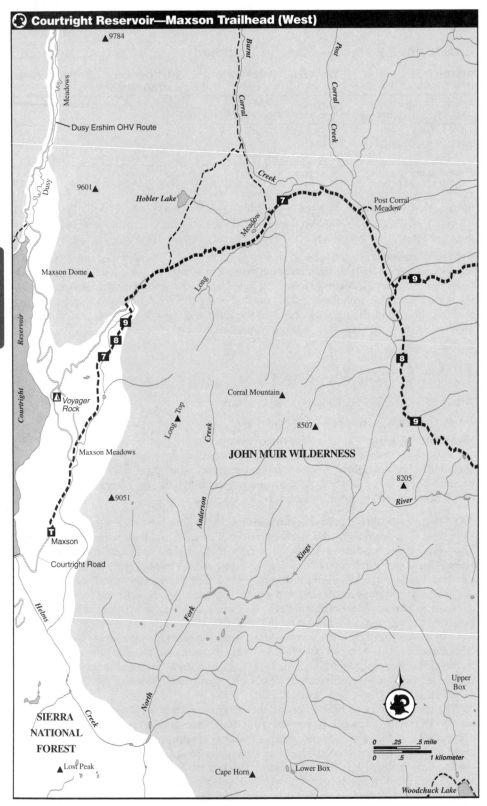

HWY 168 W

▲9784

Meadows

Dusy Ershim OHV Route

Dusy

9601▲

Hobler Lake

Burnt

Corral

Creek

Post

Corral

Creek

Creek

7

Post Corral
Meadow

Meadow

Maxson Dome ▲

Long

9

Reservoir

9
8
7

Courtright

Voyager
Rock

Long ▶ Top

Corral Mountain ▲

8507 ▲

Creek

8

9

Maxson Meadows

JOHN MUIR WILDERNESS

8205
▲

River

▲9051

Anderson

Kings

T
Maxson

Courtright Road

Helms

Fork

Creek

North

SIERRA
NATIONAL
FOREST

▲ Lost Peak

Cape Horn ▲

Lower Box

Upper
Box

0   .25   .5 mile
0   .5   1 kilometer

Woodchuck Lake

38

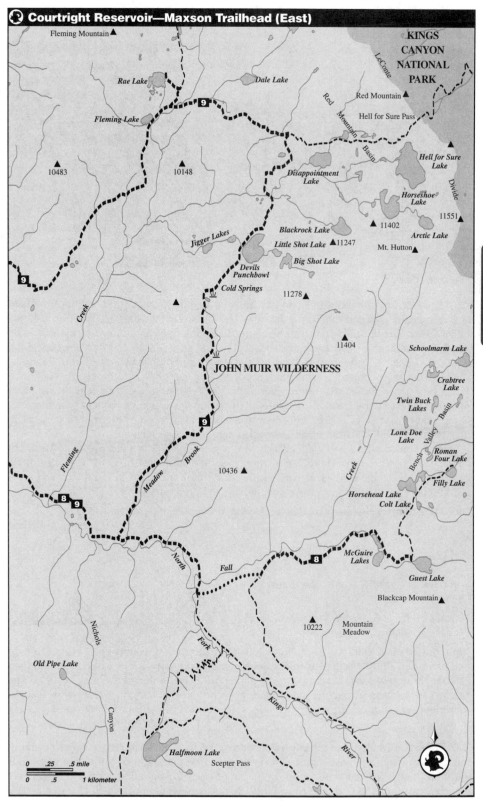

KINGS
CANYON
NATIONAL
PARK

Fleming Mountain ▲

Rae Lake

Dale Lake

LeConte

Red Mountain ▲

Hell for Sure Pass

Fleming Lake

9

Red Mountain Basin

Hell for Sure Lake ▲

▲ 10483

▲ 10148

Disappointment Lake

Horseshoe Lake

Divide

▲ 11402

11551 ▲

Jigger Lakes

Blackrock Lake

Little Shot Lake ▲ 11247

Arctic Lake

Mt. Hutton ▲

Big Shot Lake

Devils Punchbowl

Cold Springs

▲

11278 ▲

Schoolmarm Lake

11404 ▲

JOHN MUIR WILDERNESS

Crabtree Lake

Twin Buck Lakes

9

Lone Doe Lake

Bench Valley Basin

Roman Four Lake

Creek

Filly Lake

Meadow

Brook

10436 ▲

Horsehead Lake
Colt Lake

8 9

Fleming

North

Fall

McGuire Lakes

8

Guest Lake

Blackcap Mountain ▲

Nichols

Fork

10222 ▲

Mountain Meadow

Old Pipe Lake

Canyon

Kings

River

Halfmoon Lake
Scepter Pass

0   .25   .5 mile
0   .5   1 kilometer

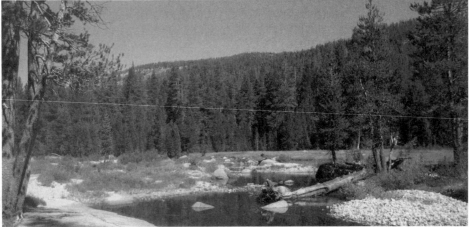

Chris Tirrell

Post Corral Creek

After reaching the mouth of Long Meadow, the route traverses the length of the field and then gently descends back into the trees. Here, reach a poorly signed junction with the Burnt Corral Creek Trail. That trail heads north and is quite faint, and the sign is easily missed when heading east along this route. Continue ahead (east) and don't be concerned if you do not see the junction. Stroll next to the stream and then ford it after about 0.75 mile.

The trail then drops back into more lodgepole pine, gradually descends, and turns toward the south. When the trail reaches a short wooden bridge and flattens, it is another mile to the Post Corral Creek ford. Although they may be difficult to spot at first, there are several quiet campsites tucked into the pines along this section of the trail. If the sites at Post Corral are full, you can backtrack to this area to find seclusion.

Just before the ford of Post Corral Creek, a granite boulder field opens on the right (west) side of the trail. There are several obvious campsites here (8200′; 11S 331535 4110014), at the edge of the encroaching forest. At the ford of Post Corral Creek, a wide granite slab eases gently into the water, making an idyllic dinner site.

DAY 2 (Post Corral Meadows to Maxson Trailhead, 7.5 miles): Retrace your steps.

8 Bench Valley Lakes

Trip Data: 11S 340056 4105107 (at Guest Lake); 40 miles; 6/1 days

Topos: *Courtright Reservoir, Ward Mountain, Blackcap Mountain, Mt. Henry*

see map on p.38

Highlights: This trip traverses the lush, forested meadows surrounding Corral Mountain and offers sweeping vistas of granite domes along North Fork Kings River. The path then ascends through serene meadows carpeted in wildflowers to the stark alpine beauty of the Bench Valley basin. The many small lakes and cliffs in this hanging valley offer fishing, rock climbing, and rich alpenglow at sunset. Since most of the trail follows marked, easy terrain, this trip makes a great choice for a longer yet moderate outing.

DAY 1 (Maxson Trailhead to Post Corral Meadows, 7.5 miles): *(Recap: Trip 7, Day 1.)* Leaving the trailhead from the west side, head north along the marked trail for 300 yards until it joins the Dusy Jeep Trail. After about 1 mile, an obvious log signed NO MOTOR VEHICLES bars vehicles; cross the log and turn right (northeast). Go generally north next to a small creek for a half mile before fording it at the entrance to Maxson Meadows. Follow a raised wood and sand trail designed to help protect the area.

After passing Chamberlain's Camp, the trail climbs about a mile of rocky switchbacks. Beyond, the trail levels off in a dense stand of lodgepole pine and comes to the signed Hobler Lake/Post Corral Meadows junction (8872´; 11S 327623 4110278). Take the right fork (east).

The trail is briefly wide and flat and then begins to descend short switchbacks. Where the sandy trail leaves the forest, cross a seasonal creek and enter Long Meadow. Late-starters will find several campsites (8544´; 11S 329085 4110671) on the small, short rise to the north of the meadow.

Traverse Long Meadow and then descend to a poorly signed junction with the Burnt Corral Creek Trail (easily missed when heading east along this route; don't worry if you don't see it). Continue ahead (east) next to the stream and then ford it after about 0.75 mile.

The trail then gradually descends while turning south. When the trail reaches a short wooden bridge and flattens, it is another mile to the Post Corral Creek ford. There are several quiet, hard-to-spot campsites tucked into the trees along this section of the trail. (If the sites at Post Corral Creek are full, backtrack to this area.)

Just before the ford of Post Corral Creek, a granite boulder field opens on the right (west) side of the trail. There are several obvious campsites here (8200´; 11S 331535 4110014).

DAY 2 (Post Corral Meadows to North Fork Kings River, 5.6 miles): Shortly after fording Post Corral Creek (wet in early season), the Hell For Sure Pass Trail heads left at a signed junction. Go right (south), following a sandy trail. After a half mile, the trail climbs out of the pines and passes larger granite boulders and sandy open flats. The route than makes a short descent and winds through more meadow and sandy forest for the next 2 miles.

After the trail gains a ridge and turns to the southeast, the vista opens dramatically, with sweeping views through the trees across the granitic North Fork Kings River's canyon. The trail follows a sandy wash down short switchbacks and then meets low-angle granite slabs near the river. There are many relaxing lunch spots here, along with plenty of water and several refreshing swimming holes farther down the trail to the south. There are many campsites near this juncture if a short day is in order. Fishing along the river is good for brook, brown, and rainbow trout.

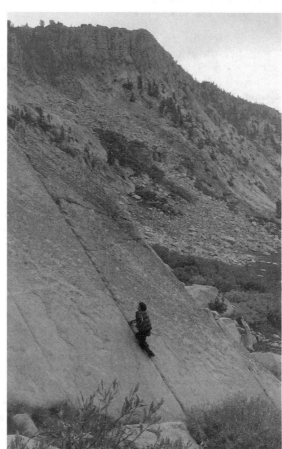

Bouldering below Blackcap Mountain

Chris Tirrell

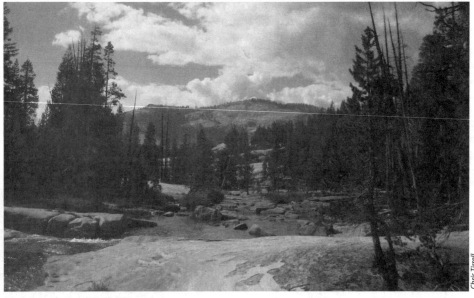

Chris Tirrell

The majestic North Fork Kings River

From here, the trail continues southeastward and reenters the ubiquitous pine forest. On the left side of the path, yellow-green lichen coats house-sized granite boulders nestled among the trees, while ferns and dense thickets of manzanita carpet the forest floor.

After a meandering half mile, the trail comes to a moderate clearing with a California Cooperative Snow Survey log cabin next to a waterfall and a large pool in the river. The trail exits the left side of this clearing to the southeast and continues on another half mile to the signed Devils Punchbowl/Big Maxson Meadow Trail junction (8183'; 11S 334724 4105551). There are several superb campsites just before the signed junction, across the granite slabs, next to the river on the west side of the trail.

DAY 3 (North Fork Kings River to Guest Lake, 6.9 miles, part cross-country): The trail leaves the signed Devils Punchbowl/Maxson Meadow junction by the right fork (southeast), staying parallel with North Fork Kings River. After crossing several small branches of Meadow Brook, the tread heads up a short set of stone stairs and crosses open granite slabs near a large pool. The normally rough granite has been worn down by the passage of the water, and several of the pools make for great swimming holes.

The path continues southeast and climbs gently up dirt and loose rock for about a mile until reaching the rocky ford of Fall Creek (wet in early season). Follow the trail 300 yards after the last ford of the creek to the point where a faint trail turns to the left (east) from the main trail; from here, the main trail goes far out of your way. So take the angler's use trail. It's indistinct near the bottom, but many ducks become apparent as it climbs higher. If you lose the trail, head cross-country generally east-northeast up the hill parallel with the creek, keeping Fall Creek about 200 yards away on your left side. The trail is steep and occasionally loose, so exercise caution while ascending. At the top, find expansive views all the way back down the valley.

Once it reaches the low-angle granite slabs at the top, the route levels off and once again enters dense lodgepole forest. Shortly thereafter, the route joins the main trail ascending from Big Maxson Meadow and begins a lazy traverse through 2 miles of beautiful foliage and dense ferns. In the spring, shooting star, penstemon, larkspur, monkshood, monkeyflower, columbine, wallflower, and paintbrush line the path. In late season, the ferns turn yellow, carpeting the forest floor with broad brushstrokes of color.

HWY 168 W

After traversing the forested meadow, the trail starts to climb again and culminates with a short but steep climb to the rim of the McGuire Lakes. The meadow-lined banks of the lake appear suddenly and make a welcome rest stop after the strenuous climb. From the vantage of the lake's shores, it becomes apparent that this point is the entrance to a hanging valley. Rising proudly to the southeast is Blackcap Mountain; its granite summit blocks sit outlined like a dark sentinel against the vibrant red alpenglow at sunset.

HANGING VALLEYS

Hanging valleys occur when a tributary glacier carves its valley more slowly than does the larger glacier of which it is a tributary. In time, the larger glacier's valley floor will be well below the tributary glacier's. The tributary's valley is left "hanging" high on the wall of the main valley after the glaciers melt, and the tributary's stream drops, often from a lake, into the deeper main valley in the form of cascades and waterfalls. Yosemite's Bridalveil and Yosemite falls are classic examples of this process. McGuire Lakes sit in one of a series of such hanging valleys that line the flanks of the LeConte Divide.

The trail skirts the lake, curving north and then south along the lake through sparse pine and large granite boulders. After the footpath veers east and crosses a short ridge, Guest Lake is visible straight ahead. There are comfortable campsites on the south side of Guest Lake among the large boulders and more sites along the north bank in the trees (10,195´; 11S 340056 4105107). If these sites are crowded, consider continuing on the fisherman's trail another mile north to Horsehead Lake, where a few campsites dot the southeast shore. There is good fishing at Guest Lake for brook trout.

EXPLORING BENCH VALLEY

If your itinerary allows time for a layover day, Guest Lake makes a fantastic base camp from which to explore the rest of the Bench Valley lakes. A wonderful dayhike follows the angler's use trail northward to Horsehead Lake, and then explores Roman Four Lake, Twin Buck Lakes, and Schoolmarm Lake. Anglers will encounter brook and rainbow at Horsehead Lake, brook at Roman Four Lake, rainbow at West Twin Buck Lake (East Twin Buck Lake is barren), and small rainbow at Schoolmarm Lake. There is also wonderful bouldering on the granite outcroppings surrounding Guest Lake. Rock climbers will be tempted to explore the inviting cracks bisecting the towering granite walls overhead. The climbing here is of such quality that the walls would surely be crowded, were it not for the high price of admission.

DAYS 4–6 (Guest Lake to Maxson Trailhead, 20 miles): Retrace your steps.

9 Red Mountain Basin

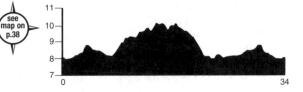

Trip Data: 11S 337471 4110684
(at Devils Punchbowl); 5/2 days;
34 miles

Topos: *Courtright Reservoir, Ward Mountain, Blackcap Mt.,*
Mt. Henry

Highlights: This trip takes an old sheepherder's route, known as the Baird Trail, from the subalpine meadows at Post Corral Creek to the stunning alpine scenery surrounding Devils Punchbowl, a lake in remote Red Mountain Basin and a good spot from which to explore the basin. The trek then descends via Meadow Brook, one of the Sierra's most picturesque subalpine meadows, to take in spectacular views of the North Fork Kings River.

DAY 1 (Maxson Trailhead to Post Corral Meadows, 7.5 miles): *(Recap: Trip 7, Day 1.)* Leaving the trailhead from the west side, head north along the marked trail for 300 yards until it joins the Dusy Jeep Trail. After about 1 mile, an obvious log signed NO MOTOR VEHICLES bars vehicles; cross the log and turn right (northeast). Go generally north next to a small creek for a half mile before fording it at the entrance to Maxson Meadows. Follow a raised wood and sand trail designed to help protect the area.

After passing Chamberlain's Camp, the trail climbs about a mile of rocky switchbacks. Beyond, the trail levels off in a dense stand of lodgepole pine and comes to the signed Hobler Lake/Post Corral Meadows junction (8872'; 11S 327623 4110278). Take the right fork (east).

The trail is briefly wide and flat and then begins to descend short switchbacks. Where the sandy trail leaves the forest, cross a seasonal creek and enter Long Meadow. Late-starters will find several campsites (8544'; 11S 329085 4110671) on the small, short rise to the north of the meadow.

Traverse Long Meadow and then descend to a poorly signed junction with the Burnt Corral Creek Trail (easily missed when heading east along this route; don't worry if you don't see it). Continue ahead (east) next to the stream and then ford it after about 0.75 mile.

The trail then gradually descends while turning south. When the trail reaches a short wooden bridge and flattens, it is another mile to the Post Corral Creek ford. There are several quiet, hard-to-spot campsites tucked into the trees along this section of the trail. (If the sites at Post Corral Creek are full, backtrack to this area.)

Just before the ford of Post Corral Creek, a granite boulder field opens on the right (west) side of the trail. There are several obvious campsites here (8200'; 11S 331535 4110014).

DAY 2 (Post Corral Meadows to Rae Lake, 5.5 miles): Top off water supplies here; today's route gains 1600 feet in 5 miles with no reliable water.

After leaving the campsites, head east to ford Post Corral Creek (wet in early season) and shortly find the signed Blackcap/Red Mountain Basin junction. Turn left (east). The trail then begins to climb the ridge separating Post Corral Creek and Fleming Creek. The first mile is moderate under shady pine cover, but shortly thereafter the trail steepens over dynamited slabs.

Continue up the obvious path to the small, wooded flat before reaching the switchbacks that lead up the last few hundred feet to the ridgeline. The trail turns toward the northeast and begins a more gentle ascent up the forested north flank of Fleming Creek's canyon.

After 1.5 miles, the track turns north and ascends steep, rocky switchbacks to gain the meadows surrounding small, photogenic Fleming Lake. Here, the landscape takes on a definite subalpine character with less tree cover and more exposed granite boulders and slabs.

The path crosses Fleming Lake's outlet and soon meets a junction with the Hell For Sure Pass Trail at the foot of a long meadow dotted with colorful wildflowers. Turn left (north) here and climb to a shaded hillside junction with the short spur trail leading to Rae Lake (9889´; 11S 335881 4113427). Idyllic campsites lie beneath the trees on the north banks of the lake, and there is good fishing for brook trout.

DAY 3 (Rae Lake to Devils Punchbowl, 4 miles): Return to the Hell For Sure Trail junction. Turn left (east) and shortly ford Fleming Creek. The path then begins a 500-foot ascent that starts on a tree-covered slope with patches of meadow and wildflowers. With the terrain growing dry and sandy, the trail gains a ridgetop and briefly turns south to cross open meadows and seasonal creeks before heading east again.

In another mile, find the unsigned junction with a trail to Devils Punchbowl next to a five-foot gray fence post. Turn right (south) and pass a small lake before dropping 300 feet to reach East Fork Fleming Creek. The trail crosses at a rocky ford (wet in early season) and then climbs 300 feet to the low ridge on the north side of Devils Punchbowl. The turnoff to the lake is an indistinct trail on the left just before you start up this ridge. Good campsites are located on the east side of the lake (10,098´; 11S 337471 4110684). The lake is popular with hikers and fishermen, so please make an effort to minimize your impact. This ideal location makes a great spot for a layover day, as the rugged terrain of Red Mountain Basin on all sides begs for exploration.

DAY 4 (Devils Punchbowl to Post Corral Meadows, 9.5 miles): From the north side of the lake, the trail heads south along the granite walls that dam the lake. Midway along the ridge, you can spy the small Jigger Lakes below and to the west. At the southwest corner of Devils Punchbowl, the trail makes several short switchbacks to gain a saddle before turning to the south and beginning a 2000-foot descent to North Fork Kings River.

The descent begins with a 200-foot sandy slope leading to lush meadows at the head of Meadow Brook. In the next mile, the path skirts the west side of the meadows, threading past lavender shooting star, purple Sierra gentian, and monkeyflower. The views from this section of trail are breathtaking: With the meadow in the foreground, you can see all the way to the far side of the North Fork Kings River drainage. Cattle may be run in this drainage; if present, they certainly detract from the natural beauty of the meadows. There are many idyllic spots to lunch and take in this meadow's beautiful setting.

After this pleasurable mile, the grade steepens and turns southwest away from the creek, angling down a forested moraine. The next mile descends continuously, and stands of red fir, Jeffrey pine, and quaking aspen welcome you back to lower elevation. The path levels out on open granite slabs at the bottom of the grade and reaches a signed junction with the Blackcap Mountain Trail. Turn right (west) along North Fork Kings River, soon curving northwest and shortly fording Fleming Creek. Cross a forested flat, descend a little to slabs near the river, and then climb an open hillside to a ridgetop with fine views over North Fork Kings River.

GLACIERS AND EXPLORERS ON NORTH FORK KINGS RIVER

The entire granitic North Fork Kings River's canyon was covered with glacial ice many times during the past million years, and the most recent glacier retreated up-canyon only about 11,000 years ago. At this spot, it is interesting to speculate on the route followed in this area by Capt. John C. Frémont, the "Pathfinder." Historians are unsure of the exact route, but they do agree that Frémont's party got lost high in this drainage in during Frémont's second great expedition of 1843-44. They were caught in an early winter storm, were forced to eat their saddle stock, and finally retreated.

HWY 168 W

Descend from the ridge and follow the sandy, undulating trail as it winds through forest and small meadows for 2 miles to a ford of an unnamed creek. Meet the Blackcap Mountain/Red Mountain Basin Trail at the junction near Post Corral Creek. Turn left (northwest) here and ford Post Corral Creek to find the good campsites of Day 1 (8200´; 11S 331535 4110014). The loop part of this trip ends here.

DAY 5 (Post Corral Meadows to Maxson Trailhead, 7.5 miles): Retrace your steps to the trailhead.

HWY 168 W

Courtright Reservoir—Cliff Lake Trailhead   8454; 11S 323436 4108468

DESTINATION/ UTM COORDINATES	TRIP TYPE	BEST SEASON	PACE (HIKING/ LAYOVER DAYS)	TOTAL MILEAGE
10 Cliff Lake 11S 318673 4112363	Out & back	Mid	2/1 Leisurely	10
11 Dinkey Lakes 11S 323436 4108468 (Island Lake)	Semiloop	Mid	3/1 Leisurely	20

Information and Permits: This trailhead is in Sierra National Forest: 1600 Tollhouse Road, Clovis, CA 93611, 559-297-0706, www.fs.fed.us/r5/sierra/. Permits are required for overnight stays, and quotas apply; reserved permits and on-demand permits are available.

Driving Directions: From Clovis (near Fresno), take Hwy. 168 northeast for 42 miles; in Shaver Lake, turn right onto Dinkey Creek Road and follow it 26 miles to the Courtright/Wishon Y. Take the left fork to Courtright Reservoir, 7.5 more miles north. Drive along the left (west) side of the reservoir past Trapper Springs Campground until the road ends at Cliff Lake Trailhead. There are four bear boxes and room for a dozen cars at this Dinkey Lakes Wilderness trailhead (no water or toilets).

10 Cliff Lake

Trip Data: 11S 318673 4112363; 10 miles; 2/1 days

Topos: *Courtright Reservoir, Dogtooth Peak, Ward Mtn.*

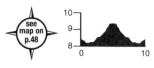

Highlights: Splendid alpine scenery keeps hikers company as they enjoy this easy trip to a lake nestled under sheer granite cliffs and ledges. An optional climb of Dogtooth Peak adds to the scenery and adventure.

DAY 1 (Cliff Lake Trailhead to Cliff Lake, 5 miles): Leaving the trailhead, the path descends gradually northwest toward Courtright Reservoir, travels a half mile under the scattered shade of red fir and lodgepole pine, and passes a spur trail on the right (east). Continue ahead (generally northwest) and traverse two marshy and mosquito-rich areas along a wooden boardwalk.

THE ORIGIN OF "DINKEY"

One might assume that the name "Dinkey" refers to the dozens of small, unnamed, and unrecognized lakes within the wilderness area. But locals will tell you the 1863 legend of a tiny dog named Dinkey. On an outing with its owner, an aggressive grizzly bear charged. Dinkey, reportedly "no bigger than a rabbit," attacked, biting the hind leg of the massive grizzly. The bear swiped, and, in a flash, Dinkey was lifeless. Yet Dinkey's bravery was not in vain. Dinkey saved its owner, distracting the grizzly and allowing its owner enough time to grab his gun and kill the bear. Local legend and Dinkey Lakes Wilderness honor small but mighty Dinkey to this day.

From the northwest finger of Courtright Reservoir, the trail crosses Nelson Creek (difficult in early season) and turns left (northwest) at a junction, leaving Courtright Reservoir. Three miles from the trailhead, the path reaches a signed junction (8570'): A lightly traveled route leads right (north) to Helms Meadow, and another route leads left (southwest) to Nelson Lakes. Your route along the Cliff Lake Trail continues straight (northwest) through a dense forest of lodgepole, red fir, and western white pine.

see map on p.48

HWY 168 W

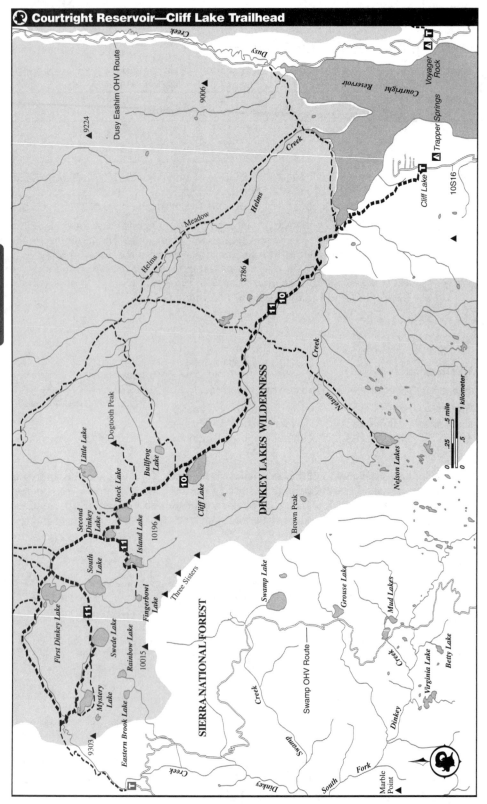

The trail's grade steepens over switchbacks as it passes through the filtered sunshine of a south-facing slope cloaked with red-barked manzanita shrubs and large western white pine. Enjoy views of Courtright Reservoir and the surrounding granite domes bordering its shores. Brown Peak (10,349´), Nelson Mountain (10,218´), and Eagle Peak (10,318´) tower on the southern skyline, while farther east, the desolate, sawtooth, granite peaks of the LeConte Divide can be seen breaking the seemingly endless expanse of sky.

Above the switchbacks, the trail returns to a more moderate grade and soon reaches an unmarked junction (9430´) with a spur trail left. Go left (west-northwest) to the banks of Cliff Lake (the right branch continues just above Cliff Lake toward Dogtooth Peak and Rock Lake). Descend this spur trail to the lower end of the lake and the first of six campsites that are nestled along the eastern shore, with a backdrop of sheer 400-foot granite walls that tower above the boulder-studded forest (9430´; 11S 318673 4112363).

DAY 2 (Cliff Lake to Cliff Lake Trailhead, 5 miles): Retrace your steps.

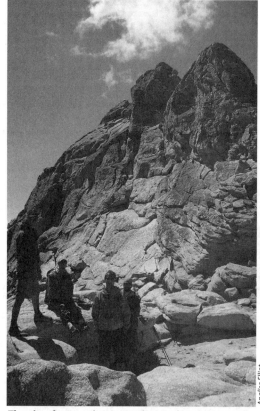

Andlise Elliot

The view from a minor summit reveals another peak dividing the "tooth" of the Dogtooth in two.

BAGGING DOGTOOTH PEAK

To begin this trip, return to the previous junction (9430´) and turn left (northwest) directly above Cliff Lake. The trail meets a junction (9760´) 0.1 mile farther, with a right-branching trail east to Bullfrog Lake. Continue northwest along the left branch for a moderate, 500-foot climb to the prominent saddle and an unmarked junction with a use trail to Dogtooth Peak; here, enjoy views of the granite cliffs that lend their name to Cliff Lake, 400 feet below.

From the saddle and junction (9860´), turn right and follow the lightly traveled route east along the south side of the ridge. This expanse offers tremendous views of the varied and colorful southern Sierra landscape—sapphire alpine lakes bordered by forested mountains bearing granite peaks, spires, and domes. The level route traverses large granite slabs between two diminutive domes.

At a notch, the route turns steeply northeast to the base of Dogtooth Peak. Hiking cross-country to Dogtooth's east side requires careful bouldering across large granite slabs. The view from a minor summit reveals another peak dividing the "tooth" of the Dogtooth in two.

At 10,302 feet, Dogtooth Peak, defined by jagged and glistening white-quartz chunks, resembles the finest ivory. At the summit, a relatively small expenditure of energy rewards peakbaggers with encompassing views of the myriad of high Sierra summits, including some of North America's highest peaks along LeConte Divide. A host of barren granite domes encircle Courtright Reservoir to the southeast, while a short distance to the west, the 10,612-foot Three Sisters soar high above the thickly forested Dinkey Lakes basin.

11 Dinkey Lakes

Trip Data: 11S 323436 4108468 (Island Lake);
20 miles; 3/1 days

Topos: *Courtright Reservoir, Dogtooth Peak*

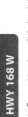

Highlights: Dinkey Lakes Wilderness receives
far less traffic than its eastern neighbor, John Muir Wilderness. This well-graded route
leads past nearly a dozen alpine lakes that are set amid granite spires and sawtooth ridge-
lines. The shallow lakes are relatively warm for swimming.

DAY 1 (Cliff Lake Trailhead to Island Lake, 7 miles): Follow the trail northwest to Courtright
Reservoir. Near the reservoir's northwest end, ford Nelson Creek (difficult in early season.
At a signed junction (8570´), continue straight (northwest) through a dense forest of lodge-
pole, red fir, and western white pine.

The trail's grade steepens over switchbacks. Above the switchbacks, the route returns
to a more moderate grade and soon reaches an unmarked junction (9430´). Take the right
fork (northwest) toward Dogtooth Peak and Rock Lake.

Ascend along switchbacks, climbing 110 feet to a junction right (east) to Bullfrog Lake.
Go left (northwest), climbing another 200 feet to a saddle and unmarked trail junction to
Dogtooth Peak (see page 49 for directions on how to bag Dogtooth Peak). From the saddle,
descend north-northwest to Rock Lake (9590´). The first of several large campsites is nestled at the southeast shore, with more open south-facing sites along the northwest bank
(fishing for brook). The path skirts Rock Lake's eastern bank, crosses the outflow, and soon
reaches a marked junction with a right-branching side trail (northeast) to Little Lake
(9640´).

LITTLE LAKE

From this junction (9640´), the 0.8-mile side trail to Little Lake turns right (northeast) and
descends along rocky switchbacks just northwest of the outflow that links Rock Lake and
Little Lake. The descent quickly drops 300 feet through dense lodgepole pine before arcing
northeast onto the grassy, mosquito-rich banks of shallow Little Lake. Little Lake is backdropped by the towering, serrated ridgeline of Dogtooth Peak. Come dusk and dawn, small
rainbow and brook trout aggressively feed on the myriad of insects.

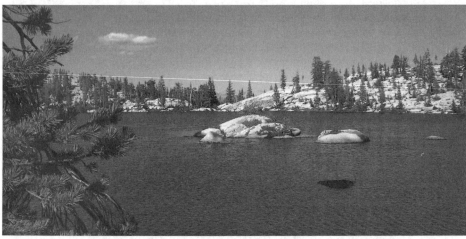

Several rocky, sun-drenched islands are surrounded by the blue waters of Island Lake.

Andlise Elliot

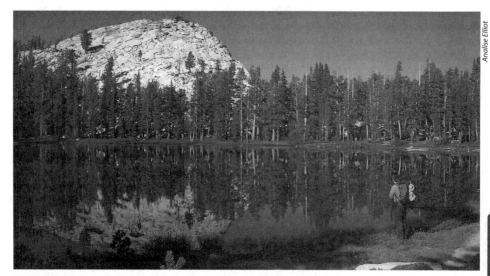

Analise Elliot

The trail arcs along the northeastern shore of Second Dinkey Lake.

This trip's route follows the left fork west, gently climbing 0.2 mile before dropping into the Dinkey Lakes basin and shortly reaching a Y-junction (9590´) with a trail left (south) to Island Lake. Take this path; en route to Island Lake, the path skirts Second Dinkey Lake's west shore and then ascends a brief but steep 200 feet. The climb offers views of the wilderness's highest peaks, the three towering granite monoliths of the Three Sisters: 10,436 feet, 10,438 feet, and 10,612 feet.

After the climb, the trail descends moderately and southwest to Island Lake (9815´; 11S 323436 4108468), the crown jewel of Dinkey Lakes Wilderness. As a result, several campsites rim its shores. True to the lake's name, there are several rocky, sun-drenched islands; they support mature lodgepole and are a popular destination for swimmers braving the frigid water. Fishing is fair for rainbow and brook trout.

> **BEYOND ISLAND LAKE**
>
> The terrain surrounding Island Lake, bare granite slabs and broad open forests, is excellent for cross-country exploring. Fingerbowl Lake (9680´), nestled west of Island Lake, can be reached easily by following the granite wall northwest to a south-trending ridge. From the ridge, westward views reveal a half-dozen lakes within a relatively small area. Fingerbowl Lake (less than a quarter mile away) is a small, deep, round lake fringed on one side by a marshy outlet and on the other by snow-covered scree. The Three Sisters are visible beyond the lake's eastern shore.

DAY 2 (Island Lake to South Lake, 5 miles): From Island Lake, return to the Y-junction at Second Dinkey Lake (9580´). Turn left and head north, closely following the western banks of Dinkey Creek as it quietly cascades from Second Dinkey Lake to First Dinkey Lake. After a moderate, 0.6-mile descent, the track reaches a junction (9280´), at which this trip's loop section begins.

While the loop can be taken in either direction, this trip takes hikers to the lakes in order of the lakes' increasing scenic beauty. So continue straight ahead (west-northwest) to the broad, marshy, east end of First Dinkey Lake (9239´), bound by bogs and meadows that host a vigorous population of mosquitoes well into summer. The barren ridge of the Three Sisters is visible beyond its southern shore.

The trail arcs around the lake's north shore, meeting a junction just past the large boulders by the lake's outlet (9270´). Turn left (generally west) and begin a gradual descent, once again following Dinkey Creek (brook trout) as it gains in volume and velocity the farther it flows from its headwaters.

After 1.6 miles, bear left (south) across Dinkey Creek and climb gradually to Mystery Lake (8963´). Near the lake's outlet, the trail becomes difficult to spot, as use paths diverge in all directions around this heavily used lake. Your main path skirts the lake's north side and the boggy area east of it before crossing Swede Lake's outlet. Now the route climbs about a dozen switchbacks and refords the outlet just prior to reaching Swede Lake's north shore. Swede Lake (9224´), bordered by smooth granite slabs on its southeast shore, presents fine swimming and angling opportunities.

Past Swede Lake's north end, the trail immediately climbs 150 feet, ending in a mellow traverse and slight descent to South Lake in 0.7 mile. South Lake (9294´; 11S 316454 4114249), with its deep, alluring, emerald waters, is fed by a waterfall rushing over an exposed granite ledge on its south side.

DAY 3 (South Lake to Cliff Lake Trailhead, 8 miles): Beyond South Lake, the main trail crosses the lake's outlet and traverses gradually above bogs to ford Dinkey Creek and reach the junction where you began the loop on Day 2. At this junction, close the loop and turn right (east). Retrace your steps to the next junction, and instead of going back to Island Lake, head left (east and then south) along Second Dinkey Lake's east shore to Rock Lake. From there, retrace this trip's route to the trailhead.

Potter Pass Trailhead

7855´; 11S 309230 4126844

DESTINATION/ UTM COORDINATES	TRIP TYPE	BEST SEASON	PACE (HIKING/ LAYOVER DAYS)	TOTAL MILEAGE
12 George Lake 11S 307566 4129484	Out & back	Mid to late	2/1 Moderate	9.4

Information and Permits: This trailhead is in Sierra National Forest: 1600 Tollhouse Road, Clovis, CA 93611, 559-297-0706, www.fs.fed.us/r5/sierra/. Permits are required for overnight stays, and quotas apply; reserved permits and on-demand permits are available.

Driving Directions: From Clovis (near Fresno), take State Hwy. 168 northeast for 42 winding, slow miles to its end at a T junction on the east shore of Huntington Lake at the community of Lakeshore. Turn right, away from Lakeshore, on Kaiser Pass Road, and go 2.7 more miles to a junction with a dirt road on the left (north). Turn left and go 0.2 mile to its end at the Potter Pass Trailhead for Kaiser Wilderness.

12 George Lake

Trip Data: 11S 307566 4129484; 9.4 miles; 2/1 days

Topos: *Kaiser Peak*

Highlights: In the heart of the Sierra National Forest, little Kaiser Wilderness boasts 35 square miles of pristine forests, emerald lakes, and rugged alpine terrain. Despite its immediate proximity to Huntington Lake, Kaiser Wilderness lures relatively few hikers compared to neighboring John Muir and Ansel Adams wildernesses. This short trip samples its solitude and ample swimming and fishing opportunities.

DAY 1 (Potter Pass Trailhead to George Lake, 4.7 miles): From the Potter Pass Trailhead, the trail briefly parallels Potter Creek before steeply climbing its west fork. The path bears east as it ascends southeast-facing slopes that offer views southeast toward the highest peaks of neighboring Dinkey Lakes Wilderness—10,000-plus-foot Three Sisters (seen as a series of rounded granite studs) and barren, serrated, 10,302-foot Dogtooth Peak. The strenuous climb culminates 2.5 miles from the trailhead at Potter Pass (8970´), where your trail converges with the California Riding and Hiking Trail, coming up from a trailhead farther east on Kaiser Pass Road.

> **VIEWS FROM POTTER PASS**
>
> Epic views await at the pass! In the north, Balloon Dome stands alone as a prominent granite knob jutting from the enormously visible San Joaquin River valley. Farther north, the Minarets of the Ritter Range are easily identified as the dark, jagged peaks, remnants of volcanoes that erupted some 100 million years ago. East-southeast, South Fork San Joaquin River drains the mountains of northern Kings Canyon National Park, while Middle Fork San Joaquin River curves north below distant Mammoth Crest, which separates the river from the Mammoth Lakes basin.

KAISER PASS RD

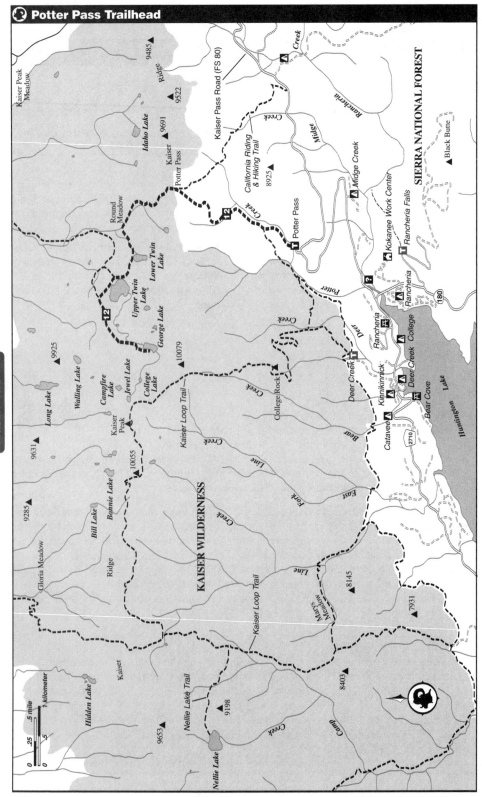

KAISER PASS RD

54

From the junction at Potter Pass, the merged trails continue ahead (north) as one and descend 0.7 mile to Round Meadow and a junction with the George Lake Trail (8650´). Turn left (generally west) and skirt the broad meadow, which offers wildflowers in summer and fall colors in autumn, thanks to aspens fringing it.

The trail briefly joins Lower Twin Lake's outlet before reaching that lake's shallow, sedge-lined shores. Lower Twin Lake (8610´) is a snow-fed lake set in 800-foot granite cliffs that rise toward a rugged 9559-foot peak to the south. The lake has a gentle, mature feel, with large trees and smooth, lichen-covered cliffs. Small brook trout are plentiful. Although there are a few campsites, better ones lie ahead at Upper Twin Lake and George Lake.

Continuing to Upper Twin Lake, the trail skirts a diminutive seasonal pond and traverses an easy half mile to exquisite Upper Twin Lake's east shore (8601´; yes, Upper Twin Lake is lower than Lower Twin Lake). The lake's sparkling blue waters are interrupted by smooth granite slab islands that host surprisingly large Jeffrey pine, red fir, and lodgepole pine. But that's not the lake's only peculiar feature: It has no outflow. A few steps north, a conspicuous boulder masks a rocky pit that indicates water moving underground from the lake toward Kaiser Creek.

As the path leads 100 feet north around the lake, it meets a marked junction with a trail branching right (8650´) and another 0.1 mile farther (8680´). Take the left fork at each junction, first north and then west, as the trail climbs above the Twin Lakes' northwestern basin, passing towering juniper pine among sugary, quartz-white granite.

Curve southwest as the trail weaves under massive western white pine to and from the creek that connects George Lake to Upper Twin Lake. The tread eventually crosses the creek and in 70 feet reaches the first of several campsites along George Lake (9100´; 11S 307566 4129484). The most scenic sites are located along the western shore between the inlet and the large granite wall that rims the northwest shore.

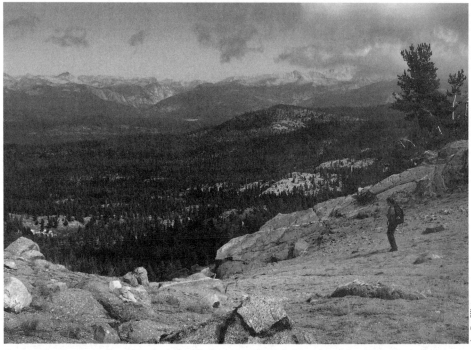

A cross-country route from George Lake climbs past College Lake to meet the Kaiser Loop Trail.

KAISER PASS RD

Analise Elliot

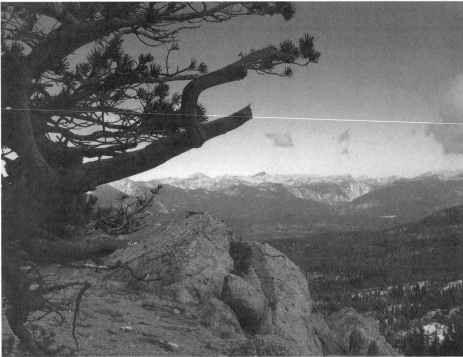

High above George Lake on the Kaiser Loop Trail, look east for views deep into the headwaters of the San Joaquin drainage.

SIDE TRIP: CROSS-COUNTRY DAYHIKE TO COLLEGE LAKE AND THE KAISER LOOP TRAIL

From George Lake, an adventurous cross-country route leads to College Lake and, with a bit of scrambling suitable for a daypack but not a full backpack, to a saddle where your route can join the Kaiser Loop Trail (Trip 13) to Kaiser Peak. Follow a use trail counterclockwise around George Lake and ascend approximately west-northwest from the scenic campsites mentioned in the main text. Loosely follow the creek connecting College and George lakes. From College Lake (9520'; 11S 307025 412955), bear south toward a visible, rocky saddle. The last 150 feet of the ascent is a loose, rocky scramble to the saddle, where this route joins the Kaiser Loop Trail (9770'; 306958 4128973). If you are venturing for a grander tour of the wilderness, turn right (north and then west) at this unmarked and unofficial junction to go 1 mile farther to 10,310-foot Kaiser Peak.

DAY 2 (George Lake to Potter Pass Trailhead, 4.7 miles): Retrace your steps to the trailhead.

Deer Creek Trailhead

7240′; 11S 307375 4125871

DESTINATION/ UTM COORDINATES	TRIP TYPE	BEST SEASON	PACE (HIKING/ LAYOVER DAYS)	TOTAL MILEAGE
13 Nellie Lake 11S 300888 4128413	Loop	Mid to late	2/0 Strenuous	21

Information and Permits: This trailhead is in Sierra National Forest: 1600 Tollhouse Road, Clovis, CA 93611, 559-297-0706, www.fs.fed.us/r5/sierra/. Permits are required for overnight stays, and quotas apply; reserved permits and on-demand permits are available.

Driving Directions: From Clovis (near Fresno), take State Hwy. 168 northeast for 42 winding, slow miles to its end at a T junction on the east shore of Huntington Lake at the community of Lakeshore. Turn left (west) on Huntington Lake Road and, in 0.9 mile, turn right at the posted turnoff for the D&F Pack Station (just before the entrance to Deer Creek Campground). Turn right on Upper Deer Creek Lane after 0.1 mile and right again onto Deer Lane after another half mile. Park in the small dirt lot before the road horseshoes over the creek and enters the pack station. This trailhead for Kaiser Wilderness is at the north end of the pack station's customer parking lot.

13 Nellie Lake

Trip Data: 11S 300888 4128413; 21 miles; 2/0 days

Topos: *Kaiser Peak*

Highlights: This demanding trip's highlight is the ascent of Kaiser Peak, with its spectacular views that encompass the central Sierra Nevada and the San Joaquin River's watershed. Note the shuttle alternative for Day 2, given on page 60.

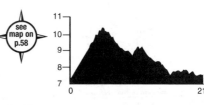

see map on p.58

HEADS UP! *For an easier trip, take this trip in reverse. Whichever way you go, take plenty of water, for long stretches of this strenuous trip are usually dry (watercourses are seasonal). The rugged terrain means that mapped lakes are often impossible to reach, so campsites are almost nonexistent unless you are prepared to dry camp. Nellie Lake is the exception.*

DAY 1 (Deer Creek Trailhead to Nellie Lake, 11 miles): From the trailhead, two trails diverge. Your route turns left (northeast) toward Kaiser Peak and reaches another junction in 100 yards, where you continue straight ahead (northeast). Ascending under mature and fragrant Jeffrey pines, the trail narrows and steadily rises 400 feet in the first half mile to meet Deer Creek on the right. Paralleling the creek, the trail begins a long series of switchbacks ascending to College Rock. After a steep 2.5 miles, College Rock (9055′) is an ideal resting spot.

> **THE VIEWS FROM COLLEGE ROCK**
> College Rock can be reached with a little scrambling that's rewarded by encompassing views of the Huntington Lake basin. To the southwest, views reach into the Central Valley, and, on an exceptionally clear day, the silhouette of the Coast Range often appears more than 100 miles along the western horizon.

Continuing, the path narrows and continues its switchbacking ascent a half mile farther before leading to a broad meadow where wildflowers abound in season, including

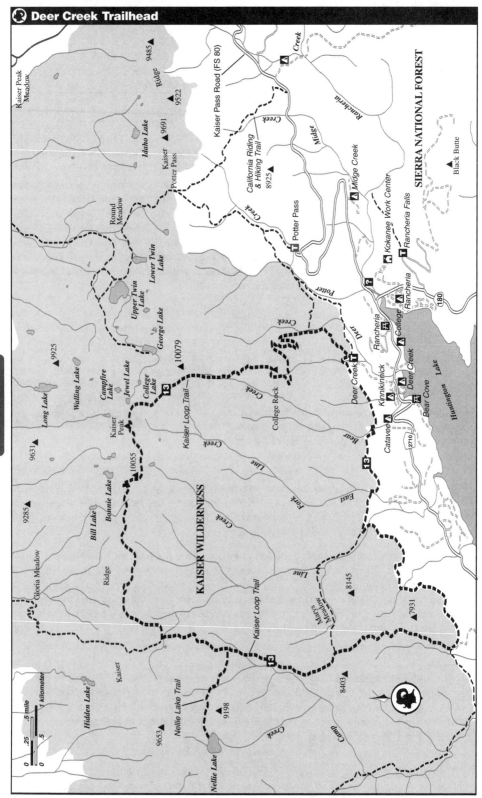

lupine, Indian paintbrush, and hound's tongue. The path meanders toward and away from seasonal Bear Creek, through lodgepole and western white pine as it ascends a massive granite crest (9800'). Past a false summit, the tread reaches a gap; Kaiser Peak is visible as the trail descends from the gap. Jewel Lake (larger) and Campfire Lake (smaller and farther away) can be seen nearly 400 feet below to the northeast.

Gain Kaiser Peak's summit by taking a short, signed spur trail (10,250') on the right that leads northward a short distance.

VIEWS FROM KAISER PEAK

Atop lone Kaiser Peak (10,310'), a western spur of the Sierra ridge, ambitious hikers get outstanding views of the central Sierra, whose highest peaks bound the San Joaquin River. Gaze around you at this great river's watershed. In the north, the serrated Minarets of the Ritter Range rim North Fork San Joaquin River, while Middle Fork San Joaquin wraps east below Mammoth Crest, and South Fork San Joaquin drains the distant, barren, granite peaks visible along the east-southeast skyline. From here, the San Joaquin continues to flow west to the trough of the Central Valley, where it joins California's other great rivers and is either diverted for agriculture, power, and people, or follows its historical route north to the Sacramento–San Joaquin Delta and then out through San Francisco Bay.

Retrace your steps down the spur trail to the junction and turn right (west) along Kaiser Ridge. Immediately below and north of the sheer granite ledge is Bonnie Lake, while the small twin disks of Bobby Lake lie northward nearly 1000 feet below.

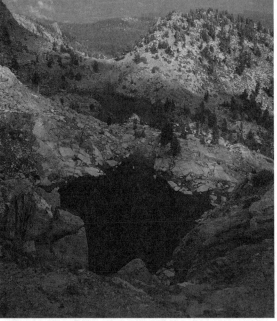

Analise Elliot

Continuing, the trail traverses west through moonscape terrain devoid of obvious plant life except the occasional gnarled whitebark pine. Diminutive and barren Line Creek Lake is nestled along the exposed southern slopes. The trail descends slowly along Kaiser Ridge, offering expansive views north that include Balloon Dome—a prominent, granite knob jutting nearly 3000 feet above the banks of the San Joaquin River, which carves its way through Ansel Adams Wilderness.

Initially heading west, the trail gently leads downslope along the exposed, sun-drenched ridge and bends south-southeast to meet a junction 3 miles from the summit (8780'). Curve west across the headwaters of Line Creek, and, in 0.9 mile, reach a junction with the Nellie Lake Trail (8430').

Turn right (west) onto the Nellie Lake Trail; Nellie Lake is the only site for established

Jewel Lake (larger) and Campfire Lake (smaller) lie nearly 400 feet below Kaiser Ridge.

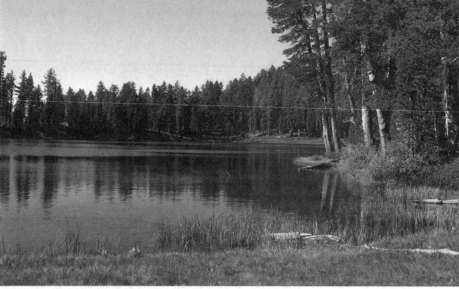

Andlise Elliot

Nellie Lake is the only site for established camps along this loop.

camps along the entire 21-mile loop. The path initially climbs 500 feet, crossing upper Home Camp Creek in 0.4 mile. It then skirts the northern flanks of Peak 9198 and drops the remaining half mile into the Nellie Lake basin. To find the best campsites, from Nellie Lake's east shore (8900´; 11S 300888 4128413), follow a use trail right 200 feet across the inlet, through a shoreline forest of mature lodgepole, red fir, and the occasional western white pine and droopy-topped mountain hemlock.

DAY 2 (Nellie Lake to Deer Creek Trailhead, 10 miles): From Nellie Lake, retrace your steps eastward to the Kaiser Loop Trail. Turn right (south) to descend under dense stands of red fir and lodgepole. The trail briefly parallels Home Camp Creek's western branch before veering southeast below Peak 8403.

Continuing, the trail descends a viewless stretch into the Billy Creek drainage and reaches a junction where an eastbound trail joins the Kaiser Loop Trail (7270´).

SHUTTLE ALTERNATIVE

If you have two cars, a possible alternative to the 21-mile loop trek is to leave one car at the Deer Creek Trailhead and the other at the Upper Billy Creek Trailhead, 150 feet south of the junction with the eastbound trail and the Kaiser Loop Trail (7230´; 11S 302413 4124099). In doing so, it will bypass the next 4.5 miles, turning this loop into a 16.5-mile shuttle.

Turn left and head east along the Kaiser Loop Trail, traversing the densely forested slopes above Huntington Lake. Look for the red cones of snow plant, a saprophyte that obtains its nutrients from forest litter instead of through photosynthesis; it protrudes from the dense layer of downed debris on the forest floor. Farther east, the forest changes from dark, shady fir stands to more open Jeffrey pine stands that allow views southward across Huntington Lake and into Dinkey Lakes Wilderness.

The route undulates across the lush, steep canyon of Line Creek (7630´) and then, in 1.4 more miles, across Bear Creek (7300´), to arrive in another 0.8 mile at the Deer Creek Trailhead.

Florence Lake Trailhead

7360'; 11S 324899 4127475

DESTINATION/ UTM COORDINATES	TRIP TYPE	BEST SEASON	PACE (HIKING/ LAYOVER DAYS)	TOTAL MILEAGE
14 Martha Lake 113 345061 4106896	Out & back	Mid to late	6/1 Leisurely	38/46
15 Red Mountain Basin 1150370824 1184859	Out & back	Mid to late	6/1 Leisurely	43.5/51.5

Information and Permits: This trailhead is in Sierra National Forest: 1600 Tollhouse Road, Clovis, CA 93611, 559-297-0706, www.fs.fed.us/r5/sierra/. Permits are required for overnight stays, and quotas apply; reserved permits and on-demand permits are available.

Driving Directions: From Fresno, take State Hwy. 168 northeast for 42 winding, slow miles toward its end at a T junction on the east shore of Huntington Lake at the community of Lakeshore. Just before reaching Lakeshore, turn right onto the Kaiser Pass Road at the Eastwood Forest Service Center. The road quickly becomes very steep, narrow, and bumpy before Kaiser Pass and is even worse beyond the pass. Blind curves and reckless drivers are problems on this stretch. Allow time to drive very slowly (about 10 mph). As the road descends north and then east from the pass, find seasonally open High Sierra Ranger Station, where you can get on-demand permits. One mile beyond is the Lake Edison/Florence Lake Y junction. Turn right (east) on the Florence Lake Road for another 6 miles to the overnight parking lot. Beyond the far end of the lot, look leftward to the store and water taxi or rightward to the trailhead.

14 Martha Lake

Trip Data: 11S 345061 4106896; 38/46 miles; 6/1 days

Topos: *Florence Lake, Ward Mountain, Blackcap Mountain, Mt. Henry, Mt. Goddard*

see map on p.62

Highlights: Beyond Muir Trail Ranch, this trip visits remote backcountry in the northwestern corner of Kings Canyon National Park. The scenery along South Fork San Joaquin River is stunning, with a parade of thrilling cataracts, cascades, and waterfalls visible from the trail. The long journey up the river culminates in a splendid crescendo at Martha Lake, a large alpine lake cradled in a rocky cirque basin nearly surrounded by craggy peaks and ridges. Along the way, sore backpackers can soak their weary bones in the soothing waters of Blayney Hot Springs.

HEADS UP! *You can save a total of 8 miles of uninspiring hiking along the shore of Florence Lake with arrangements for a water-taxi ride across the lake. The different distances shown above and in the Day headers below reflect this (with water taxi/without).*

> **WATER TAXI**
>
> Rather than backpack the first 4 miles, you could purchase a ticket at the store and take advantage of the ferry ride across Florence Lake. From 8:30 A.M. to 5 P.M., the ferry makes a minimum of five scheduled trips (more on weekends) across the lake and back. From the ferry dock at the far end of the lake, climb uphill over barren granite slopes for a half mile to the junction with the trail around Florence Lake. For your return, there's a radiophone near the dock, from which you can call the store for your ride back.

KAISER PASS RD

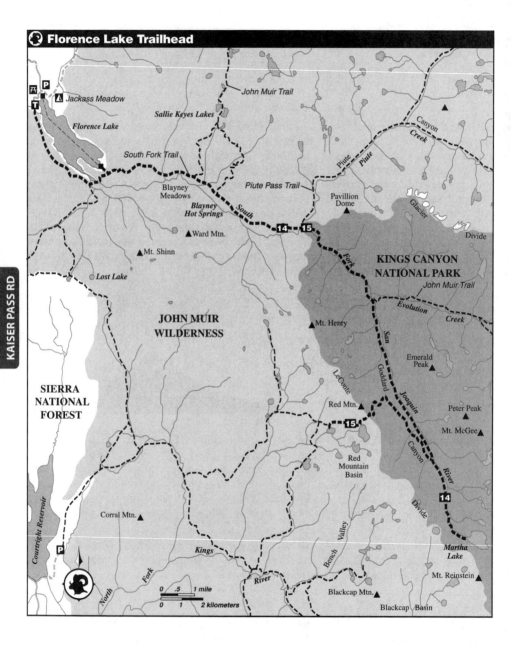

KAISER PASS RD

Jackass Meadow

John Muir Trail

Sallie Keyes Lakes

Florence Lake

Canyon

Creek

South Fork Trail

Piute

Piute

Blayney
Meadows

Piute Pass Trail

Pavillion
Dome

Blayney
Hot Springs

South

14 15

Glacier

Divide

Ward Mtn.

Mt. Shinn

Fork

KINGS CANYON
NATIONAL PARK

John Muir Trail

Lost Lake

JOHN MUIR
WILDERNESS

Mt. Henry

Evolution

Creek

San Goddard

Emerald
Peak

SIERRA
NATIONAL
FOREST

LeConte

Red Mtn.

Joaquin

Peter Peak

Mt. McGee

15

Canyon

Red
Mountain
Basin

River

Courtright Reservoir

Corral Mtn.

Divide

14

Kings

Fork

Bench Valley

Martha
Lake

North

River

Mt. Reinstein

0   .5   1 mile

0   1   2 kilometers

Blackcap Mtn.

Blackcap Basin

DAY 1 (Florence Lake Trailhead to PCT/JMT Junction, 5.5/9.5 miles): If you've elected not to take the ferry, follow the paved road through the picnic area, down to the lake, and along the west shore to the beginning of single-track trail. Enter John Muir Wilderness and proceed generally south across gently rolling terrain beneath mixed forest for 2 miles to a junction with the Burnt Corral Meadows Trail. Continue ahead (southeast) at the junction, traveling above the southwest arm of the lake for another mile to a junction with a lateral to the Burnt Corral Meadow Trail. Go ahead (southeast) here.

From there, head downhill to a bridge over a stream. A short stroll leads to another bridge, this one spanning South Fork San Joaquin River at 3.5 miles from the trailhead. Lodgepole-shaded campsites are spread along both banks of the river and a pit toilet is up the north hillside. From the bridge, head upstream and briefly follow the trail along the river until a moderate, half-mile climb over granite slabs leads to the ferry dock lateral.

JEEP ROAD

Keen eyes will spy a primitive jeep road beyond the southeast end of the lake. Muir Trail Ranch, 2.5 miles upstream, uses an old Army personnel carrier to transport guests along this road, which parallels and occasionally coincides with the route of the hiking trail. Such activity would seem incompatible with the idea of wilderness, but the family-owned operation has been in business for more than 50 years and was grandfathered into the 1964 Wilderness Act.

From the ferry junction, turn right (east) and climb over granite slabs and up dry gullies for a mile to the edge of pastoral Double Meadow. There is an ancient, fallen Jeffrey pine next to the trail here, and a cross-section of the tree is labeled with a chronology of human events. After skirting the meadow, the trail crosses a seasonal stream lined with grasses and wildflowers and then makes a gradual descent to a crossing of Alder Creek, where sheltered campsites are found on the far bank. A short distance past the creek is a lateral to better campsites near the river at Lower Blayney Campground. Past this junction, the broad expanse of Blayney Meadows momentarily springs into view, but the path quickly veers away in favor of a forested route that bypasses the meadows.

About 2.5 miles from the ferry dock, you pass through a gate at the fenced boundary of privately owned Muir Trail Ranch. The route across the ranch property may be difficult to distinguish amid a maze of dusty stock trails and the churned-up jeep road. Farther down the road, pay close attention to makeshift signs that direct you away from the road and onto single-track trail to the left. Proceed southeastward through open terrain and light forest on gently graded trail to crossings of Sallie Keyes and Senger creeks. A moderate climb of a hillside, followed by a lightly forested traverse, leads to a chain gate.

MUIR TRAIL RANCH

Although the presence of a resort seems inconsistent with a designated wilderness area, Muir Trail Ranch is hiker-friendly. For a small fee, packages can be held at the ranch for John Muir and Pacific Crest through-hikers. On the rare occasion when the ranch is not completely booked, usually only in early June, backpackers can purchase an overnight stay complete with three meals. Unfortunately, single meals are not available to non-guests. For more information, check out the ranch's website at www.muirtrailranch.com.

Beyond the gate, you continue across an open hillside in cadence to the rhythmic sound of a Pelton wheel that generates electricity for the ranch below. Reach an open knoll and then drop to a signed junction of a lateral accessing the ranch and Blayney Hot Springs.

BLAYNEY HOT SPRINGS

To visit the hot springs, turn right (south) and proceed a mere 50 feet, where the trail divides again—follow the path on the left marked HOT SPRINGS and pass overused campsites to the north bank of South Fork San Joaquin River. Ford the broad stretch of the river (difficult in early season) and reach more overused campsites on the far bank. Beyond the campsites, a use trail crosses Shooting Star Meadow to access the public pool at Blayney Hot Springs. Please enter and exit carefully, as the muddy pool is very susceptible to erosion.

Just beyond a patch of willows is "Warm Lake," a magical little gem of a swimming hole that is the result of an unlikely combination of beaver dams, moraines, and springs having come together far below the usual elevations common for Sierra lakes. This area is very fragile, so please minimize your impact by being a good steward of this healing place.

Return to the junction and head southeast on gradually rising trail through light forest to a well-signed junction with a steep lateral to the PCT/JMT climbing northbound toward Selden Pass. Go ahead (southeast) and upstream as the main trail continues to parallel the river through a scattered forest of aspens, lodgepole pines, and Jeffrey pines. Pass by a stagnant pond and reach an extensive camping area that occupies a forested bench above the river, 5.5 miles from the ferry dock, just prior to a junction with the John Muir Trail (8025´; 11S 334845, 4121555).

DAY 2 (PCT/JMT Junction to Goddard Canyon Trail Junction, 5.75 miles): Now on the southeast-trending JMT, follow the course of the river through a mixture of granite and conifers, with fine views of the South Fork San Joaquin over the next couple of miles or so. Just prior to the confluence of Piute Creek with the river is a junction with the Piute Pass Trail, 7.75 miles from the ferry dock. Go ahead (briefly east) and immediately find a steel bridge that spans the tumultuous creek and crosses the border into Kings Canyon National Park. A number of good campsites can be found on a flat near the junction, bordered by chaparral and partially shaded by widely scattered Jeffrey pines.

Hike upstream on a gradual, exposed climb around John Muir Rock and then draw nearer the river as it flows through a narrow channel of dark rock. About 1.5 miles from the Piute Pass Trail junction, enter the cool forested glade of aspens and pines misnamed Aspen Meadow. While there is no semblance of a meadow here, but there are a few sheltered campsites.

Leave Aspen Meadow behind and continue to follow the river upstream on a gradual, mile-long climb of a narrow and exposed section of the canyon. Cross a steel bridge over the river to a small, forested flat, where a use trail leads shortly downstream to campsites. Now on the south side of the river, pass through a gate near more campsites, and walk through wildflower gardens to ford a vigorous stream draining several tarns below LeConte Divide. Reach campsites shaded by a mixed forest of aspens, lodgepole pines, and junipers near the signed junction with the Goddard Canyon Trail (10,100´; 11S 340681, 4117756).

From the junction, head either right (south) a short distance up the Goddard Canyon Trail, or left (briefly east, then north) across the river on the JMT's wooden bridge to fine campsites within sound of the soothing South Fork San Joaquin.

DAY 3 (Goddard Canyon Trail Junction to Martha Lake, 7.75 miles): If necessary, return to the junction and take the Goddard Canyon Trail southward. Climb moderately through a light forest of lodgepole pines a half mile to Franklin Meadow, where tall aspens dot a picturesque, wildflower-laden grassland bisected by gurgling rivulets. A couple of primitive campsites are near the south end of the meadow just above the river.

Follow the trail away from the meadow and the river for a while on a gradual-to-moderate climb through the trees. Soon, the narrowing walls of the canyon force the path up the hillside and along an ascending traverse above the river. Pass more campsites on a

KAISER PASS RD

narrow bench overlooking the river on the way to a lush hillside well watered by a series of rivulets and carpeted with willows, aspens, and wildflowers, including paintbrush, clover, coneflower, columbine, and heather. Visible across this verdant meadowland is Pig Chute, where a seasonal stream pours down a narrow, rocky cleft beside a dark, knife-edged protrusion of rock. Farther up the trail, a spectacular waterfall spills into an emerald pool.

For a while, the trail heads upstream with spectacular views across Goddard Canyon of the cascading river plunging down a narrow, deep, rocky cleft. Along the way, pass two more waterfalls as scenic as any to be found in the High Sierra and cross several flower-lined streams spilling across the trail.

Near the confluence with North Goddard Creek, the canyon widens, allowing the river to slow down and broaden. Stroll through meadowlands for a fine view of both river canyons separated by a low rock dome. A short, moderate climb leads to an unsigned junction with the Hell-for-Sure Pass Trail, 5 miles from the JMT junction. A few primitive campsites shaded by a grove of trees can be found a short distance beyond the junction, near a creek crossing. Go ahead (south-southeast) on the Goddard Canyon Trail.

Now the upper part of Goddard Canyon spreads out in subalpine splendor on an ascent of lush meadowlands, unbroken except for an occasional stunted pine or small clump of willows. Pockets of lupine and heather accent the green meadow as you gaze south and southeastward toward the mighty hulks of Mt. Goddard and Mt. Reinstein. Eventually, the path grows indistinct, but the route upstream along the South Fork is obvious on the way to its birthplace beneath the LeConte and Goddard divides. Flowers cover the slopes, including daisy, shooting star, and paintbrush.

After crossing the outlet stream from Lake Confusion, which is high above, begin a moderately steep, cross-country ascent over grassy benches and granite slabs to the lip of the basin holding Martha Lake. From there, a short, easy stroll leads to the west shore of the austere, rock-bound lake (11,004´; 11S 345061 4106896).

AT MARTHA LAKE

A smattering of small pocket meadows almost soften the predominantly barren, rocky shoreline of the lake. Situated above timberline near the convergence of three divides—Goddard, LeConte, and White—the lake is located in a truly alpine environment. The dark, rugged flanks of Mt. Goddard (13,368´) tower 2500 feet over the northeast shore, while Mt. Reinstein (12,604´) provides a fine backdrop to the south. Although developed campsites are virtually nonexistent, resourceful backpackers will be able to find sandy spots suitable for pitching a tent in various locations around the shoreline. Anglers can ply the waters in search of rainbow and golden trout. For cross-country enthusiasts, Martha Lake is also the western gateway into some of the most coveted off-trail terrain in the High Sierra: Directly east lies the mysterious realm of Ionian Basin, a trip through which is considered a Sierra classic. Mountaineers may want to tackle the Class 2–3 route up the southeast ridge of Mt. Goddard.

DAYS 4–6 (Martha Lake to Florence Lake Trailhead, 19/23 miles): Retrace your steps to the trailhead.

15 Red Mountain Basin

Trip Data: 11S
370824 1184859;
43.5/51.5 miles;
6/1 days

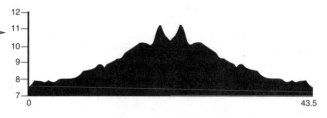

see map on p.62

Topos: *Florence Lake,
Ward Mountain, Blackcap
Mountain, Mt. Henry,
Mt. Goddard*

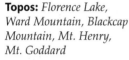

Highlights: Red Mountain Basin offers backpackers the type of scenery for which the High Sierra is famous: Alpine peaks, glacier-scoured terrain, and sparkling lakes highlight this rugged area on the west side of the LeConte Divide. A bounty of picturesque lakes—some near the trail and others a short, easy cross-country jaunt away—make excellent base camps for the exploration of the extensive basin. Travelers can expect to find solitude on this multilayer journey along the lightly used trails necessary to reach Red Mountain Basin.

HEADS UP! You can save 4 miles of uninspiring hiking along the shore of Florence Lake by arranging for a ferry ride across the lake (see details on page 61).

DAY 1 (Florence Lake Trailhead to PCT/JMT Junction, 5.5 miles): *(Recap Trip 14, Day 1.)* Follow the trail 4 miles generally southward around Florence Lake , or take the ferry to the dock on the far side and take the ferry dock lateral east to meet the Florence Lake Trail. From this junction, go ahead (east) over granite slabs and up dry gullies on a combination of single-track trail and jeep road around Double Meadow and across Alder Creek to a junction with a lateral that accesses campsites at Lower Blayney Camp. Follow a forested path southeastward around Blayney Meadows and continue across the private property of Muir Trail Ranch. In the midst of the ranch property, reach a crudely signed junction and follow single-track trail southeastward across Sallie Keyes and Senger creeks, past the ranch boundary, and to a junction with a lateral to Blayney Hot Springs and Muir Trail Ranch. To visit the hot springs, follow the directions in the sidebar, "Blayney Hot Springs," on page 64.

To stay or get back on the main trail, from the junction, head southeast on a gradual climb through light forest to a junction with a lateral trail north and steeply uphill to the PCT/JMT much farther north than you want to go. Don't take the lateral; go ahead here (southeast), upstream along the river, to campsites on a forested bench just before a junction with the PCT/JMT (8025´; 11S 334845 4121555).

DAY 2 (PCT/JMT Junction to Goddard Canyon Trail Junction, 5.75 miles): *(Recap Trip 14, Day 2.)* Follow the southeast-trending JMT along South Fork San Joaquin River to the junction of the Piute Pass Trail, cross a bridge over the river, and enter Kings Canyon National Park (campsites). Go ahead (briefly east and then southeast) and continue upstream around John Muir Rock to Aspen Meadow (campsites) and across another bridge over the river (campsites). Follow the south bank upstream past additional campsites to a junction of the PCT/JMT and the Goddard Canyon Trail. Good campsites can be found near the junction along either trail.

DAY 3 (Goddard Canyon Trail Junction to Disappointment Lake, 10.5 miles): Return to the Goddard Canyon Trail and turn south. Climb moderately through Franklin Meadow into a narrowing section of the canyon. Near the confluence with North Goddard Creek, the canyon widens and the grade eases as the trail passes through flower-filled meadowlands. Make a short, moderate climb to an unsigned junction with the Hell for Sure Pass Trail, 5 miles from the JMT junction (campsites).

Turn right (west) at the junction and begin a 4-mile jaunt toward Hell for Sure Pass. After a half mile, switchbacking climb, the trail follows a gentle 2-mile traverse that heads northwest across the west wall of Goddard Canyon. Near the end of the traverse, you hop across a creek draining the slopes below the pass. A short distance beyond this initial crossing, begin an 1150-foot climb that generally follows the north side of creek's drainage on the way to Hell for Sure Pass (11,297′; 11S 370845 1184746).

The views of Goddard Canyon have been stunning since you left the Goddard Canyon Trail, but they reach a climax at the pass, where views open up to the west over Red Mountain Basin. While the route from Goddard Canyon to Hell for Sure Pass has consumed 4 miles of hiking, the trail down into Red Mountain Basin plunges rapidly to Hell for Sure Lake, tightly winding 500 feet down a steep gully to the north shore of the 10,782-foot lake. Tucked into a stunning cirque immediately below LeConte Divide, the lake is surrounded by polished granite slabs that sparkle in the sunlight of a typically clear Sierra sky. Tiny pockets of meadow make feeble attempts to break up the otherwise rocky slopes of the basin. A few campsites are scattered around the north shore, and fishing is reported to be good for medium-size brook trout.

From Hell for Sure Lake, descend a hillside of granite slabs, pass by some small tarns, and step over a sparkling stream on the way to an unmarked lateral heading south that leads shortly to Disappointment Lake (10342′; 11S 370824 1184859). Backdropped by Mt. Hutton and the craggy LeConte Divide, the lake is as attractive as any in the High Sierra, with alternating sections of meadow and sandy beach ringing the north shore and rolling granite slabs along the south shore. Fine campsites with grand views of the surrounding terrain will reward tired backpackers. A healthy population of brook trout should satisfy anglers.

EXPLORING RED MOUNTAIN BASIN

Red Mountain Basin offers many alternatives for spending extra days exploring the region. Several lakes are easily accessible by connecting trails, and many other lakes can be visited via easy cross-country routes. Due to the lengthy approaches necessary to reach the basin, you're unlikely to encounter many other backpackers. For peakbaggers, Red Mountain is a straightforward Class 1 climb from Hell for Sure Pass.

DAYS 4–6 (Disappointment Lake to Florence Lake Trailhead, 21.75/25.75 miles): Retrace your steps to the trailhead. A radiophone is available near the ferry landing for arranging your return via the water taxi across Florence Lake.

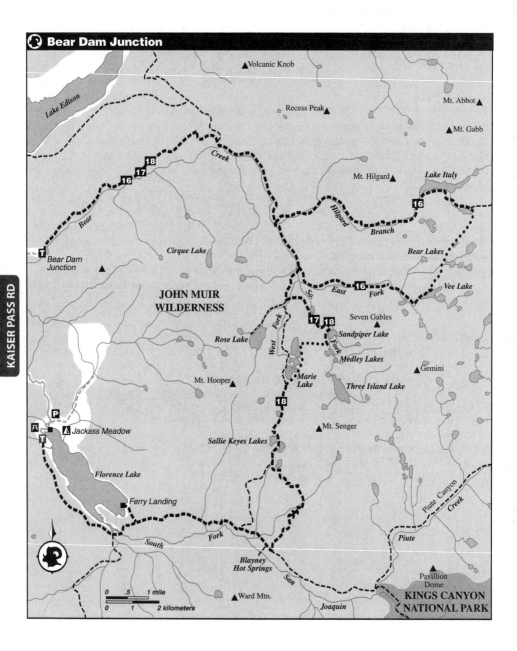

Bear Dam Junction
7017'; 11S 322442 4134284

DESTINATION/ UTM COORDINATES	TRIP TYPE	BEST SEASON	PACE (HIKING/ LAYOVER DAYS)	TOTAL MILEAGE
16 Bear Lakes 11S 339738 4132346 (at Vee Lake)	Semiloop	Mid to late	5/1 Moderate-strenuous, part cross-country	39
17 Medley Lakes 11S 335324 4130348	Out & back	Mid to late	4/1 Moderate	33
18 Florence Lake 11S 325091 4127479	Shuttle	Mid to late	4/1 Moderate, part cross-country	28.5/32.5

Information and Permits: This trailhead is in Sierra National Forest: 1600 Tollhouse Road, Clovis, CA 93611, 559-297-0706, www.fs.fed.us/r5/sierra/. Permits are required for overnight stays, and quotas apply; reserved permits and on-demand permits are available.

Driving Directions: From Fresno, take State Hwy. 168 northeast for 42 winding, slow miles toward its end at a T junction on the east shore of Huntington Lake at the community of Lakeshore. Just before reaching Lakeshore, turn right onto the Kaiser Pass Road at the Eastwood Forest Service Center. The road quickly becomes very steep, narrow, and bumpy before Kaiser Pass and is even worse beyond the pass. Blind curves and reckless drivers are problems on this stretch. Allow time to drive very slowly (about 10 mph). As the road descends north and then east from the pass, find seasonally open High Sierra Ranger Station, where you can get on-demand permits. One mile beyond is the Lake Edison/Florence Lake Y junction. Turn left to remain on Kaiser Pass Road and head toward Lake Edison. Bypass the turnoff left to Mono Hot Springs, and go 2.5 miles from the Y junction to the Bear Diversion Dam Road junction, on the right. This is the "Bear Dam Junction" from which these trips start and whose elevation and UTM are given at the start of this section. Most vehicles can go no farther, so park near this junction and walk 2.5 more miles east on a rough 4WD road, to the dam proper and to the true trailhead above the reservoir. (A high-clearance 4WD vehicle, not the average, urban SUV, can travel this road those 2.5 more miles to the true trailhead above the reservoir.)

16 Bear Lakes

Trip Data: 11S 339738 4132346 (at Vee Lake); 39 miles; 5/1 days

see map on p.68

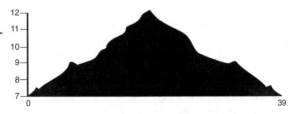

Topos: *Mt. Givens, Florence Lake, Mt. Hilgard*

Highlights: This spectacular hike tours a wide variety of High Sierra delights. Starting from the forested depths of Bear Creek Canyon, this trip climbs to the picturesque and secluded Bear Lakes through glacially carved valleys and lush meadows. Although several parts of the terrain are strenuous, solitude and breathtaking beauty richly reward the determined hiker.

HEADS UP! This trip is for experienced hikers only. The route involves some cross-country travel.

DAY 1 (Bear Dam Junction to Twin Falls, 5.5 miles): From the junction with the paved road, the unmaintained 4WD road to Bear Dam heads east. The dusty road first descends to cross open granite slabs, and then it climbs for 2 miles before reaching the trailhead above Bear Diversion Dam (7400'; 11S 325053 4134161).

Here, the rocky road becomes a wide, northeast-bound trail that soon passes the sign for John Muir Wilderness. For the first mile, the path is gentle and easy, with many inviting pools and fine campsites to be found next to the creek and among the live oaks. Once past the unmapped cutoff for the Bear Ridge Trail, the path branches east up the hill and parallels the course of Bear Creek. The creek here runs over short, rocky falls and swift rapids, and it collects in long, quiet pools shaded by aspens.

After ascending at a gentle but continuous grade for a mile, the trail passes out of the last of the live oak trees, and you will encounter damp ground conditions in early season. Skirt these patches, beyond which Twin Falls appears ahead to the north. The twin cascades flow over silver-flecked granite slabs, and the waters collect in an inviting pool at the base.

While the water may be chilly in the swimming hole, the small, sandy beach and sun-warmed rocks make idyllic spots to rest and dry off. A well-used campsite is located several hundred feet farther along the trail, near a grove of aspens (8000'; 11S 328338 4136603). There are less obvious campsites located across the creek below the falls.

DAY 2 (Twin Falls to Lake Italy, 11.5 miles): The path leading away from Twin Falls begins with a steep climb northeast for the first 2 miles, and then rapidly levels off to a gentler grade. The route travels sections of steep, stony trail interspersed with stands of aspen. Rocky outcrops and steep ravines testify to the glacial forces that hewed the valley through the granite, leaving the boulders and other debris in the bottom of the canyon. The trail climbs up the north side of the canyon wall here to skirt this difficult landscape.

Following 1000 feet of elevation gain, clear vistas begin to appear to the south and southeast. As the route climbs, the Jeffrey pine and aspen of the lower canyon are left behind. The ubiquitous lodgepole pine begins to make her appearance, and will provide shade and company along the remainder of the trek. The route traces the natural curve along the north side of the canyon and follows this contour as it curves east.

After crossing a ridge, the trail turns back toward Bear Creek and heads down the hill, leveling off after reaching the creek. Well-used campsites begin to appear along the banks of the water. As you continue east, Old Kip Camp appears after a wet, muddy area. Just beyond is the junction with the PCT/JMT (8975'; 11S 332792 4137402).

Turn right on the PCT/JMT, now heading south. This section of trail parallels Bear Creek, running at the bottom of the canyon, for the next mile. Several granite slabs rise from the rushing water, providing relaxing lunch spots along the banks. The path jogs west briefly before entering a narrow section of canyon, and then it levels off while heading away from the creek.

Soon after the trail levels, reach the Italy Pass Trail junction (11S 333831 4134908). Here, this trip turns left (east), leaving PCT/JMT and heads east up open granite slabs. The trail may be faint here, but it becomes quite definite under the trees. Pass a drift fence and a welcome sign announcing that Hilgard Meadow is closed to grazing. From here, the trail threads gently under lodgepole pine for an easy mile to reach the grassy expanses of Hilgard Meadow (9600'). Mt. Hilgard looms almost 4000 feet above, and the meadow underfoot supports thousands of purple Indian paintbrush plants in mid-season. Excellent campsites border the northwest side of this subalpine meadow.

Skirting the north side of Hilgard Meadow, the trail stays near Hilgard Branch as it climbs moderately over slabs and crosses the outlet of Hilgard Lake before passing another drift fence. The path then rapidly crosses several small creeks before leaving tree cover behind. Here, the route may become faint as it climbs away from Hilgard Branch and crosses an open, rocky slope. The path then passes through a wet meadow and becomes indistinct. Descend slightly before meeting the edge of the forest, where the trail becomes more obvious and resumes climbing. The track passes a nice campsite near the main creek before crossing another spring-fed rill.

Now far from the main creek, the trail climbs up steep slabs, following the curve in the canyon as it turns east, steepens, and narrows. Downstream, the canyon is wide and gently sloping, and beyond the narrow gorge, the canyon floor again becomes a meadow, wide and gently sloping. This variation in form is due to differences in the structure of the bedrock.

EFFECTS OF GLACIAL EROSION

Although stream erosion did most of the difficult work to carve this canyon, glaciers have also modified its shape. Before glaciers come, stream canyons usually have a V-shaped cross-section. After the passing of glaciers, the canyons usually have a pronounced U-shaped cross section.

Glaciers, then, tend to do most of their erosion horizontally for several reasons. Primarily, Sierra glaciers are wet based: They ride along on a thin layer of water between the ice and the rock. (Water occurs there due to heat and pressure trapped under the heavy, insulating river of ice.) With this kind of lubrication, the ice tends to slide over, rather than dig deeply into, the bedrock. However, out at the margins of the glacier, colder air and thinner ice allow the glacier to freeze to the ground. Being "glued" to the sides of the valley, the passing glacier tears out pieces of bedrock and carries them away. This action is called glacial quarrying.

In order to account for the variations in canyon slope and width, you can look at how erosion reflects bedrock structure. In this canyon, the primary variable of structure is joints—cracks in the bedrock. Since joints are planes of weakness, then the more there are, the faster the rock is weathered (broken down) and carried away.

Where joints are mostly oriented vertically, glaciers break off column-like pieces from the valley sides, thereby undermining the canyon walls above. In such a place, the valley will be exceptionally flat-bottomed and steep-sided, like Yosemite Valley.

Where jointing is primarily horizontal, the glaciers of course flow parallel to the joints. In such a place, glaciers tend to just slide along the surface, eroding less and leaving more of the original V-shaped profile. This is the process that shaped the narrow, steep sections of Hilgard Branch's canyon.

Continuing along this beautiful meadow, the trail climbs over smooth bedrock. It swings near the creek, which has carved a miniature, gorge-like channel since the glaciers left. Don't follow the trail across the creek. Rather, go 200 yards east up this channel to Teddy Bear Lake's outlet, which comes in on the other side. Cross just above this confluence and climb east across slabs and meadow.

The route then veers north across slabs into the canyon before suddenly arriving at Lake Italy (11,154´) and great vistas of Mt. Gabb, Mt. Abbot, Bear Creek Spire, and Mt. Julius Caesar. This large lake (124 acres) gets its name from its similarity in shape to the European peninsula; consider this west end of it to be the "boot top." Some illegal campsites are found by the outlet, but much better, legal camping lies across the outlet and up the hill a bit (11S 339697 4136421).

More legal camps can be made near the creek from Jumble Lake, which comes into Lake Italy 1 mile along the south shore—but anywhere in this incredible basin can be a sublime campsite. The best way to get to the "toe" of Lake Italy (it's east end), is via the north shore. There are golden trout in the nearby lakes, and alpine wildlife is all around.

DAY 3 (Lake Italy to Vee Lake via the Bear Lakes, 5 miles, part cross-country): The next section of trail is demanding yet glorious. The path tours some very high and wild places along this stretch.

Following the rocky south shore of Lake Italy, the trail reaches the inlet from Jumble Lake at a small meadow; this is considered Lake Italy's "heel." Turn south at the "heel," ascending along the inlet's west side. Near rocky slabs, the trail veers east, picking up the now-distinct Italy Pass Trail at the base of the moraine that dams Jumble Lake. The Italy Pass Trail climbs east around this moraine.

Staying far above the chaotic north shore of aptly named Jumble Lake, the trail crosses a sandy bench. There is a nice rest area here, especially if the meadowy little creek is flowing just beyond. The high point of this trip can be seen to the south, at the saddle between peaks 12756 and 12710, as shown on the 15′ *Mt. Abbott* topo. (On the 7.5′ topo, they are the two peaks bracketing the long, skinny pond south of Jumble Lake and northeast of White Bear Lake. The long, skinny pond is in the saddle. On the 15′ topo, these peaks are labeled 12769 (11S 341207 4134347), southeast of Jumble Lake, and 12716 (11S 340592 4134760), southwest of Jumble Lake. The peaks aren't labeled on the 7.5′ topo. A waypoint on the saddle at the northeast end of the pond is at 12,152′; 11S 340855 4134359.)

From this bench, the trail climbs straight up the hill toward a sandy gully to the left of some bedrock slabs. Leave the main trail at the base of those slabs and head southeast, going cross-country. Climb steadily in order to attain the steep slope above Jumble Lake. You may encounter much snow up here, so exercise caution.

Leveling off at the saddle, a use trail heading south becomes distinct as your cross-country route passes that long, skinny pond, which is seasonal. Pick up that trail; shortly, the route arrives at the lip of East Fork Bear Creek's basin. This is an awe-inspiring location in which to rest and drink in the view.

GLACIAL SCENERY

The lip of East Fork Bear Creek's basin marks the upper limit of glaciers that flowed over the top of the dome to the south and then through the pass to the right of White Bear Lake, just below. Most of this basin was under ice many times during the Pleistocene Epoch, 2 million to 10,000 years ago. Indeed, ice caps covered most of the High Sierra, from Mt. Whitney to Lake Tahoe.

To tell which areas remained above the ice, note the jagged or pointed peaks and ridges. These high points protruded above the glaciers, which eroded them from several sides, leaving them very steep but not smoothed over.

Conversely, total glacial cover produces round, domelike peaks and ridges. The sandy, bouldery areas behind you were never glaciated (or at least, not recently), and they show no clean or fresh bedrock, such as glaciers uncover in places where they scrape away surface debris. If glaciers never come, then, over hundreds of thousands of years, the rock cracks into angular boulders, which, in turn, weather into gravel and sand.

From this majestic vantage point, look beyond the outlet of White Bear Lake to the southeast. There lies a shallow valley with two ponds that run in a line of sight connecting you and the outlet of White Bear Lake (shown on the 15′ map, but not the 7.5′ map, as flowing south into Big Bear Lake). This valley is your route to Vee Lake. The descent to White Bear Lake follows the steep, sandy gully below. The path skirts White Bear Lake's west shore and follows the west side of the outlet to Big Bear Lake. Ursa and Bearpaw lakes are an easy detour east from Big Bear Lake, as these three lakes virtually form one body of water in wet seasons.

The best path follows the outlet of Big Bear Lake west-southwest through a gorge to Little Bear Lake. Follow the south shore of Little Bear Lake from its inlet, climbing over a small outcrop by the water. A sort of meadowy corridor then appears, veering east away from the lake, heading toward Seven Gables. Follow this and descend to cross a wet area where the corridor continues away from the lake southwest to a low saddle. Now on a faint trail, you pass two ponds. By now, this corridor has become a small valley, and the path turns south toward Vee Lake. The last pond above Vee Lake offers good camping with wonderful views.

From the seasonal outlet of this pond, thread east a short distance to find a cleft path through the cliff below, and descend to the meadowy shore of Vee Lake's north arm (11,163'; 11S 339738 4132346), where wonderful campsites abound. Feather Peak (13,242'; north of Royce Peak) dominates the eastern skyline, and hikes in that direction are full of opportunities to find secret places in this secluded glacial wonderland. This is a perfect place to spend a well-deserved rest day.

DAY 4 (Vee Lake to Bear Creek, 6.5 miles): The unmapped trail traverses the north shore west-southwest to Vee Lake's bedrock dam. From the outlet, head east and descend a grassy swale for several hundred feet. The small dome that is separated from the ridge in front of you provides great views, as the existence of a trail up it testifies. The path passes north of this dome before heading down the gully that cuts through this ridge. Your goal is to pick up the use trail from the PCT/JMT to the Seven Gables Lakes.

From wherever you pick it up, turn north on the use trail connecting the PCT/JMT and the Seven Gables Lakes. The twisting trail follows the lakes' outlet, passes a pond, and fords the outlet of Little Bear Lake. Several hundred feet beyond is a small gorge. Cross East Fork Bear Creek to a small stand of whitebark pines. The trail stays along the south side of the creek, usually far from the water, until it begins a steep descent under the imposing northern ramparts of Seven Gables. The trail becomes indistinct at times before crossing the creek at the base of a long cascade down slabs. Partway down this gorge, cross the creek, and then recross it at the lower end.

The grade eases now as the shady trail winds away from the creek to the northwest. Soon, campsites appear and a scarcity of downed wood reveals the obvious: The PCT/JMT is nearby. At a signed junction with the PCT/JMT, turn right (north) and stroll through open stands of lodgepole pine to ford Hilgard Branch. A little beyond Hilgard Branch is the Italy Pass Trail junction, where you close the loop part of this trip by going ahead (north) on the PCT/JMT.

Now back on familiar trail, travelers soon arrive at the obvious campsites lining Bear Creek. They may appear in a different light after the adventure in the land above the trees.

DAY 5 (Bear Creek to Bear Dam Junction, 10.5 miles): Retrace your steps to the trailhead (half of Day 2 and all of Day 1).

17 Medley Lakes

Trip Data: 11S 335324 4130348;
33 miles; 4/1 days

Topos: *Mt. Givens,*
Florence Lake, Mt. Hilgard

see map on p.68

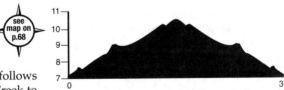

Highlights: This moderate hike follows almost the entire course of Bear Creek to the beautiful and serene Medley Lakes. While the hike joins the PCT/JMT for a busy but relatively short section, opportunities abound to find solitude and quiet campsites just off the trail. The alpine campsites found around the Medley Lakes can serve as idyllic base camps for side trips that explore the rugged terrain surrounding the basin.

DAY 1 (Bear Dam Junction to Twin Falls, 5.5 miles): *(Recap: Trip 16, Day 1.)* From the junction with the paved road, the unmaintained 4WD road to Bear Dam heads east. Cross open granite slabs and then climb for 2 miles before reaching the trailhead above Bear Diversion Dam (7400'; 11S 325053 4134161).

Here, the rocky road becomes a wide trail and enters John Muir Wilderness. For the next mile, the path is gentle and easy. Go ahead (northeast) at the cutoff north for the Bear

Ridge Trail, paralleling Bear Creek. In another mile, skirt damp ground and then see Twin Falls ahead to the north. A well-used campsite is located several hundred feet farther along the trail, near a grove of aspens (8000´; 11S 328338 4136603). There are less obvious campsites located across the creek below the falls.

DAY 2 (Twin Falls to Medley Lakes, 11 miles): Climb steeply away from Twin Falls for the first 2 miles, and then rapidly level off on a gentler grade. The trail climbs up the north side of the canyon wall here to skirt this difficult landscape. The route traces the natural curve along the north side of the canyon and follows this contour as it turns from the northeast to the east.

After crossing a ridge, the trail turns back toward Bear Creek and heads down the hill, leveling off after reaching the creek. Well-used campsites begin to appear along the banks of the water. Reach the junction with the PCT/JMT (8975´; 11S 332792 4137402).

Turn right on the PCT/JMT, now heading south; this section of trail parallels Bear Creek. The path jogs to the west briefly before entering a narrow section of canyon, and then it levels off while heading away from the creek. Soon after the trail levels, reach the Italy Pass Trail junction. That faint trail heads east up granite slabs but peters out near Lake Italy.

This trip goes ahead (south) along the PCT/JMT, soon crossing the multiple channels of Hilgard Branch. The track is nearly level now, and the walls of Bear Creek's canyon open wide.

At the signed junction with the Seven Gables and Vee Lake Trail, go right (south-south-west) on the PCT/JMT, ford Bear Creek (wet in early season), and begin a shaded ascent that steepens quickly when approaching Rosemarie Meadow. The path turns left (south-east) at the signed junction to Sandpiper and Three Island Lake near the bottom of the meadow. Having left the PCT/JMT, the trail ascends a low ridge and reaches the western shore of Lou Beverly Lake. The marshy banks of this lake support Brewer's blackbirds, and the pond is stocked with golden trout.

The trail hugs the south shore of Lou Beverly Lake and clambers over boulders at the inlet. Now heading east, the track goes straight uphill, with Seven Gables towering straight ahead. This strenuous climb is brief and temporarily eases as the route jogs toward the south. After passing a tumbling waterfall, the trail veers sharply north and makes a final, steep ascent to gain the lip of the glacial bench above.

Upon reaching the lip, open meadows and lakes stretch away before you. The trail follows the contour of the hillside south and presently arrives at the outlet of Sandpiper Lake. Several overused campsites appear here. Better sites can be found by fording the outlet and skirting the northwest shore.

On the west bank of Sandpiper Lake, the now faint trail turns south and climbs toward a small cleft in the bedrock. Once past the cleft, the Medley Lakes appear to the southwest, and the trail disappears near the westernmost lake. Wonderfully secluded campsites abound on all sides, especially by the last lake (10,550´; 11S 335324 4130348). While theses lakes are not stocked with fish, the Medley Lakes that lie farther to the south do contain golden trout, and more idyllic campsites can be found along their banks. The vistas from the ridge to the west at sunset are well worth the climb.

DAYS 3–4 (Medley Lakes to Bear Dam Junction, 16.5 miles): Retrace your steps to the trail-head.

18 Florence Lake

Trip Data: 11S 325091 4127479;
28.5/32.5 miles; 4/1 days

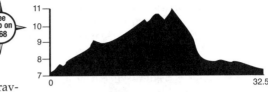

see map on p.68

Topos: *Mt. Givens,*
Florence Lake, Mt. Hilgard,
Ward Mountain

Highlights: This popular shuttle trip traverses the length of Bear Creek's canyon, takes in pristine alpine scenery at Medley Lakes, descends past alpine lakes, and eventually reaches Blayney Hot Springs. The last miles of the trip tour wildflower-carpeted meadows before arriving at Florence Lake. It's an excellent longer trip for the intermediate or advanced hiker.

HEADS UP! This route involves several miles of cross-country travel and is not recommended for beginners.

Shuttle Directions: From the Lake Edison/Florence Lake Y junction, head east on Florence Lake Road for 6 miles to the overnight parking lot.

DAY 1 (Bear Dam Junction to Twin Falls, 5.5 miles): *(Recap: Trip 16, Day 1.)* From the junction with the paved road, the unmaintained 4WD road to Bear Dam heads east. Cross open granite slabs and then climb for 2 miles before reaching the trailhead above Bear Diversion Dam (7400´; 11S 325053 4134161).

Here, the rocky road becomes a wide trail and enters John Muir Wilderness. For the next mile, the path is gentle and easy. Go ahead (northeast) at the cutoff north for the Bear Ridge Trail, paralleling Bear Creek. In another mile, skirt damp ground and then see Twin Falls ahead to the north. A well-used campsite is located several hundred feet farther along the trail, near a grove of aspens (8000´; 11S 328338 4136603). There are less obvious campsites located across the creek below the falls.

DAY 2 (Twin Falls to Medley Lakes, 11 miles): *(Recap: Trip 17, Day 2.)* Climb steeply away from Twin Falls for the first 2 miles, after which the trail levels. The path passes through sections of steep, rocky trail interspersed with stands of aspen. Following 1000 feet of elevation gain, clear vistas begin to appear to the south and southeast. After crossing a ridge, the trail turns back toward Bear Creek and heads downhill. The track levels off after reaching the creek, and well-used campsites begin to appear along the banks of the water. Just above Old Kip Camp is the junction with the PCT/JMT (8975´; 11S 332792 4137402).

Turn right (south-southeast) on the PCT/JMT, following Bear Creek for the next mile. At the Italy Pass Trail junction, go ahead (south-southeast) on the PCT/JMT. Immediately cross Hilgard Branch and, in another 2 miles, find the signed junction with the Seven Gables and Vee Lake Trail. Go right (southwest) and ford Bear Creek (wet in early season) to begin a shaded ascent that steepens quickly when approaching Rosemarie Meadow. This trip turns left (southeast) at the signed junction to Sandpiper and Three Island lakes near the bottom of the meadow.

The trail to Sandpiper becomes fainter and presently reaches Lou Beverly Lake. The track hugs the south shore of this lake and clambers over boulders at the inlet. Make a strenuous, brief, eastward climb that eases as the route jogs toward the south. Beyond a waterfall, the trail veers sharply north and makes a final, steep ascent to the glacial bench above.

On the bench, the trail follows the hillside south to the outlet of Sandpiper Lake. Several overused campsites appear here, but better sites can be found by fording the outlet and skirting the northwest shore.

From the west bank of the lake, the faint trail turns south and climbs toward a small cleft in the bedrock. Beyond the cleft, the Medley Lakes appear to the southwest, and the faint trail disappears near the westernmost lake. Campsites abound on all sides, especially by the last lake (10,550´; 11S 335324 4130348).

DAY 3 (Medley Lakes to Blayney Hot Springs, 8 miles, part cross-country): Stock up on drinking water before starting today's hike, as the first few miles involve waterless cross-country travel. The objective, Marie Lake, lies on the west side of the ridge to the west of the Medley Lakes. Your goal is to work your way to Marie Lake while avoiding the cliffs on the ridge's north end. Climb only as high as needed to miss the cliffs; climbing higher will make your descent needlessly steeper and more difficult.

Here is a possible route: From your campsite, first head to the north side of the three small Medley Lakes lying just southwest of larger Sandpiper Lake. From between the two lakes nearest the ridge, head northwest toward a low point between the ridge and the low dome west of Sandpiper Lake. Bear left (more toward the west) toward the ridge to reach slabs and climb the ridge toward the ridgeline. Gain the ridge and enjoy expansive views.

Once at the east side of Marie Lake, find a faint use trail. Turn left on it and follow it south along the reed- and flower-lined shore. After rounding the south end of the lake, the faint trail climbs briefly to rejoin the PCT/JMT.

Turn left (south) on the PCT/JMT and begin a short climb to Selden Pass (10,873´; 11S 333956 4128650). From the pass, descend a short series of switchbacks to Heart Lake (golden trout.) Continuing south, descend to the Sallie Keyes Lakes (campsites), winding through small alpine meadows with patches of bright, colorful wildflowers highlighted against the green grass.

The path turns east before reaching the bank of Upper Sallie Keyes Lake, descends on the east shore, and then enters a dense stand of lodgepole pine. The trail crosses the outlet of the second lake but bypasses the third before swinging east and crossing several small creeks. Once again, the trail beings to climb, skirting a moraine before reaching South Fork San Joaquin River. There is an overlook of the valley here a few yards off the trail, and the stunning view from it, of South Fork San Joaquin River's U-shaped, glacially carved valley, is well worth the short detour.

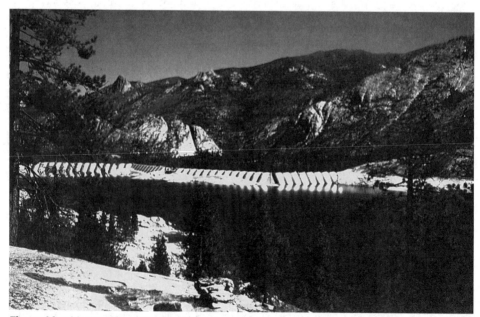

The goal for this shuttle trip is Florence Lake.

After crossing a meadow, the trail turns south and descends to ford Senger Creek. The canyon below is open and sunny, filled with manzanita and sagebrush. On this part of the descent, look for a small lake lying at the base of the opposite canyon wall. Blayney Hot Springs is just north of this lake.

More switchbacks descend into a forest of aspen, juniper, and pine, and the trail becomes steep and dusty for the next mile. At long last, the descent eases. Turn right (northwest) at the signed junction with the Florence Lake Trail. Strolling more or less along the river, you presently find the lateral trail to the hot springs, just past the eastern edge of private Muir Trail Ranch.

Turn left (southwest) and follow a winding use trail past obvious campsites to a wide ford of South Fork San Joaquin (dangerous in early season). More obvious and overused campsites lie on the opposite side (7660'; 11S 333022 4122571). Beyond is the trail crossing Shooting Star Meadow to the public pool at Blayney Hot Springs. Since the muddy pool is very susceptible to erosion, please enter and exit the pool carefully. Just beyond the willows is a magical little lake where you can go swimming. "Warm Lake" is the result of beaver dams, moraines, and springs that come together to form this body of water, far below the usual elevation of Sierra lakes. The entire meadow and hot springs area is fragile; please try to minimize your impact.

MUIR TRAIL RANCH

Muir Trail Ranch is a family-owned guest ranch. The ranch provides a food-drop service, and they can be reached at P.O. Box 176, Lakeshore, CA 93635, in the summer, and P.O. Box 269, Ahwahnee, CA 93601, in the winter. For information, send a self-addressed, stamped envelope and allow plenty of time for your correspondence and your food to arrive there.

DAY 4 (Blayney Hot Springs to Florence Lake, 8 miles, or 4 miles with a ferry ride): Return to the signed trail toward Florence Lake. Turn left (northwest) on this trail and pass through a gate onto Muir Trail Ranch property. No camping is allowed on the property without a fee. Follow the dusty livestock trail for the next 1.25 miles. While many trails diverge to the side, follow the main track, which occasionally coincides with the road to the ranch.

Ford an unnamed creek and then Senger Creek, where you leave the main road for a while, only to rejoin it near the gate at the western edge of the private land. Past the gate and back on public land, go ahead (generally west) at a signed junction with a lateral leading right (south) to Lower Blayney Public Camp, and continue west.

Weaving in and out of dense pine forest, the track ascends gently before crossing the Sallie Keyes Lakes' outlet. After 2 miles of easy climbing, the trail levels off and skirts the north side of Double Meadow before rejoining the main road.

The trail continues west, wandering away from the valley bottom. After crossing open granite slabs and sandy gullies, the trail reaches a signed junction with a spur trail going right (west) to the ferry landing (see sidebar "Water Taxi," on page 61 for details on taking the ferry).

If hiking to the trailhead, continue ahead (west and then south) from the last junction to the bridge across South Fork San Joaquin River. Once over a low ridge, cross Boulder Creek, and turn right (northwest) at the trail to Thompson Lake. Now high above Florence Lake, the trail eventually joins the Southern California Edison Company road and then arrives at the Florence Lake Trailhead (7360'; 11S 324899 4127475).

Lake Edison Trailhead

7790'; 11S 321717 4139068

DESTINATION/ UTM COORDINATES	TRIP TYPE	BEST SEASON	PACE (HIKING/ LAYOVER DAYS)	TOTAL MILEAGE
19 Graveyard Lakes 11S 325667 4146195	Out & back	Mid to late	4/1 Leisurely	16.8
20 Mosquito Flat 11S 345426 4144580	Shuttle	Mid to late	3/2 Moderate	19

Information and Permits: This trailhead is in Sierra National Forest: 1600 Tollhouse Road, Clovis, CA 93611, 559-297-0706, www.fs.fed.us/r5/sierra/. Permits are required for overnight stays, and quotas apply; reserved permits and on-demand permits are available.

Driving Directions: From Fresno, take State Hwy. 168 northeast for 42 winding, slow miles toward its end at a T junction on the east shore of Huntington Lake at the community of Lakeshore. Just before reaching Lakeshore, turn right onto the Kaiser Pass Road at the Eastwood Forest Service Center. The road quickly becomes very steep, narrow, and bumpy before Kaiser Pass and is even worse beyond the pass. Blind curves and reckless drivers are problems on this stretch. Allow time to drive very slowly (about 10 mph). As the road descends north and then east from the pass, find seasonally open High Sierra Ranger Station, where you can get on-demand permits. One mile beyond is the Lake Edison/Florence Lake Y junction. Turn left to remain on Kaiser Pass Road toward Lake Edison, bypass the turnoff left to Mono Hot Springs, and go left for 7 more miles, past the dam and bypassing Vermilion Valley Resort, to Vermilion Campground. To reach the trailhead, go past the turnoff to the campground and follow the dirt road 0.15 mile to a parking area. Don't part here; instead, turn right up the hill and go past the turnoff to the pack station (on the left) to a parking area at a Forest Service sign.

VERMILION VALLEY RESORT

This resort, powered by its own generators, is on the west shore of Lake Edison and isn't exactly the epitome of a quaint mountain getaway. But what it lacks in charm it more than makes up in hospitality—the rooms, tent cabins, store, and restaurant are a haven for PCT/JMT through-hikers, who are treated like kings and queens here. Traditionally, the resort buys the through-hiker's first beverage and offers her/him a free stay in the (shared) hikers' tent cabin. It's a good opportunity to share information about trail conditions and exchange trail tips.

Through-hiking or not, VVR is a nice stop on an extended trip, and daily ferry service from June to October makes for easy access to the resort from main trails across the lake. The ferry (fee) leaves the resort at 9 A.M. and 4 P.M., and departs the Mono Creek landing at 9:45 A.M. and 4:45 P.M. Call the resort for updated information or to make reservations in a room or tent cabin: 559-259-4000. The resort website has good hiking links, food drop details, and driving directions: www.edisonlake.com.

KAISER PASS RD

19 Graveyard Lakes

Trip Data: 11S 325667 4146195; 16.8 miles; 4/1 days

Topos: *Sharktooth Peak, Graveyard Peak*

Highlights: Phantom, Murder, Headstone, and Ghost lakes: Don't let the ominous names fool you—the granite-covered Graveyard Lakes basin is one of the loveliest and most regal in the Silver Divide country.

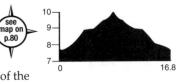

DAY 1 (Lake Edison Trailhead to Graveyard Meadows, 5.2 miles): Head east from the trail-head and, after 0.3 mile, reach a signed junction with the trail to Quail Meadows. Turn right (east) onto it and descend to the bridge across Cold Creek. The route then reaches a junction; take the Goodale Pass Trail left, proceeding north under Jeffrey pines, white firs, and junipers into Ansel Adams Wilderness.

Soon, the trail begins a long, dusty ascent, passing a meadow and, very near the top, offering good views of Lake Edison and the peaks of the Mono Divide. From the crown of the climb, it is a short distance to a ford of Cold Creek. Continue, now northeastward, into John Muir Wilderness. Graveyard Meadows (8850´; 11S 325951 4141992) is on the right, and secluded camping can be found at the head of the meadows. Or, if you prefer, stay at the more popular sites near the ford.

DAY 2 (Graveyard Meadows to Lower Graveyard Lake, 3.2 miles): The trail skirts the north edge of the meadows under a dense cover of lodgepoles and red firs—a wonderful bird habitat. At the north end of the meadows, the trail begins climbing moderately, and soon it fords Cold Creek again (difficult in early season). Continue the ascent on forested, duff trail.

At Upper Graveyard Meadow, find a junction (9370´; 11S 326657 4145558) with the trail to Graveyard Lakes. Turn left (west) and ford Cold Creek yet again. Beyond the ford, the trail enters a cover of lodgepole and hemlock and begins a steep, rocky climb to the basin above, where there are lush meadows at the eastern fringes of beautiful Lower Graveyard Lake (9950´; 11S 325667 4146195). Good though heavily used campsites are in the trees where the trail first meets the lake, or along the east side of the lake between this point and the inlet stream.

From any of these places, there are marvelous views of Graveyard Peak and the tumbled granite cirque wall that surrounds the entire Graveyard Lakes basin. Graveyard Peak—reminiscent of a tombstone with its salt-and-pepper granite—lives up to its name. Lower Graveyard Lake makes an excellent base camp from which to fish and explore the remaining five lakes in the basin. The three small lakes directly above offer prettier and cleaner camping. Follow the trail around to the head of the lake and climb the hill to reach them. Fishing is good on lower Graveyard Lake for brook trout.

Days 3–4 (Graveyard Lakes to Lake Edison Trailhead, 8.4 miles): Retrace your steps.

KAISER PASS RD

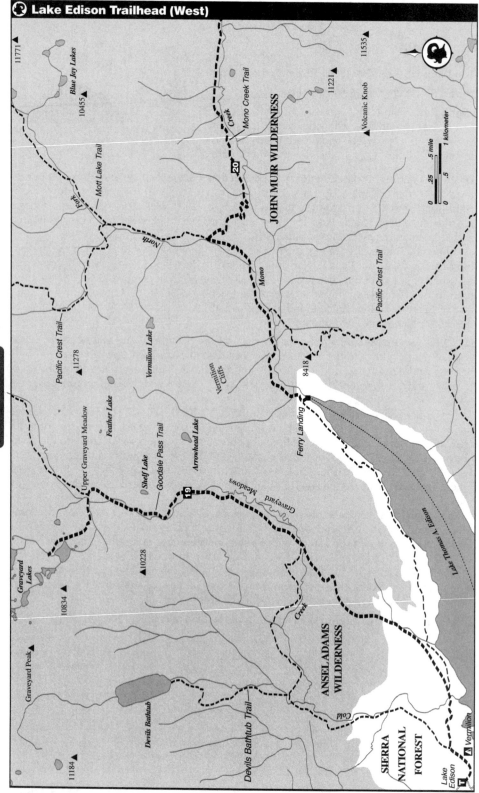

KAISER PASS RD

JOHN MUIR WILDERNESS

ANSEL ADAMS WILDERNESS

SIERRA NATIONAL FOREST

11771

Blue Jay Lakes

10455

Mott Lake Trail

North Fork

Mono Creek Trail

Creek

20

Mono

11221

Volcanic Knob

11535

Pacific Crest Trail

Pacific Crest Trail

11278

Upper Graveyard Meadow

Feather Lake

Vermilion Lake

Vermilion Cliffs

8418

Ferry Landing

Shelf Lake

Goodale Pass Trail

Arrowhead Lake

Graveyard Meadows

19

10228

Graveyard Lakes

10834

Graveyard Peak

11184

Devils Bathtub

Devils Bathtub Trail

Cold Creek

Lake Thomas A. Edison

Vermilion

Lake Edison

0   .25   .5 mile
0   .5   1 kilometer

80

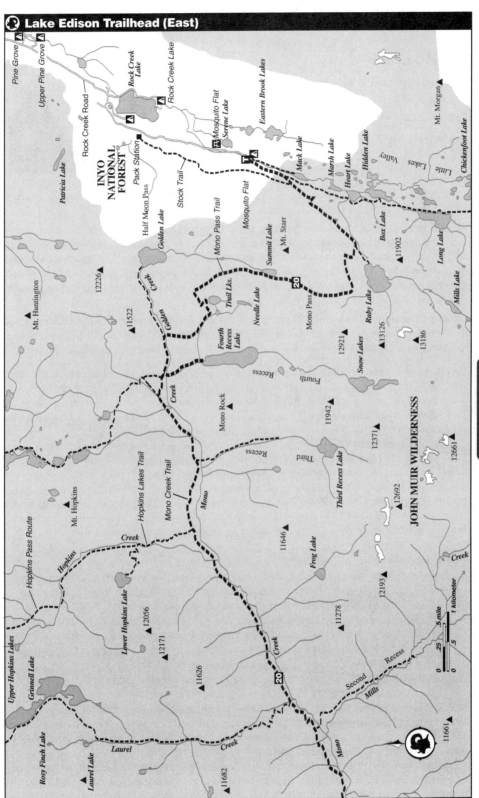

KAISER PASS RD

81

20 Mosquito Flat

Trip Data: 11S 345426 4144580; 19 miles;
3/2 days

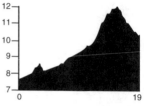

Topos: *Graveyard Peak, Mt. Abbot, Mt. Morgan*

Highlights: From the gentle landscape around
Lake Edison, follow pretty Mono Creek into the High Sierra
on a trail that offers access to several lake basins as well as
to the famed Mono Recesses, four glacier-sculpted hanging
valleys that invite exploration. This trip is not only beautiful, it is just about the shortest
trans-Sierra backpack possible.

HEADS UP! *The trip's first-day mileage starts at the northeast end of Lake Edison and assumes you've taken the ferry from Vermilion Valley Resort across the lake. See the sidebar "Vermilion Valley Resort" on page 78. If you hike from the Lake Edison Trailhead, add 5.5 miles to the trip. Setting up the shuttle is a two-day job; on the other hand, the trip is short enough that simply retracing your steps to Lake Edison is a reasonable option. In the upper Mono Creek and Rock Creek drainages, fires are prohibited above 10,000 feet.*

Shuttle Directions: From Hwy. 395 at Tom's Place, turn southwest onto Rock Creek Road and drive to its end, about 13 miles up-canyon, at Mosquito Flat. You'll pass numerous campgrounds, a couple of resorts, Rock Creek Lake, and another trailhead on the way.

DAY 1 (Lake Edison Trailhead to Second Recess, or "Fish Camp," 6 miles): From the ferry landing, which varies as the lake level drops over the season, make an easy ascent of about 1.5 miles generally northeast through forest and meadow to a T-junction with the PCT/JMT. Go ahead (northeast) onto the PCT/JMT. Cross North Fork Mono Creek and then climb to meet the Mono Creek Trail.

At this junction, turn right (southeast) onto the Mono Creek Trail. Leaving the PCT/JMT, traverse a southwest-trending ridge, and presently drop back to creekside to begin the pleasant hike generally eastward up Mono Creek's valley. Under evergreen cover, stroll for about 3 more miles past the mouth of trailless First Recess to Fish Camp, a traditional camping area where Mono Creek meets the Second Recess and Mills Creek (8500´; 11S 335731 4143573) trails. While Fish Camp is a convenient area for today's landmark, it is badly overused. It's best to camp farther upstream or downstream.

LAKE BASINS ABOVE MONO CREEK

The Mono Creek Trail offers access to the marvelous Mono Recesses south of Mono Creek and to several more beautiful basins north of the creek. The temptation to stay in Mono Creek's valley to visit these many basins is almost irresistible.

In the Fish Camp area, adventurous hikers will want to spend a layover day exploring (or camping in) the Second Recess high country. Follow the trail along the banks of Mills Creek. It can be difficult to follow, but a use trail beyond does lead to beautiful Lower Mills Lake (10840´; 11S 339602 4140719).

Trips 50, 52, 55, and this trip explore some of these magnificent basins.

DAY 2 (Second Recess to Fourth Recess Lake, 5.5 miles): This day's journey is a gorgeous, ever-opening hike up-valley, heading generally east and northeast. The route is sheltered by whispering aspens and features tempting pools in Mono Creek, which is framed by Mono Rock and surrounding high peaks.

Less than half a mile from Second Recess, meet a lateral going left (north) to Laurel and Grinnell lakes. Stay on the Mono Creek Trail east-northeastbound, ford Laurel Creek, and continue to a ford of Hopkins Creek. At a junction, the trail to the Hopkins Lakes heads left (north). Stay northeastbound on the Mono Creek Trail. Next, bypass a neglected track left (south) into Third Recess.

At a junction with the Pioneer Basin Trail (left, north), go ahead (east) on the Mono Creek Trail; just 0.1 mile more is the signed lateral right (south) to Fourth Recess Lake (10,150´; 11S 342007 4145440). Camping is limited on this long lake, bounded on three sides by 1000-foot walls and fed by an 800-foot waterfall. A camp near the outlet stream is a good option.

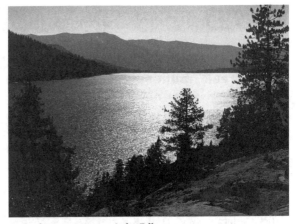

Late afternoon sun on Lake Edison

OTHER CAMPING OPTIONS IN THE FOURTH RECESS AREA

If you've planned another layover day and don't mind a few extra miles, take the lateral to stunning Pioneer Basin (see Trip 55 for details). Good camping can also be found at Golden Lake: Stay on the Mono Creek Trail (ahead, east) as it trades Mono Creek proper for Golden Creek, one of the three principal tributaries that create Mono Creek here. At a ford of Golden Creek, don't ford; instead, take a use trail east-northeast up Golden Creek to Golden Lake, a total of 1.5 more miles.

DAY 3 (Fourth Recess Lake to Mosquito Flat, 7.5 miles): Regain the Mono Creek Trail and turn east on it. Those who camped at Fourth Recess or Pioneer Basin will soon find a junction with the use trail northeast up Golden Creek to Golden Lake.

Stay on the Mono Creek Trail and ford Golden Creek as the trail hooks right (south) to begin a rocky ascent of almost 3 miles to Mono Pass. On the way to the pass, the route skirts the Trail Lakes (overused campsites). Barren Summit Lake lies a little north of (before) Mono Pass in the moonscape of decomposed granite around the 12,060-foot pass (11S 343164 4143539).

The descent is a bit dizzying, as switchbacks drop 1000 feet in less than 2 miles to a junction near a pretty pond with the lateral right (southwest) to Ruby Lake. Go ahead (northeast) to stay on the main trail, now the Mono Pass Trail, which descends moderately as it traverses the east slope of Mt. Starr, offering excellent over-the-shoulder views of Little Lakes Valley (Trip 54).

Near the end of the descent, go right (briefly south, down a switchback) where a stock trail takes off ahead (northeast). Shortly beyond, find a junction with the trail into Little Lakes Valley (the Morgan Pass Trail) near a high point with a splendid view south to the great peaks at Little Lakes Valley's head. Go left (ahead, northeast), roughly paralleling Rock Creek downstream. In a half mile, find the Mosquito Flat Trailhead and your shuttle car (10,255´; 11S 345426 4144580; tiny one-overnight campground for those beginning a trip here, with a valid wilderness permit; toilet).

Lewis Creek Trailhead

4570'; 11S 349196 4074031

DESTINATION/ UTM COORDINATES	TRIP TYPE	BEST SEASON	PACE (HIKING/ LAYOVER DAYS)	TOTAL MILEAGE
21 East Kennedy Lake 11S 352651 4082693	Out & back	Mid to late	4/1 Strenuous	26
22 Volcanic Lakes 11S 354221 4084613	Shuttle	Mid to late	6/1 Strenuous, part cross-country	31/33

Information and Permits: The Lewis Creek Trailhead is in Kings Canyon National Park: 47050 Generals Hwy., Three Rivers, CA 93271, 559-565-3341, www.nps.gov/seki/. Permits are required, there is a fee for them, and quotas apply. Some areas have fire restrictions and bear-canister requirements. You may reserve a permit in advance for trips between mid-May and through September by mail or fax only, no earlier than March 1 and no later than three weeks before the start of your trip. Permit quotas are in effect from mid-May to September. On-demand permits are available beginning at 1 P.M. the day before your trip starts at the Cedar Grove Visitor Center (559-565-3793), which is near Cedar Grove Village (campgrounds, store, lodging, cafe, showers, laundromat, pack station; www.nps.gov/seki/cgf&s.htm) and next to Sentinel Campground on Hwy. 180, about 6 miles west of Road's End. On-demand permits are also available seasonally at Road's End Station (at the east end of Hwy. 180, 6 miles east of Cedar Grove Village). Call the Sequoia-Kings Canyon Wilderness Office (559-565-3775) for days and operation hours.

Driving Directions: From Fresno, take Hwy. 180 east into the Grant Grove unit of Kings Canyon National Park. The road curves north through Grant Grove and Sequoia National Forest before bending east along a long, winding descent into Kings Canyon proper. Now on the canyon's floor and roughly paralleling South Fork Kings River, continue east and head back into Kings Canyon National Park. About a quarter mile east from the boundary, find the Lewis Creek Trailhead parking lot on the north (left) side of the road. It's 77 miles from Fresno. The Lewis Creek Trailhead is also 1.5 miles west of Cedar Grove Village.

21 East Kennedy Lake

Trip Data: 11S 352651 4082693; 26 miles; 4/1

Topos: *Cedar Grove, Slide Bluffs*

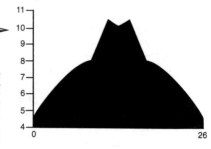

see map on p.86

Highlights: Ascending the Lewis Creek drainage, the trail passes through many different habitats and plant communities. Since much of this drainage has experienced fire in recent decades, the trip is an exceptional tour of fire ecology and forest succession. The geologically and scenically varied lakes in this region are favored by anglers, but the route to them from South Fork Kings River challenges even the most fit.

HEADS UP! *This brutally steep, little-used route climbs over 6000 feet to well-named Monarch Divide. The exposed trail radiates heat, baking hikers from below, while the sun fries them from above. Reward yourself with some layover days!*

84

DAY 1 (Lewis Creek Trailhead to Frypan Meadow, 6 miles): The trail heads north from the parking lot, bypassing a use trail leading off to the right, and it immediately begins to climb short switchbacks in the shade of incense-cedar, ponderosa pine, and black oak. This cover diminishes shortly after leaving the mouth of Lewis Creek's canyon, for much of this drainage has been burned over repeatedly. The legacy of those fires is evident by the lack of cover and the presence of charred stumps. Conifers, especially pines, benefit from fires because the heat helps open the cones so seeds can reach the soil, and fire also clears the ground so young trees can get enough sun.

Climbing at a moderate angle, the trail makes two more sets of switchbacks before the grade eases in a Jeffrey pine forest. The trail passes a junction with the Hotel Creek Trail; go ahead (northeast) here before descending to cross a small stream. Beyond the creek, the trail climbs over uneven ground to ford larger Comb Creek (wet in early season). After this ford, make a shadeless climb through short stands of young Jeffrey pines. The larger, shade-giving trees appear just prior to the ford of Lewis Creek (can be difficult in early season).

The track continues to climb generally north up the divide after the ford and passes Jeffrey pines with burn marks low on the truck as evidence of a ground fire. Wide vistas of Comb Spur appear to the east, and the Great Western Divide is visible in the far distance from this dusty, steep section of trail. The trail curves west for a half mile before again bearing north. Continue ahead (north) past the junction with the trail to Wildman Meadow.

The grade finally eases as the trail enters Frypan Meadow. There is a fine campsite near the upper end of the glade under towering white firs (7800´; 11S 348575 4080090).

DAY 2 (Frypan Meadow to East Kennedy Lake, 7 miles): It is imperative that you fill water bottles and hydration packs before this next section of trail, which climbs 3000 feet in 4 miles; the last 1600 feet are waterless and very steep.

Leaving Frypan Meadow behind, the trail begins a leisurely climb eastward under tall pines, fording two small creeks and then Lewis Creek. There are several fair campsites at the creek fords. The path then makes several switchbacks before beginning a traverse around the south side of Kennedy Mountain. In a short half mile, the forest diminishes, and soon you are climbing on a sunny, manzanita-choked slope. After about a mile of steep terrain, the trail enters an extensive grove of aspens, where several small creeks encourage a rest stop and a water refill.

The ford of East Fork Lewis Creek appears at around 9300 feet. This is the largest ford and the last one on the ascent. There are many obvious good campsites here; this is the last opportunity to rest before the final 1600 feet to the pass. The foliage decreases noticeably at this elevation, and the end of the climb passes only under cover of sparse whitebark pines.

The reward upon reaching Kennedy Pass is the view over the Middle Fork Kings River's canyon into northern Kings Canyon National Park. From the pass, hikers can spot several tarns to the north where there are excellent campsites. These tarns are not displayed on the topo.

The descent to the first tarn (10,600´; 11S 352054 4082725) is very steep and is difficult and dangerous if there is a lot of snow. Above this first tarn lies a regal campsite perched like a throne, from which you can view Kennedy Pass above and the tarns below. More campsites of exceptional quality may be found northwest of the tarns, about 100 feet below the first campsite. During late season, a spring originates below the east side of the second tarn and provides fresh drinking water.

Past these sites, the trail turns sharply eastward and disappears over the edge of Kennedy Canyon. The path is faintly visible down steep switchbacks, but exercise caution. Leave the trail when the steep grade eases, and aim for the level area just above the little lake northwest of East Kennedy Lake. Follow the north bank of this lake until you can go

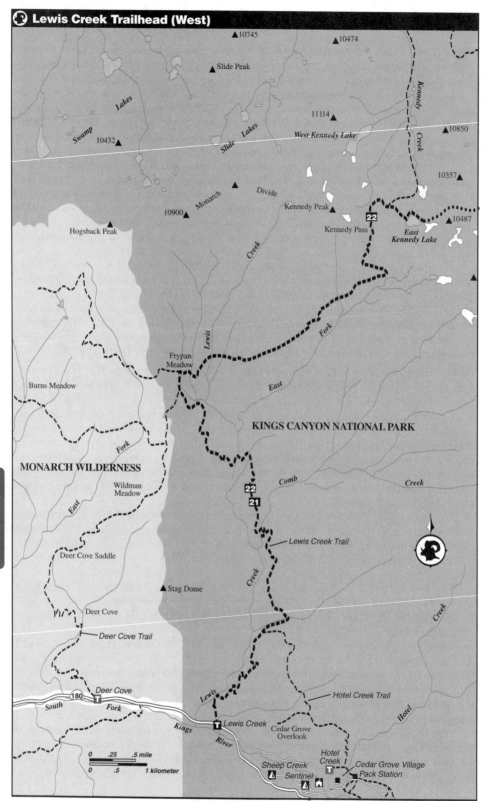

▲10745

▲10474

▲ Slide Peak

Lakes

Swamp

Slide

Lakes

10432▲

11114▲

West Kennedy Lake

▲10850

10357▲

▲

Monarch ▲ *Divide*

10900▲

Kennedy Peak ▲

▲10487

Hogsback Peak ▲

Kennedy Pass

22

East Kennedy Lake

▲

Creek

Fork

Lewis

Frypan Meadow

Burns Meadow

East

KINGS CANYON NATIONAL PARK

Fork

MONARCH WILDERNESS

Wildman Meadow

Comb

Creek

22
21

East

— *Lewis Creek Trail*

Deer Cove Saddle

▲ Stag Dome

Creek

Deer Cove

— *Deer Cove Trail*

Deer Cove

180 T

— *Hotel Creek Trail*

South

Fork

Lewis

Hotel

Kings

T *Lewis Creek*

Cedar Grove Overlook

River

Hotel Creek

Cedar Grove Village Pack Station

Sheep Creek ▲ Sentinel

T

▲ ⌂ ■

HWY 180

0   .25   .5 mile
0   .5   1 kilometer

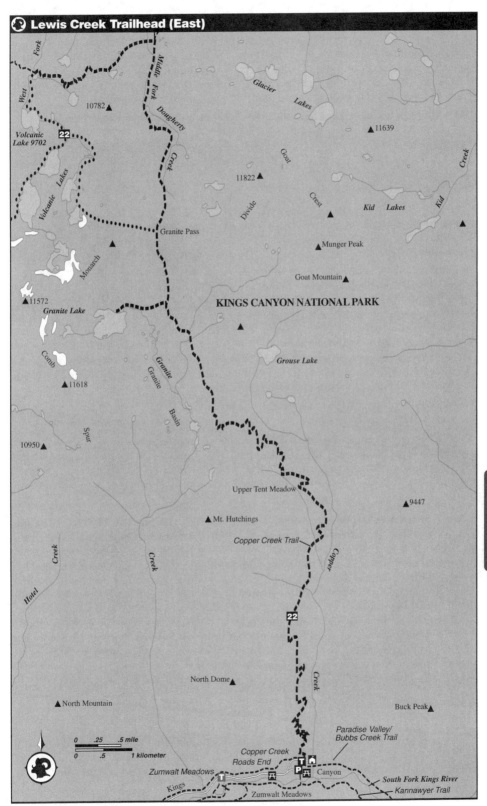

straight uphill to East Kennedy Lake. There are good, protected campsites in the trees below the lake and poor, exposed sites on the north shore (10,200′; 11S 352651 4082693).

Layover days spent here can be used to explore the Kennedy Canyon Creek Trail to West Kennedy Lake or to head cross-country toward the lower Volcanic Lakes.

DAYS 3–4 (East Kennedy Lake to Lewis Creek Trailhead, 13 miles): Retrace your steps.

22 Volcanic Lakes

Trip Data: 11S 354221 4084613; 31/33 miles; 6/1 days

Topos: *Cedar Grove, Slide Bluffs, Marion Peak, The Sphinx*

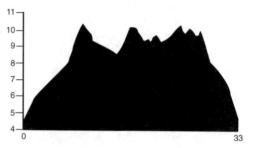

Highlights: This adventurous trip climbs steeply from lush subalpine forest to the stark alpine beauty of the Monarch Divide. Upon climbing to the ridge, you are rewarded with wide views of the gigantic chasms formed by South and Middle Fork Kings rivers. For a short distance in a section west of the park boundary, Kings Canyon is one of the deepest canyons in North America (from 2260 feet to 10,051 feet). The many lakes found on this trip afford fine camping, wonderful fishing, rock climbing, and solitude.

HEADS UP! *This is a very demanding route, with more than 6000 feet of elevation gain and a fair amount of cross-country travel. This trip should be attempted by strong, experienced hikers only.*

Shuttle Directions: From the Lewis Creek Trailhead, continue east for 7.5 miles through Cedar Grove to Roads End. Park at the Copper Creek Trailhead on the parking loop's north side. Near the parking area are vault toilets and picnic tables. The wilderness cabin near the trailhead offers backcountry information, wilderness permits, and bear-canister rentals.

DAY 1 (Lewis Creek Trailhead to Frypan Meadow, 6 miles): *(Recap: Trip 21, Day 1.)* The trail heads north from the parking lot, bypassing a use trail leading off to the right, and it climbs switchbacks before the grade eases among a Jeffrey pine forest. Go ahead (northeast) at a junction with the Hotel Creek Trail before descending to cross a small stream. Beyond this creek, climb to the ford of larger Comb Creek (wet in early season). After this ford, climb through young Jeffrey pines and then mature ones to the ford of Lewis Creek (can be difficult in early season).

The track continues to climb after the ford, and the views are impressive. The trail turns west for a half mile before again bearing north. Continue ahead (north) at the junction with the trail to Wildman Meadow. The grade finally eases at Frypan Meadow, where there is a fine campsite under towering white firs (7800′; 11S 348575 4080090).

DAY 2 (Frypan Meadow to East Kennedy Lake, 7 miles): *(Recap: Trip 21, Day 2.)* It is imperative that you fill water bottles and hydration packs before this section of trail: It climbs 3000 feet in 4 miles, and the last 1600 feet are waterless and very steep.

Leaving Frypan Meadow, climb eastward, fording two small creeks and then Lewis Creek (fair campsites at the creek fords). Switchback to begin a traverse around the south side of Kennedy Mountain, and soon you are climbing on a sunny, manzanita-choked slope. After about a mile of steep terrain, find a grove of aspens and several small creeks.

Ford East Fork Lewis Creek at around 9300 feet; this is the largest ford and the last one on the ascent (good campsites and last chance to rest before the final 1600 feet to the pass). The view at Kennedy Pass is your reward.

Tarns not on the map but north of the pass offer excellent campsites. The descent to the first tarn (10,600´; 11S 352054 4082725) is very steep and is difficult and dangerous if there is a lot of snow. During late season, a spring originates below the east side of the second tarn and provides fresh drinking water.

Past these sites, the trail turns sharply east and disappears over the edge of Kennedy Canyon; use caution on the steep switchbacks. Leave the trail when the steep grade eases and, rambling cross-country, aim for the level area just above the little lake northwest of East Kennedy Lake. Follow the north bank of this lake until you can go straight uphill to East Kennedy Lake (10,200´; 11S 352651 4082693).

DAY 3 (East Kennedy Lake to Volcanic Lake 9702, 3 miles, part cross-country): Continuing cross-country, head to the north shore of East Kennedy Lake and skirt around to the northeast to a grassy gully. Boulder-hop several hundred feet and then head uphill toward the obvious saddle. Just left of the shallow saddle is an excellent viewpoint, where you can see Mt. Gardiner, Arrow Peak, the Palisades, and the Sierra Crest beyond.

The route makes an eastward descent down another grassy gully whose upper end is about 50 feet south of that viewpoint, toward the south end of Volcanic Lake 10,199, the largest of the Volcanic lakes. The slabs by the lake can be avoided by heading south about 200 feet before reaching them. Clamber over large boulders to reach the outlet of this stark lake on the west bank.

Continue along the west bank and then follow the outlet downhill to Volcanic Lake 10,077, also devoid of tree cover. There are several excellent campsites on the west shore of this lake by the outlet. Following the watercourse generally north, ford the main stream and continue to descend, now on the northwest side, to a small tarn. From here, make a gentle descent westward to Volcanic Lake 9702. Spectacular campsites may be found on the east and north sides of the lake, under lodgepole pines (9700´; 11S 354221 4084613). Colorful shooting stars line the inlet and outlet of this lake, adding dashes of color to the otherwise stark alpine scenery. These sites provide a wonderful base camp for a layover day spent exploring the rest of the Volcanic Lakes. Abundant fishing, untouched rock climbing, colorful wildflowers, and solitude abound in this remote location.

DAY 4 (Volcanic Lake 9702 to Granite Lake, 5.5 miles by trail or 3.5 miles cross-country): To reach Granite Lake by trail: Follow the north outlet of Volcanic Lake 9702 approximately half a mile downhill to a small lake at about 9500 feet, where the trail appears, ending the cross-country part of this trip. This is a continuation of the Kennedy Pass Trail left at East Kennedy Lake. Turn right to head east along the path. The trail encounters short switchbacks in half a mile and then turns to the northeast for another mile to reach the signed junction with the Middle Fork Dougherty Creek Trail.

Turn right (south) onto this trail toward Granite Pass. The track fords Middle Fork Dougherty Creek several times in the next mile as it climbs gently through open pine. When the trail turns southwest, it encounters rocky switchbacks, passes a drift fence, and then reaches a small alpine meadow where the trail levels.

Continuing south, the trail heads up a small canyon for another mile before making the final climb to Granite Pass (10,673´; 11S 356440 4082574), where panoramic vistas abound. It is as difficult to capture these views on camera as it is to describe them on paper.

The trail, now the Copper Creek Trail, makes an easy quarter-mile descent before encountering steep switchbacks that lead down a narrow gully. At the base, a colorful alpine meadow dotted with specks of lavender provides excellent campsites. After reentering forest cover, the path descends to the meadow east of Granite Lake, and shortly thereafter reaches a signed lateral. Turn right (west) on the lateral, cross a creek, and then wind up the slope to the north side of beautiful Granite Lake. Good campsites can be found above the lake here (10,673´; 11S 355699 4081776)

To reach Granite Lake by a cross-country route: From the Volcanic Lakes, head east up the inlet stream of Volcanic Lake 9702 to meet the outlets of Volcanic Lakes 10,077 and 10,284. Continue ascending east and then south up the waterway to Volcanic Lake 10,284. Cross the low saddle to the southeast of that lake to reach Volcanic Lake 10,288, the highest of the Volcanic Lakes. The east side of the lake boasts a sandy beach and two points of rock jutting into the clear water, calling out for a swimming stop.

Beyond the lake, a grassy gully heads east and up to the top of the ridge. From this windblown ridgetop, contour generally east, maintaining your elevation, to Granite Pass (10,673´; 11S 356440 4082574). Meet the Copper Creek Trail here, ending the cross-country section of this trip. Turn right on the trail, heading south, and follow the above directions to the fine campsites at Granite Lake.

DAY 5 (Granite Lake to Lower Tent Meadow, 7 miles): *(Recap in Reverse: Trip 23, Day 2.)* Retrace your steps on the lateral to the main trail—now the Copper Creek Trail—on which you descended from Granite Pass. Turn right (south-southeast) on the mail trail, above Granite Basin. Climb eastward over a forested moraine before descending eastward and then southward on 1300 feet of switchbacks on this moraine, which divides Granite and Copper creeks.

In an avalanche swath near a creek, tank up on water before dropping on a moderate grade to Lower Tent Meadow Camp (7825´; 11S 359057 4077125).

DAY 6 (Lower Tent Meadow to Copper Creek Trailhead, 4.5 miles): *(Recap in Reverse: Trip 23, Day 1.)* From Lower Tent Meadow, head generally south to cross a creek and presently hop over a couple of rivulets in a clearing with a small campsite. High above Copper Creek itself, descend 2400 feet of hot, waterless, and only partly shaded trail to the trailhead on the north side of the parking loop at Cedar Grove Roadend.

Roads End—Copper Creek Trailhead

5055'; 11S 358743 4073444

DESTINATION/ UTM COORDINATES	TRIP TYPE	BEST SEASON	PACE (HIKING/ LAYOVER DAYS)	TOTAL MILEAGE
23 Granite Lake 11S 355856 4081108	Out & back	Early or late	3/1 Strenuous	23
24 South Lake 11S 360994 4114798	Shuttle	Mid to late	7/3 Moderate	51

Information and Permits: This trailhead is in Kings Canyon National Park: 47050 Generals Hwy., Three Rivers, CA 93271, 559-565-3341, www.nps.gov/seki. Permits are required, there is a fee for them, and quotas apply. Some areas may have fire restrictions and bear-canister requirements. You may reserve a permit in advance for trips mid-May through September by mail or fax only, no earlier than March 1 and no later than three weeks before the start of your trip.

Driving Directions: From Fresno, take Hwy. 180 east into the Grant Grove unit of Kings Canyon National Park. The road curves north through Grant Grove and Sequoia National Forest before bending east along a long, winding descent into Kings Canyon proper. Now on the great canyon's floor and roughly paralleling South Fork Kings River, continue east, back into Kings Canyon National Park, through Cedar Grove Village, and all the way to Roads End, with its little satellite ranger station (backcountry information, wilderness permits, bear canister rentals). It's a total of 84.5 miles from Fresno. The Copper Creek Trailhead is on the north side of the parking loop. There are three trailheads at Roads End: the Copper Creek Trailhead on its north side, the Cedar Grove Roadend Trailhead on its east side, and a trail to Zumwalt Meadows on its southwest side.

23 Granite Lake

Trip Data: 11S 355856 4081108; 23 miles; 3/1 days

see map on p.92

Topos: *The Sphinx, Marion Peak*

Highlights: The South Fork Kings River's valley is comparable to Yosemite Valley in many ways, but without the crowds. Granite Basin is perched high above the north rim of this valley, with a setting definitely worthy of a king—or a queen, for that matter. The climb out of the valley is arduous, but once you experience the matchless scenery and excellent fishing at Granite Lake, the memory of the difficult ascent will soon fade.

HEADS UP! *Because the canyon walls are so steep, the Copper Creek Trail climbs out of the canyon very quickly—5000 feet in a mere 6 miles. This ferocious ascent, often exposed to blazing sunlight, is suitable only for the backpacker in top shape. With a starting elevation just barely over 5000 feet, you should plan on a very early start to try and beat the heat.*

DAY 1 (Copper Creek Trailhead to Lower Tent Meadow, 4.5 miles): The Copper Creek Trail begins on the north side of the parking loop (5036') under tall pines, but all too soon it leaves the shady pines behind on a hot climb up the north wall of Kings Canyon. Canyon live oaks provide insufficient shade for the first 1.25 miles of ascent to the first stream. The granite walls reflect much sunlight, and on a typically hot summer's day, hiking up this trail produces the sensation of being baked in a glaring furnace. Despite the heat, this route has been well used for centuries.

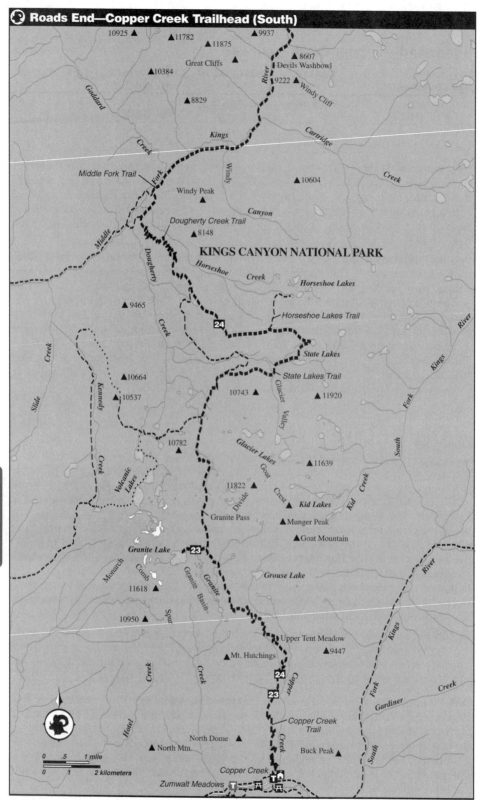

▲ 10925

▲ 11782

▲ 11875

▲ 9937

Great Cliffs ▲

▲ 8607
Devils Washbowl

▲ 10384

Goddard

9222 ▲

▲ 8829

River

▲ Windy Cliff

Creek

Kings

Cartridge

Creek

Middle Fork Trail

Fork

Windy Peak
▲

Windy

▲ 10604

Middle

Dougherty Creek Trail

▲ 8148

Canyon

KINGS CANYON NATIONAL PARK

Dougherty

Horseshoe   Creek

△ *Horseshoe Lakes*

▲ 9465

Creek

24

Horseshoe Lakes Trail

Kings

River

State Lakes

Slide

Kennedy

▲ 10664

▲ 10537

State Lakes Trail

10743 ▲

Glacier

Valley

▲ 11920

Fork

▲ 10782

Glacier Lakes

Goat

▲ 11639

South

Creek

Creek

Volcanic
Lakes

11822 ▲

Crest

Kid Lakes

Kid   Creek

Divide

Granite Lake

23

Granite Pass

▲ Munger Peak

▲ Goat Mountain

Comb

Monarch

11618 ▲

Granite

Granite

Grouse Lake

River

10950 ▲

Spur

Basin

Upper Tent Meadow

Kings

▲ 9447

Creek

Creek

▲ Mt. Hutchings

24

Copper

23

Fork

Creek

*Copper Creek
Trail*

Gardiner   Creek

North Dome ▲

▲ North Mtn.

Creek

Buck Peak ▲

South

0   .5   1 mile

0   1   2 kilometers

Copper Creek

🚻 ⛺ 🚻 ⛺

Zumwalt Meadows   🚻

HWY 180

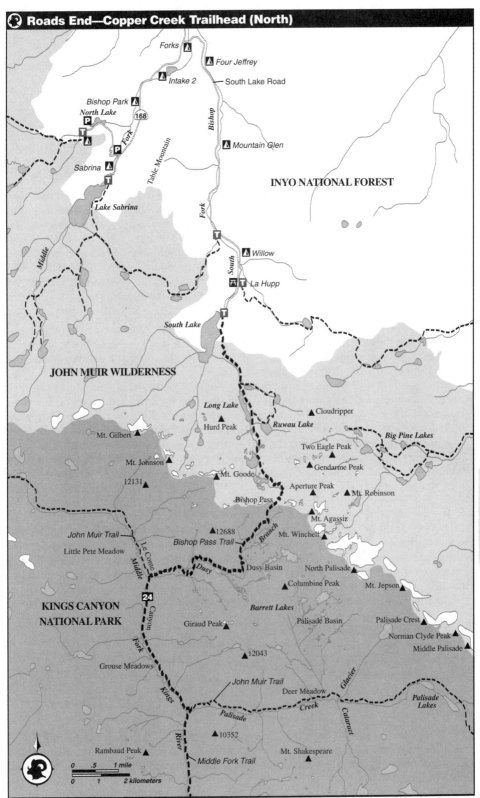

Forks

Four Jeffrey

Intake 2

South Lake Road

Bishop Park

North Lake

168

Bishop Fork

Mountain Glen

INYO NATIONAL FOREST

Sabrina

Lake Sabrina

Middle

Willow

South Fork

La Hupp

South Lake

JOHN MUIR WILDERNESS

Long Lake

Hurd Peak

Ruwau Lake

Cloudripper

Big Pine Lakes

Mt. Gilbert

Two Eagle Peak

Gendarme Peak

Mt. Johnson

Mt. Goode

Aperture Peak

Mt. Robinson

12131

Bishop Pass

Mt. Agassiz

12688

Bishop Pass Trail

Branch

Mt. Winchell

John Muir Trail

Le Conte Canyon

Middle

Little Pete Meadow

Dusy

Dusy Basin

North Palisade

24

Columbine Peak

Mt. Jepson

KINGS CANYON
NATIONAL PARK

Barrett Lakes

Palisade Basin

Palisade Crest

Giraud Peak

Norman Clyde Peak

Middle Palisade

Fork

12043

Grouse Meadows

Kings

John Muir Trail

Deer Meadow

Glacier

Cataract

Palisade
Lakes

Palisade Creek

10352

Rambaud Peak

River

Middle Fork Trail

Mt. Shakespeare

Table Mountain

0   .5   1 mile
0   1   2 kilometers

The first set of switchbacks gains 1400 feet and then the trail swings into Copper Creek's canyon, where the path is partially shaded under Jeffrey pines, sugar pines, incense-cedars, and white pines.

CHICKAREES

Along the dusty Copper Creek Trail, you might see dismantled white fir cones, chewed apart by chickarees. These small, squirrel-like rodents emit a rapid-to-slowing series of high-pitched squeaks (reminiscent of an alarm clock running down), and are more often heard than seen.

The trail crosses several previously burned slopes with a healthy covering of manzanita. So intense is the heat radiating from the sandy trail across these slopes, that imagining the forest floor is still smoldering is quite easy. Soon, the trail reaches a large, aspen- and brush-covered clearing harboring a small campsite. Hop over a couple of rivulets in this well-watered clearing and then reenter forest on the way to the next creek crossing. Just after the crossing, the path arrives at Lower Tent Meadow Camp (7825′; 11S 359057 4077125), with five designated campsites and a bear box. Be forewarned, Lower Tent Meadow is the only decent place to camp from here to Granite Basin.

DAY 2 (Lower Tent Meadow to Granite Lake, 7 miles): Continuing a northward, now moderate climb, the trail passes through an area burned in 1980. After two long switchbacks, the path nears the creek in a wide avalanche swath where only low-lying shrubs and a profusion of wildflowers are allowed to grow. The trail switchbacks again and nears the creek for the last time (9100′); fill your water bottles here.

Enter shady red fir forest and begin a long series of switchbacks that angle northwest as the trail climbs 1300 feet up a moraine dividing Copper and Granite creeks. En route, cross a belt of western white pines and then lodgepole pines along the ridgetop. From here, you see two prominent peaks to the east, Mt. Clarence King, on the left, and Mt. Gardiner.

A short, winding descent leads through a drift fence and down toward Granite Basin, filled with delightful tarns and irregular-shaped meadows. The trail avoids the floor of the basin in favor of an undulating traverse across a lodgepole-shaded hillside above. Parties interested in camping at locations within the basin other than Granite Lake must leave the trail and go cross-country.

Just beyond the large meadow at the north end of the basin, in a pocket of willows, reach a signed junction with a lateral to the lake. Turn left (west) and follow this lateral over a stream and past a couple of seldom-used campsites on a gradual ascent toward the lake. Hop over the seasonal inlet and arrive at campsites along the north shore of Granite Lake (10,093′; 11S 355856 4081108). The island-dotted lake nestles in a rocky basin below the cliffs of the Monarch Divide. Sparse pines offer little shelter for the smattering of campsites scattered around the lakeshore. Anglers can test their skill on fair-size brook trout.

DAYHIKING FROM GRANITE LAKE

A layover day at Granite Lake offers so many choices for farther wanderings that you might want to stay a week or more. Leaving your backpack behind, a day is long enough to explore several Volcanic Lakes or State Lakes, or the unnamed lakes in lower Granite Basin. Also within easy reach are the Glacier Lakes and the two unnamed lakes just northeast of Granite Pass.

DAY 3 (Granite Lake to Copper Creek Trailhead, 11.5 miles): Retrace your steps to the trailhead. Backpackers wishing to avoid the 11.5-mile, one-day hike out should plan on two days and a stay at Lower Tent Meadows, as it is the only viable campsite between Granite Basin and the trailhead.

HWY 180

24 South Lake

Trip Data:
11S
360994
4114798;
51;
7/3 days

see map on p.92

Topos: *The Sphinx, Slide Bluffs, Marion Peak, North Palisade, Mt. Thompson*

Highlights: This spectacular trans-Sierra trek is little used between Granite Lake and the JMT. The Middle Fork Kings River runs entirely through wilderness, and backpackers will follow this watercourse upstream through its mighty canyon for much of the route. Beyond the Middle Fork, the trail crosses the Sierra Crest near the north end of the Palisades, a world-renowned group of some of the most rugged alpine peaks in the entire range.

HEADS UP! *Backpackers must be in top shape for this trip. It includes a difficult, 5000-foot ascent in 6 miles along the Copper Creek Trail; a leg-brutalizing, mostly waterless, 4400-foot descent in 7 miles to Simpson Meadow; the trying hike up the Middle Fork Kings River; and a stiff climb through Dusy Basin to 11,972-foot Bishop Pass. In addition, the ford of Palisade Creek is often difficult.*

Shuttle Directions: From Hwy. 395 in the town of Bishop, turn west onto Hwy. 168 and drive southwest 15 miles to a junction with South Lake Road. Turn left onto South Lake Road and go 7 more miles to the end of the road at South Lake, where there are many day-use-only parking spaces, restrooms, the trailhead, and an overnight parking lot opposite the restrooms and trailhead. If the overnight lot is full, backtrack to additional parking 1.3 miles down the road; a footpath connects the lower and upper parking lots.

DAY 1 (Copper Creek Trailhead to Lower Tent Meadow, 4.5 miles): *(Recap: Trip 23, Day 1.)* The Copper Creek Trail begins on the north side of the parking loop (5036′). Climb away from the trailhead on a stiff, switchbacking ascent of the north wall of Kings Canyon that offers little shade. Swing into the canyon of Copper Creek and continue climbing through alternating sections of light forest and previously burned or avalanched slopes that are thick with shrubs. Just after the crossing of a tributary stream, arrive at Lower Tent Meadow Camp with five designated campsites and a bear box.

DAY 2 (Lower Tent Meadow to Granite Lake, 7 miles): *(Recap: Trip 1, Day 2.)* Climb up switchbacks on a moderate ascent across shrub-covered slopes and the last reliable steam near 9100 feet. Beyond, enter pockets of forest and continue climbing up a moraine that separates Copper and Granite creeks. A short descent leads toward Granite Basin, although the route of the trail stays off the basin floor in favor of a traverse across a hillside. Just beyond a large meadow is a junction with a lateral on the left (west) that leads to campsites on the north shore of Granite Lake.

DAY 3 (Granite Lake to Lower State Lake, 7 miles): First, retrace your steps to the junction with the Copper Creek Trail and then turn left (north), leaving the forest behind on a steep, rocky, 0.6-mile climb toward Granite Pass (10,673′) on the Monarch Divide. After enjoying the fine views, follow a zigzagging descent past a series of meadow-covered benches rimmed by granite walls, as the trail nears Middle Fork Dougherty Creek several times along the way. After a pair of drift fences, continue to wind downstream through scattered lodgepole pines, hopping over the creek three times and gaining a ridge that affords a fine view down the Middle Fork's canyon. Reach a junction with the Lewis Creek/Kennedy Pass Trail at 2.7 miles from Granite Pass.

Continue down the trail, stepping across a creek flowing toward Lake of the Fallen Moon. A short, moderate climb leads to a traverse across a forested hillside, followed by a brief descent to a pocket of lush meadow and a trail junction.

Turn right (east) at the junction, onto a lateral trail that loops through the State Lakes, and head toward the State Lakes through lodgepole pine forest. Pass a good-size meadow filled with wildflowers, including shooting star, cinquefoil, tiger lily, and aster, and then climb to the crest of a rise. Drop from the rise to a creek draining lovely Glacier Valley and then traverse to a vigorous stream plummeting downslope from Lower State Lake.

A moderately steep climb away from the stream leads up a hillside and, over the lip of the lake's basin, to gently rising, flower-dotted terrain below the lower lake. Soon, you reach the northwest shore of Lower State Lake (10,250´; 11S 359885 4087636). Backdropped by the impressive cliffs of Cirque Crest, the lower lake offers a few lodgepole pine-shaded campsites along the north shore. Fishing is usually excellent for good-size golden and rainbow trout, probably because the lake sees so few anglers.

DAY 4 (Lower State Lake to Simpson Meadow, 8 miles): This hiking day entails a 4400-foot descent in 7 miles that can put a tremendous strain on your knees.

However, instead of retracing your steps to the main trail, begin this day by taking the rest of this looping lateral trail: Make an easy, half-mile climb north from Lower State Lake and then east through lodgepole pine, currant, and gooseberry to the grassy fringes of Middle State Lake (10,450´). This seldom-visited lake is not as desirable as its lower neighbor. Hop across the outlet and stroll through boulder-strewn and lightly forested terrain on moderately ascending trail past a small meadow to the crest of a hill and a Y junction with the path to Horseshoe Lakes. From the junction, go ahead (left, west) and descend 1.25 miles to a junction with a trail (left) back to Dougherty Creek.

Turn right (north) and soon begin the giant drop into the canyon of Middle Fork Kings River. The long descent will reflect the 4400-foot elevation loss by the appearance of 11 different tree species along the way, beginning with whitebark and lodgepole pines. Continuing the descent, these trees are left behind as western white pine and Sierra juniper begin to appear. Tall red fir is plentiful by the time the trail reaches a junction with the main trail. For this trip, go right (north) on the main trail at this junction and begin to descend more steeply. (Going left here would take you down to Dougherty Creek, a year-round stream, in 0.3 mile; this is a segment of the main trail that you bypass by taking the lateral through the State Lakes.)

From here to the east end of the Simpson Meadow, the trail passes through areas that were charred to varying degrees by a lightning-caused fire that burned slowly for weeks in 1985. Park Service policy recognizes fire as a normal part of forest ecology, allowing natural fires to run their course in the backcountry. Indeed, many trees, such as the giant sequoia, require fire for reproduction. Cones of various trees, especially some pines, release their seeds if heated, and young trees usually grow better following a fire that clears the soil and opens the forest floor to sunlight.

Fire also releases nutrients from dead plant matter back into the soil. Even if most of the trees are killed in a fire, enough usually survive to reseed an area rather quickly, at least by nature's standards. (See Trip 84 for an exception.) Hardwood plants such as manzanita, aspen, and black oak, even if burned to the ground, can sprout new foliage from the crowns of their roots.

Sometimes, large trees literally explode when water in their trunks is superheated by fire. Depressions you may see along the trail mark the sites of large trees whose roots were burned below ground level. Trees with thick bark, such as Jeffrey pine and incense-cedar, usually won't burn unless fire gets under their bark and starts burning the trunk. The recuperative power of nature is clearly evident on these slopes, the result of more than two decades of revegetation following the 1985 fire.

The downward grade eases temporarily on a moraine near 8000 feet, where knees can catch a break before tackling the remaining 2000 feet down to the river. The next few hundred feet beyond the moraine are extremely steep and rocky. Soon, white fir appears, followed by aspen and incense-cedar. The grade eases again on an open slope where sugar pines join the forest and Windy Peak appears high above to the northeast.

By the time the trail levels off at 6000 feet on the floor of the canyon at huge Simpson Meadow, you can feel the warm, oxygen-rich air. Curving upstream (eastward), the trail passes through an open area on the way to a junction (5960´, 11S 354837 4093297) with a trail heading southwest toward Tehipite Valley.

THE TRAIL TO TEHIPITE VALLEY

A bridge over the Middle Fork Kings River a half mile downstream of Simpson Meadow was washed out in 1982, and the Park Service has no plans to rebuild this structure. Those who wish to visit magnificent Tehipite Valley—and those who don't mind the threat of the rattlesnakes for which Tehipite Valley is rightly known—may have to make a wet ford (difficult in early to mid-season) near this junction or farther upstream. Trails to Tehipite Valley have deteriorated, so getting there may demand cross-country thrashing through snake-filled brush.

The official, signed junction with the trail up Middle Fork Kings River, near a three-trunked incense-cedar with burnt bark, is almost hidden by a flourishing young white fir. Bear right (northeast) up-canyon from the junction. Still in Simpson Meadow, you soon cross the forks of Horseshoe Creek near a packer campsite. Fishing for rainbow trout in the Middle Fork is good.

Around Simpson Meadow, there are campsites near the trail on this east side of Horseshoe Creek, a quarter mile up-canyon, or a little farther along the river. Beyond these campsites, it's 3 miles to the next decent campsites, at Cartridge Creek. A number of use trails crisscross the meadow, leading to campsites or accessing the riverbank.

DAY 5 (Simpson Meadow to Grouse Meadows, 10 miles): Get an early start, as the temperatures are extremely hot in the canyon by mid-morning, and the trail provides little in the way of shade. In addition, access to the river is extremely limited, and trail-crossing streams may be few and far between by mid-season.

Starting at the junction with the trail to Tehipite Valley, head northeast and ford Horseshoe Creek. The multiple use trails in Simpson Meadow may make distinguishing the main trail a tad difficult, so keep working upstream until the use trails converge with the main trail. Skirt a meadow and then contour around the base of Windy Peak, opposite the cleft of Goddard Creek's canyon.

ALLUVIAL PROCESSES IN GODDARD CREEK'S CANYON

The river channel has been pushed to the south side of the canyon by the sediments deposited by Goddard Creek's debouching from its canyon. This process is widespread within the canyon of the Middle Fork Kings River: Farther upstream, the river flows on the north side of the canyon floor opposite the alluvial fan at the base of Windy Canyon.

Gradually ascend this shadeless alluvial fan, which is covered with numerous black oaks—evidence of a high water table. More black oaks appear on the approach to the forks of Windy Canyon Creek, where the water table is all the way up to the surface. Beyond this creek, the main canyon turns north, becoming steep and narrow. The trail gets steeper as well, winding through thickets of black oak. Soon, the trail crosses Cartridge Creek on a wood bridge. A packer camp is off trail beyond the bridge, north of some switchbacks— the last adequate campsite until Palisade Creek. By mid-season, Cartridge Creek provides the last reliable water source before the ford of the creek that drains Windy Cliff.

From Cartridge Creek to Palisade Creek, the rocky canyon is very steep and narrow, and the trail climbs steeply, usually high above the falls and pools of the river. Flowers seen along this stretch are generally of the dry-country variety, such as paintbrush, penstemon, Clinsia, forget-me-not, lupine, and fleabane.

Climb steeply to the flats just below Devils Washbowl. To the right, the east canyon walls provide a fascinating study in convoluted glacial polish, and the views to the west and northwest of the Great Cliffs and the heavily fractured rock of Devils Crags portend later, equally exciting views of the Black Divide. Switchbacks lead up to awesome Devils Washbowl, a wild, spectacular falls and cataract set in a granite gorge.

Leaving this tumult of water behind, the trail continues the ascent over rock to the ford of the unnamed creek draining Windy Cliff to the southeast in high, beautiful cascades. The flora around these tributary fords deserve attention for their lushness and for the presence of the water birch, a rare plant in westside Sierra canyons (although quite common on the east side). Wildflowers along these streams may include white mariposa lily, cinquefoil, tiger lily, lupine, columbine, and elderberry.

Beyond, the undulating trail is rarely at river's edge; more often, it is tens to hundreds of feet above. The underfooting is rocky until the approach to Palisade Creek, where the grade levels and then curves through a packer camp on the way to the flower-lined stream. The ford is preceded by a return to timber cover from a forest of Jeffrey, lodgepole, and western white pine and white fir. The bridge across Palisade Creek has been gone since the 1980s, and, like the bridge for the trail to Tehipite Valley mentioned earlier, it will not be replaced. Wade the swift, rolling, ice-cold waters, about 50 feet upstream from the confluence with Middle Fork Kings River. The ford is difficult at any time during the summer and may also be dangerous in early season. After successfully fording the creek, head east across the lodgepole-shaded flat (poor campsites) on a use trail to meet the JMT.

Turn left (west) onto the JMT and climb a mile upriver toward Grouse Meadows, initially on a stiff climb that soon becomes moderate. Follow the course of the river through light forest across a stream draining a trio of unnamed lakes below the southeast face of Giraud Peak, and then head across an open hillside covered with sagebrush to Grouse Meadows (8250'; 11S 358689 4103088). The meadows are quite scenic, with the Middle Fork assuming a sedate, meandering course through lush grasslands amid a scenic backdrop from the near-vertical granite walls of LeConte Canyon, a sight strikingly similar to Yosemite Valley. A couple of large, fair campsites offer fine views of the meadows and the river, although the mosquitoes can be quite bothersome in early season.

DAY 6 (Grouse Meadows to Dusy Basin, 7.5 miles): Beyond the serene grasslands of Grouse Meadows, the placid river begins to pick up speed again as the trail climbs gradually through scattered-to-light forest. Continuing the gentle ascent, the effects of an old avalanche and a past forest fire combine with natural breaks in the forest to provide occasional views of the surrounding terrain. Towering over LeConte Canyon, the mighty granite ramparts of the Citadel combine with the cascading stream from Ladder Lake to paint a dramatic mountain portrait on the west wall of the valley.

Where the trail draws nearer the Middle Fork, shooting cascades of whitewater catapult across sparkling granite slabs. Farther up the trail, watery ribbons of Dusy Branch slide gracefully down the sloping face of an extensive granite slab on the deep canyon's east wall. Near the crossing of Dusy Branch, campsites are just off the trail. A bridge leads across the creek past more campsites to a signed junction with the Bishop Pass Trail. Nearby, the LeConte Ranger Station is just a short walk up a path on the left.

Turn right (east) onto the Bishop Pass Trail and climb away from the floor of LeConte Canyon, soon leaving the cover of forest behind to scale an open, chaparral-covered slope with excellent views of towering Langille Peak across the canyon. Beyond this slope, enter scattered-to-light lodgepole pine forest and continue climbing to a bench and a pair of crossings over a multibranched stream. Good campsites are spread across the bench along the banks of Dusy Branch.

Continue the stiff, switchbacking climb up the east wall of LeConte Canyon. At various points along the ascent, there are excellent views of the Dusy Branch spilling down a near vertical wall of granite. Keep climbing to the Dusy Branch bridge, which is a fine spot to catch your breath and enjoy the superlative view of the deep declivity of LeConte Canyon. Resuming the seemingly interminable climb, the trail continues to switchback steeply until cresting the lip of the canyon at the beginning of Dusy Basin.

Moderately ascending trail along the Dusy Branch through the basin is a welcome relief after the hot climb out of the valley. Dusy Basin is a sublime mixture of flower-covered meadowlands, sparkling slabs of granite, crystal-clear rivulets, and azure-colored tarns. The lower lakes offer excellent angling. Dwarf whitebark pines are widely scattered about the open basin, decreasing in both number and stature as you gain elevation on the climb toward Bishop Pass. A number of use trails branch away from the Bishop Pass Trail at various locations, accessing view-filled campsites near the plethora of lakes and tarns sprinkled across the area, including Lake 11388 (11S 362493 4106843), in the heart of the basin directly northwest of Isosceles Peak.

DUSY BASIN SCENERY

The alpine scenery in Dusy Basin is breathtaking in its vastness. The Inconsolable Range rises behind Bishop Pass and the mountaineer's mecca, the Palisades, fills the eastern skyline. Isosceles and Columbine peaks separate Dusy Basin from rugged Palisade Basin, home to the secluded Barrett Lakes, and they are accessible to cross-country enthusiasts by a route over Knapsack Pass (see Trip 69). Dusy Basin is not only a favorite destination of backpackers; photographers are drawn to the area in almost equal numbers—the alpenglow on the western faces of the Palisades often creates a dreamlike conclusion to a beautiful sunset.

DAY 7 (Dusy Basin to South Lake Trailhead, 7 miles): From Dusy Basin, follow the Bishop Pass Trail on a moderate climb with occasional switchbacks to Bishop Pass (11,972′). Views from the pass are excellent of the Inconsolable Range to the north; Mt. Agassiz to the southeast; Dusy Basin to the south, flanked by Columbine and Giraud peaks; and the Black Divide on the distant western skyline.

Descend from the pass through rocky, above-timberline terrain. Depending on the previous winter's snowpack and the time of year, you may have to cross snowfields directly below the pass. Wind down on switchbacks through a seemingly endless sea of granite slabs and boulders until red, metamorphosed rock appears near tree line. Entering more hospitable terrain, the trail passes to the east of irregular-shaped Bishop Lake (11,230′) and continues down the canyon a short distance to Saddlerock Lake (11,128′) and the Timberline Tarns. Another descent leads past Spearhead Lake (10,750′). All these lakes offer marginal-to-fair campsites and fair fishing for brook and rainbow trout.

From Spearhead Lake, the trail continues to descend, crossing the outlet from Ruwau Lake before reaching the aptly named Long Lake (10,753′). Follow gently graded trail along the east side of the lake, bypassing the south junction with the loop trail to Ruwau Lake and the Chocolate Lakes; continue ahead (generally north) here. Since Long Lake is a very popular destination for backpackers, hikers, and anglers coming from the South Lake Trailhead, campsites abound around the overused lakeshore, particularly on the knoll near the south end of the lake. From the north end of Long Lake, a short stroll leads to the northern junction with the Chocolate Lakes loop (here, to Bull Lake); go ahead (generally north) again.

From the junction, a series of short switchbacks descend around granite outcrops and large boulders and through scattered pines to the crossing of a creek and an occasionally signed junction with the faint, partly cross-country route heading west to seldom-visited Marie Louise Lakes. Continue ahead (generally north) down the canyon to a bridged crossing of a tributary stream and proceed to the Treasure Lakes Trail junction; continue descending ahead (generally north). Beyond there, exit John Muir Wilderness and follow the trail on a gradual descent across open slopes high above the reservoir of South Lake to the trailhead (9760´; 11S 360994 4114798).

HWY 180

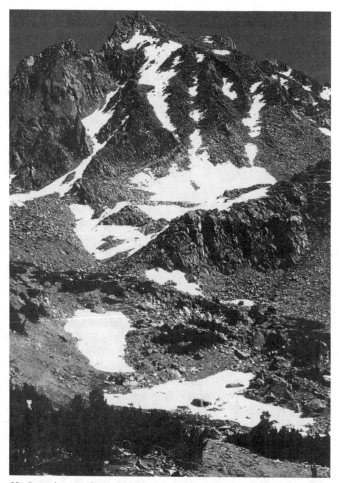

Mt. Agassiz, guardian of Bishop Pass, from Bishop Lake

Roads End—Cedar Grove Roadend Trailhead 5036'; 11S 358138 4073439

DESTINATION/ UTM COORDINATES	TRIP TYPE	BEST SEASON	PACE (HIKING/ LAYOVER DAYS)	TOTAL MILEAGE
25 Lake Reflection 11S 355856 4081108	Out & back	Mid to late	4/1 Moderate	31
26 Rae Lakes 11S 375125 407477	Semiloop	Mid to late	6/1 Moderate	41.75

Information and Permits: This trailhead is in Kings Canyon National Park: 47050 Generals Hwy., Three Rivers, CA 93271, 559-565-3341, www.nps.gov/seki. Permits are required, there is a fee for them, and quotas apply. Some areas may have fire restrictions and bear-canister requirements. You may reserve a permit in advance for trips mid-May through September by mail or fax only, no earlier than March 1 and no later than three weeks before the start of your trip.

Driving Directions: From Fresno, take Hwy. 180 east into the Grant Grove unit of Kings Canyon National Park. The road curves north through Grant Grove and Sequoia National Forest before bending east along a long, winding descent into Kings Canyon proper. Now on the great canyon's floor and roughly paralleling South Fork Kings River, continue east, back into Kings Canyon National Park, through Cedar Grove Village, and all the way to Roads End, with its little satellite ranger station (backcountry information, wilderness permits, bear-canister rentals). It's a total of 84.5 miles from Fresno. The Cedar Grove Roadend Trailhead is on the east side of the parking loop.

25 Lake Reflection

Trip Data: 11S 355856 4081108; 31 miles; 4/1 days

Topos: *The Sphinx, Mt. Clarence King, Mt. Brewer*

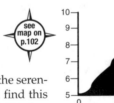

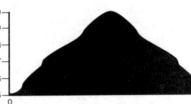

Highlights: Those who appreciate the serenity of high, alpine lake basins will find this trip to the upper reaches of East Creek a rewarding choice. Excellent fishing amid spellbinding surroundings makes this a fine trip for anglers. Non-anglers can while away the time simply soaking up the country.

HEADS UP! *Bears are a serious problem in this area; use bear canisters when hiking out of Cedar Grove. The area around Lake Reflection can be quite windy.*

DAY 1 (Cedar Grove Roadend Trailhead to Charlotte Creek, 7.5 miles): Since the climb is hot and dry, an early start is highly recommended. From the paved roadend loop (5036´), the wide, sandy trail heads generally east through a mixed forest of ponderosa pines, incense-cedars, black oaks, sugar pines, and white fir. Soon, the shade is left behind amid a sparse cover of ponderosa pines.

> **EARLY HISTORY**
> The balmy climate characteristic of the gently sloping canyon floor made Kings Canyon a favorite of Native Americans, who camped here from spring to fall. Foraging parties of Yokuts established spur camps along Bubbs Creek at many of the same spots currently used by modern-day backpackers.

HWY 180

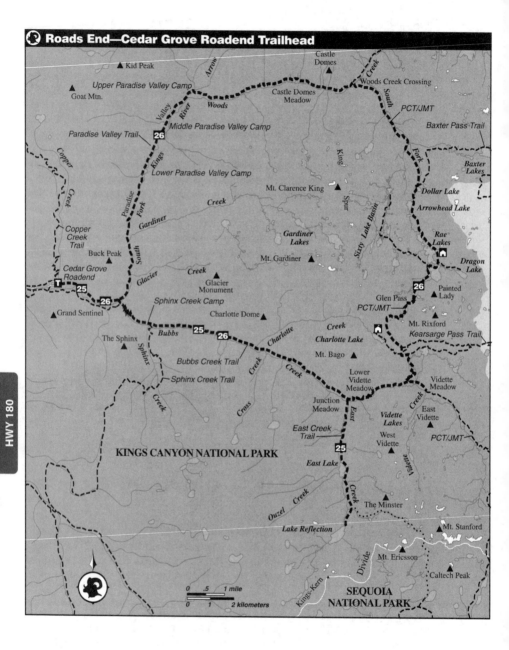

Roads End—Cedar Grove Roadend Trailhead

Soon, the trail enters a cool, dense forest of alders, white firs, ponderosa pines, and sugar pines on the way to a junction with the Paradise Valley/Woods Creek Trail, branching north. Head right (southeast) at the junction and cross a steel bridge over South Fork Kings River just below its confluence with Bubbs Creek. Past the bridge is another junction, where the Kanawyer Loop and Bubbs Creek trails meet. Continue ahead (southeast) up the Bubbs Creek Trail and follow a series of short, wood bridges across braided Bubbs Creek.

A moderate climb leads to the first of many switchbacks that climb away from the floor of the canyon and up the Bubbs Creek drainage.

PINYON PINES

Along the climb up Bubbs Creek, you may notice a rarity for this side of the Sierra—pinyon pines. This single-needle pine, quite common to the lower elevations on the east side of the Sierra, has a distinctive spherical cone, the fruit of which is the tasty pine nut. Most noticeable about the cone is the very thick, blunt, four-sided scale.

The stiff ascent offers fine views for the panting backpacker down into the dramatic, U-shaped South Fork Kings River's canyon. On the south wall of Bubbs Creek canyon, the dominating landmark is the pronounced granite point named the Sphinx. To the east, Sphinx Creek cuts a sharp-lipped defile on the peak's east shoulder.

Above the switchbacks, moderately ascending trail heads into the cool shade of tall conifers on the way to a junction with the southbound Sphinx Creek Trail. Continue ahead (east) here and cross Bubbs Creek on a wood plank bridge, and then continue to Sphinx Creek Camp (6280′). Excellent campsites with bear boxes are here on either side of Bubbs Creek.

From Sphinx Creek Camp, continue ahead, eastbound on the Bubbs Creek Trail, traveling in and out of mixed forest for the next few miles. Well past the crossings of a trio of tiny brooks, ford Charlotte Creek and reach a path that leads to pleasant, tree-shaded campsites (about 7320′; 11S 367450 4070534) near the bank of Bubbs Creek. Fishing is good for brown, brook, rainbow, and golden-rainbow hybrid.

DAY 2 (Charlotte Creek to Lake Reflection, 8 miles): Alternating stretches of lush foliage and dry slopes greet you for the next couple of miles on a steady ascent away from Charlotte Creek. Across periodic clearings, Mt. Bago looms above the north side of Bubbs Creek's steep-walled canyon. Reach some campsites, stroll through a gap in a drift fence, and pass a horse camp on the way to lengthy Junction Meadow (8190′), carpeted with lush grasses, wildflowers, and ferns. Near the far end of the meadow is a signed junction with the East Creek Trail.

Turn right (south) and follow the East Creek Trail across the dense foliage of the meadow to a wet ford of Bubbs Creek (difficult in early season). Past the creek, the trail ascends East Creek's canyon via rocky switchbacks that zigzag through a sparse-to-moderate cover of lodgepoles, western white pines, firs, and aspens. The red, metamorphic rocks of Mt. Bago dominate the view to the north, with Mt. Gardiner coming into view just behind. As you reach the top of the first rise, look for the peaks of the Kings-Kern Divide, which join the vista. Anglers trying their luck along East Creek may find small rainbow and brook trout; the fish in East Lake may be a bit larger.

Following a brief stretch of moderate climbing, the trail crosses East Creek (wet in early season) and then climbs steadily along the east bank. The grade gets steeper where the trail enters a forest of pines and firs. After the ford of an unnamed, fern-lined stream, the grade eases near the outlet of East Lake. Lucky hikers may spot one of the many mule deer that frequent East Lake's picturesque, grass-fringed waters. The trail rounds the east shore to good campsites in dense forest near the head of the lake. The barren, unjointed granite

HWY 180

walls rising on either side—especially Mt. Brewer on the west—provide an impressive backdrop for those leisurely moments you'll want to take to enjoy the views from the shores of this mountain gem.

Beyond the head of East Lake, the trail climbs steadily south past a drift fence and through rock-broken stands of lodgepole and foxtail pine. Just before crossing a 50-yard rockpile, bypass an unsigned junction with the route toward Harrison Pass (no real trail). Beyond this talus slope, the easy grade traverses many wet areas along the east side of East Creek to good campsites beside the little lake below and at the northeast end of Lake Reflection (10,005´; 11S 371171 4063204). Anglers should find good fishing for golden, rainbow, and hybrids. When breezes fail to stir the lake's surface, the tableau of peaks reflected in the mirrored waters is a memorable scene of a scope seldom matched in the Sierra. At the head of the cirque basin, all side excursions are straight up, but your effort is repaid by great views and a sense of achievement shared by many mountaineers.

DAYS 3–4 (Lake Reflection to Cedar Grove Roadend Trailhead, 15.5 miles): Retrace your steps to the trailhead.

26 Rae Lakes

Trip Data: 11S 375125 407477; 41.75 miles, 6/1 days

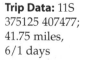

Topos: *The Sphinx, Mt. Clarence King*

Highlights: This fine trip circles King Spur. The scenery en route is dramatic enough to challenge the most accomplished photographer or artist as the trail ascends the glacially carved canyon of South Fork Kings River, visits the exceptionally beautiful Rae Lakes, makes a breathtaking ascent of Glen Pass, circles beneath the towering ramparts of the Videttes and Kearsarge Pinnacles, and returns down the canyon of dashing Bubbs Creek.

HEADS UP! See www.nps.gov/seki/raelakes.htm for the latest information on and regulations affecting this extremely popular area. Bears are a serious problem in the Cedar Grove area; use bear canisters when hiking out of Cedar Grove. Due to heavy use, camping at Charlotte Lake, Arrowhead Lake, Dollar Lake, and each of the Rae Lakes is restricted to a maximum of two nights. In Paradise Valley, camping is limited to designated sites at three camps (two-night limit). Crafty bears have made the use of approved bear canisters mandatory on this route. Along the Rae Lakes, the permanent metal food-storage boxes are for use by through-hikers on the PCT and JMT only. Campfires are not permitted above 10,000 feet.

DAY 1 (Cedar Grove Roadend Trailhead to Middle Paradise Valley Camp, 7.25 miles): From the paved roadend loop (5036´), the wide, sandy trail heads east through a mixed forest of ponderosa pines, incense-cedars, black oaks, sugar pines, and white firs. Soon, the shade is left behind amid a sparse cover of ponderosa pines. The trail enters a cool, dense forest of alders, white firs, ponderosa pines, and sugar pines on the way to a junction with the Bubbs Creek Trail on the right, where, in a few days, you'll close the loop.

For now, turn left (north) on the Paradise Valley/Woods Creek Trail along the river, which, in this stretch, is broad and peaceful, and ascend moderately under a cover of conifers, alders, black oaks, and live oaks. In sunny spots, slopes are covered with chaparral, including plants such as silk-tasseled mountain mahogany and manzanita. Soon, the river swirls, leaps, and pools through a narrow channel, and the canyon walls soar on both sides. Open granite slabs offer opportunities for rest stops with excellent views downcanyon to the Sphinx and Avalanche Peak. Soon reach Mist Falls, a spectacle of tumbling whitewater in early season that becomes sedate and subdued by late season.

The trail continues climbing to the lower end of Paradise Valley, where the river dashes straight down the canyon. The grade eases to gentle once the trail curves into Paradise Valley (6640´), beneath a mixed forest cover of lodgepole pine, red fir, Jeffrey pine, and a smattering of aspen and juniper. Soon arrive at Lower Paradise Valley Camp, with designated campsites, a pit toilet, and bear boxes. Proceed on a gentle stroll alongside the sedate river to Middle Paradise Valley Camp (6670´; 11S 363631 4080134), with more designated campsites and bear boxes.

DAY 2 (Middle Paradise Valley Camp to Woods Creek Crossing, 7 miles): Continue upstream (north) on easy trail through alternating stands of mixed conifers and clearings with awesome views of the steep-walled canyon. A moderate stretch of climbing followed by another gentle stroll near a flower-filled meadow leads to Upper Paradise Valley Camp (6190´), with more designated sites and bear boxes. Immediately beyond the camp, a new bridge crosses to the east side of South Fork Kings River, upstream from its confluence with Woods Creek.

Now on the north side of Woods Creek, the trail curves east as it rises steeply at first and then follows an undulating ascent eastward on a moderate grade up the canyon, crossing two unnamed tributaries along the way. Wind through Castle Domes Meadow (campsites, bear box at east end), named for the obvious landmarks to the north. Stands of water-loving quaking aspen dot the banks of Woods Creek.

Away from the meadow, the underfooting is alternately sandy and rocky as the trail climbs, and the forest cover includes more and more lodgepole pines, corresponding to the increase in altitude. Where the path meets the PCT/JMT, turn right (south) onto the PCT/JMT and soon cross roaring Woods Creek on a swaying suspension bridge, built in 1988 and dubbed the "Golden Gate of the Sierra." Obviously, this crossing would be extremely difficult without the bridge. On the creek's south side, find overused but welcome, fair-to-good campsites beneath Jeffrey and lodgepole pines with bear boxes nearby (8555´; 11S 371762 4081835). Although campfires are legal, most of the available firewood is gone by midsummer at this popular stop along the PCT/JMT.

DAY 3 (Woods Creek Crossing to Rae Lakes, 6.5 miles): Follow the PCT/JMT southeast to begin the long climb up South Fork Woods Creek. Juniper and red fir provide forest cover on the way past several adequate campsites along the creek to the left.

SHORTY LOVELACE

To the left (northeast) of the trail near Woods Creek, hidden by foliage, is one of Shorty Lovelace's pigmy log cabins. Shorty ran a trap line through this country during the years before the establishment of Kings Canyon National Park. Remains of some of his other miniature cabins nearby are located in Gardiner Basin and along Bubbs Creek.

Presently, the trail rounds the base of King Spur, leaves forest cover, and begins a hot, exposed climb up South Fork Woods Creek, staying well above the stream. Legal campsites are almost nonexistent along this stretch of the PCT/JMT up to the junction with the trail to Baxter Pass, and they are similarly absent along the Baxter Pass Trail until the Baxter Lakes basin. Resist the temptation to pitch a tent on the inviting patches of alpine grass along the way: These pockets of grass can live for decades—some clumps are known to be more than 50 years old—but can't survive repeated use by campers.

Jump over the rivulet that hurries down from Lake 10296 and enter an open, rocky area. Beyond, a wooden span provides an easy crossing of a boggy meadow. Pass through a drift fence, ascend a rocky ridge, and then pass by a pair of fair campsites near the crossing of a willow-and-flower-lined stream that drains Sixty Lake Basin. Across the canyon, Baxter Creek stitches a ribbon of water down a rock-ribbed slope.

A mile-long ascent through diminishing forest cover affords fine views ahead of the peaked monolith of Fin Dome, heralding the approach to the beautiful Rae Lakes. To the right (southwest) are the impressive steel-gray ramparts of King Spur. In contrast, the massive, sloping Sierra Crest in the east is made up of dark metamorphic rocks. Finally, ascend a low, rounded spur and reach a junction with the Baxter Pass Trail, just north of Dollar Lake, where an old post is all that marks the unsigned junction. The setting of jewel-like Dollar Lake is magnificent; lodgepoles crowd the shore amid granite outcroppings, and Fin Dome, along with some blackish spires beyond, provides a jagged backdrop for the mirrored surface of the lake.

Go ahead (south) at the junction, pass west of Dollar Lake and some small ponds, and then ford South Fork Woods Creek below Arrowhead Lake. Continue up the canyon on the east side of the lake chain. The long black striations seen along the face of Diamond Peak and the ridge that extends to the north are metamorphosed lava—one of the few remaining bits of volcanic evidence to be found in this area.

With the familiar landmark of distinctive Fin Dome in sight, pass a lateral to campsites with a bear box on the north side of Arrowhead Lake and continue above the east side of the lake. Climb high above the creek through widely scattered lodgepole pines past a small, unnamed lake on the way to the Rae Lakes. Campsites and bear boxes are found near the lower two lakes, and a summer ranger station tucked into the trees above the second lake (10,560´; 11S 375125 407477) sometimes provides emergency services. The highest lake's shores are rocky-marshy and offer no good camping, but higher Dragon Lake offers campsites (see Day 4).

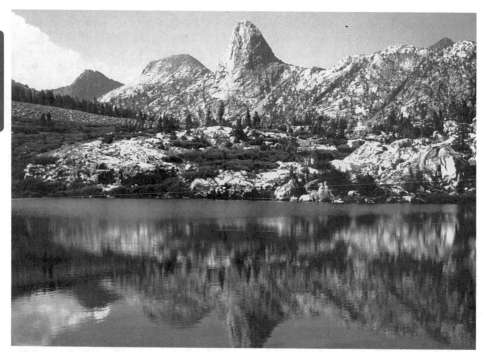

Fin Dome over Dollar Lake

RAE LAKES

A camp at one of the Rae Lakes should be among the best and longest remembered of the trip, simply because of the extraordinary views: The rugged granite Fin Dome reflected in the still waters of the lake; the jagged King Spur beyond; and, if you are camped at one of the higher lakes, multicolored Painted Lady to the south. Glistening slabs of granite and pockets of verdant, flower-sprinkled meadow surround the island-dotted lakes. Despite the area's popularity, fishing should be good for brook and rainbow trout.

DAY 4 (Rae Lakes to Vidette Meadow Camp, 8 miles): The gently ascending trail goes south from the middle lake toward the highest of the Rae Lakes (10,541´), where a use trail heads east to more secluded camping around Dragon Lake. Stay on the PCT/JMT here. The path then bends west around the north shoreline of the upper lake, fords the creek at the narrow "isthmus" separating the near-rockbound highest lake from the rest of the chain, and comes to a junction with a well-trod use trail into Sixty Lake Basin, an extremely worthy destination for a layover day (also see Trip 77).

From the Sixty Lake Basin junction, turn left (south) on the PCT/JMT and begin the climb toward Glen Pass, following switchbacks through diminishing pockets of vegetation to a tarn-filled bench covered with talus. A winding ascent leads to the crest of a ridge and then a short traverse to 11,978-foot Glen Pass. The view from the pass is somewhat disappointing when compared to other High Sierra passes, but there is a fine, farewell glimpse of the Rae Lakes.

A winding, rocky descent switchbacks past a pair of green, rockbound tarns on the way to a crossing of a seasonal stream with a pair of poor campsites nearby. The trail continues the descent through an extensive boulder field until more hospitable terrain appears where the trail veers southeast. The grade eases on a descending traverse across a lodgepole pine-covered hillside above Charlotte Lake. Gaps in the pines allow brief views of the lake and Charlotte Dome father down Charlotte Creek. At 2.3 miles from the pass, reach a junction with a connecting trail to Kearsarge Pass. Go right (south), staying on the PCT/JMT, and soon breaking out of the forest to fine views of Mt. Bago. Stroll across a sandy flat to a four-way junction. From here, the Kearsarge Pass Trail heads northeast and the Charlotte Lake Trail heads northwest 0.8 mile to the lake, with excellent campsites (two-night limit) and a seasonal ranger station.

Go left on the PCT/JMT and climb east, away from the sandy flat and over a low rise. Follow tight switchbacks downhill through dense forest to a junction with the Bullfrog Lake Trail, which climbs northeast to the picturesque lake (no camping). Continue ahead (southeast) on the descent, crossing Bullfrog Lake's outlet twice on the way to Lower Vidette Meadow and a junction with the Bubbs Creek Trail. At the junction, turn left (east), remaining on the PCT/JMT, ford the outlet of Bullfrog Lake again, and arrive at a junction with an unmapped path to the good and possibly crowded campsites at Vidette Meadow Camp (bear box; about 9542´; 11S 374414 4069089) along Bubbs Creek and near beautiful Vidette Meadow. Fishing for brook and rainbow trout is reported to be fair.

DAY 5 (Vidette Meadow Camp to Charlotte Creek, 5.5 miles): Retrace your steps a half mile to the junction of the PCT/JMT and the Bubbs Creek Trail. Turn left (west), make a short descent, and pass to the north of Lower Vidette Meadow. Excellent campsites with a bear box are nestled beneath lodgepole pines along the fringe of the meadow. Leaving the gentle grade near the meadows, the trail begins a more pronounced descent along the now tumbling creek plunging down the gorge. Break out into the open momentarily near a large granite hump that provides an excellent vantage point for surveying the surrounding terrain.

Head back into the trees and continue down the canyon, generally west, stepping over numerous meadow-lined streamlets along the way. Periodic switchbacks mark the

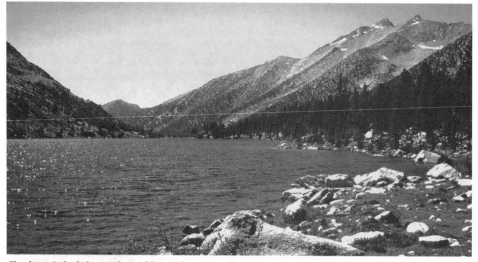

Charlotte Lake is just a short side trip from Day 4's route.

descent, along with occasional views of the topography above East Creek, including such notable landmarks as Mt. Brewer, North Guard, and Mt. Farquhar. The stiff, protracted descent eventually eases near the grassy, fern-filled, and wildflower-covered clearing of Junction Meadow (8190′). Reach the signed junction with the East Creek Trail heading south to East Lake and Lake Reflection. Overnighters can find passable campsites a short way down the trail on either side of the ford of Bubbs Creek; additional campsites are farther down Bubbs Creek past the large horse camp at the west edge of Junction Meadow.

Go right (ahead, northwest) at this junction. Away from the meadow, the moderate descent resumes, as you stroll alongside turbulent Bubbs Creek through a moderate forest, composed primarily of firs. After nearly 2 miles of steady descent, Bubbs Creek mellows, and gently graded trail leads through a grove of aspens on the way to the ford of Charlotte Creek. Just before the ford, a path leads to pleasant, tree-shaded campsites (about 7320′; 11S 367450 4070534) near the bank of Bubbs Creek. Fishing is good for brown, brook, rainbow, and golden-rainbow hybrid to 10 inches.

DAY 6 (Charlotte Creek to Cedar Grove Roadend Trailhead, 7.5 miles): The trail continues descending gradually for a while past Charlotte Creek, as you hop across a trio of streams and stroll through shoulder-high ferns, before Bubbs Creek returns to its tumultuous course down the gorge. A steady, moderate descent follows the tumbling stream over the next several miles before arriving at Sphinx Creek Camp and a junction with the Sphinx Creek Trail.

From here, continue ahead (west, downstream) on the Bubbs Creek Trail to a lengthy series of switchbacks that drop to the floor of Kings Canyon. At the bottom of the canyon, follow a series of short, wood bridges over multibranched Bubbs Creek, go ahead (northwest) at the next junction, cross a steel bridge over South Fork Kings River, and soon reach a signed junction with the Paradise Valley/Woods Creek Trail. The loop closes here.

From the junction, go left (west) to retrace your steps 1.9 miles to the trailhead.

Big Meadows Trailhead

7615'; 11S 336134 4065221

DESTINATION/ UTM COORDINATES	TRIP TYPE	BEST SEASON	PACE (HIKING/ LAYOVER DAYS)	TOTAL MILEAGE
27 Jenny Lakes 11S 336134 4065221	Semiloop	Early to mid	3/0 Leisurely	18.2

Information and Permits: This trailhead is in Sequoia National Forest. Permits are not required, but you must have a California Campfire Permit in order to have a campfire or use a stove. If you plan to go into Sequoia or Kings Canyon national parks for an overnight stay, you must have a valid permit from them.

Driving Directions: From Fresno, take Hwy. 180 generally eastward for about 54 increasingly slow and windy miles into Kings Canyon National Park to the junction with the Generals Hwy. Turn right (south) and proceed on Generals Hwy. 6.4 miles to Big Meadows Road. Turn left (northeast) and drive 3.5 miles to the Big Meadows Trailhead parking lot, equipped with vault toilets.

27 Jennie Lakes

Trip Data: 11S 336134 4065221; 18.2 miles; 3/0 days

Topos: *Muir Grove, Mt. Silliman*

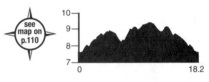

see map on p.110

Highlights: A peaceful alternative to the popular backcountry in adjacent Kings Canyon National Park, this stroll through Jennie Lakes Wilderness leads backpackers along rushing streams, through shady forests, and across flower-filled meadows to a pair of pleasant lakes with craggy backdrops.

DAY 1 (Big Meadows Trailhead to Weaver Lake, 3.2 miles): A sign near the restroom points the way to the start of the trail heading southeast up a wooded hillside and across the paved access road. A short descent leads to a wood bridge across a sluggish stretch of Big Meadows Creek to a trail register. From there, gradually traverse across the base of a granite hump, and then curve along a delightful, spring-fed tributary of Big Meadows Creek. Through a mixed forest of red firs, lodgepole pines, and Jeffrey pines, briefly follow this stream south before fording it.

Away from the crossing, the trail makes a moderate climb around an exposed ridge with a momentary view over lupine and manzanita of Monarch Divide and Shell Mountain. Continuing the arc around the ridge, you pass by verdant Fox Meadow and then climb to a streamside junction, 2 miles from the trailhead, where the loop part of this trip begins.

Head straight (northeast) across the stream from the junction into signed Jennie Lakes Wilderness and follow the path eastward through alternating sections of scattered to light forest and shrub-covered clearings. After 1.1 miles, reach a junction with the lateral to Weaver Lake.

Turn right (east and then south) onto the lateral and wind uphill through mixed forest sprinkled with boulders 0.2 mile to Weaver Lake (8707´; 11S 339423 4063618). Lodgepoles and firs shade the shoreline and the boulder-studded forest floor is carpeted with patches

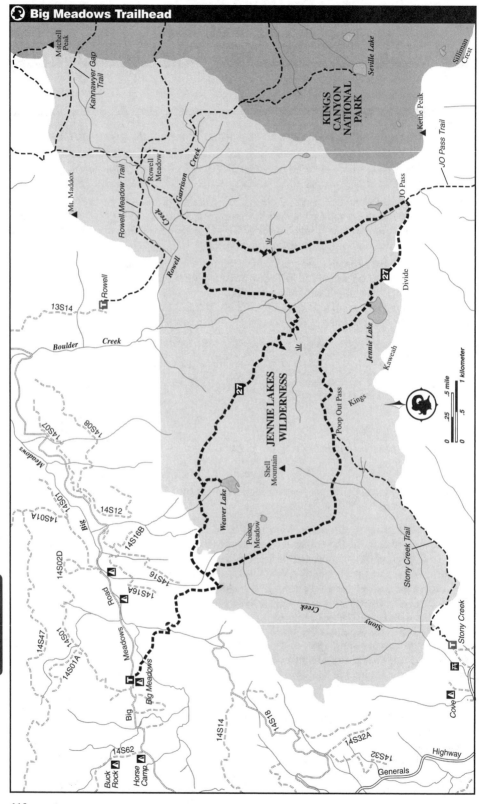

Mitchell Peak

Kannawyer Gap Trail

Silliman Crest

Seville Lake

KINGS CANYON NATIONAL PARK

Kettle Peak

JO Pass Trail

Rowell Meadow Trail

Rowell Meadow

Garrison Creek

JO Pass

Mt. Maddox

Creek

Rowell

27

Divide

Rowell

13S14

Jennie Lake

Kaweah

Boulder   Creek

Kings

JENNIE LAKES WILDERNESS

Poop Out Pass

27

1 kilometer

.5 mile

.25   .5

0   .5

Meadows

14S07

14S08

Shell Mountain

Weaver Lake

14S12

14S01A

14S07

Big

Poison Meadow

Stony Creek Trail

14S16B

14S02D

14S16

14S16A

14S47

14S01

14S01A

Road

Meadows

Stony   Creek

Big Meadows

Stony Creek

Big

14S14

14S18

Cove

Buck Rock

14S62

Horse Camp.

14S32A

14S32

Generals   Highway

of azalea, red heather, and Labrador tea. The whitish granite of Shell Mountain creates a fine backdrop, mirrored in the lake's usually placid surface. An array of campsites pepper the shoreline, the least crowded of which seem to be above the south shore amid a grove of conifers. Anglers will be tempted by the resident brook trout, but the easily reached lake appears to be heavily fished.

DAY 2 (Weaver Lake to Jennie Lake, 8.7 miles): Retrace your steps 0.2 mile from Weaver Lake to the junction, and turn right (northeast) to follow less-used tread on a moderate climb toward Rowell Meadow. Proceed through a mixed forest of firs, lodgepole pines, and western white pines across a pair of saddles and then down to the head of Boulder Creek's canyon. After multiple crossings of the creek's tributaries, follow a moderate climb northward up the west-facing wall of the canyon. Shade from a scattered to light forest greets you where the path bends east over the crest of a ridge and then descends to a Y-junction with the trail to Rowell Meadow.

Turn sharply right at the junction to head south on a gradual climb to the crest of a rise. From the rise, descend gently, then moderately, enjoying occasional glimpses of Shell Mountain through the trees and crossing back over a lushly lined tributary of Boulder Creek. A lengthy climb follows, past slabs and boulders and across a small stream draining a hidden pond 0.1 mile east of the trail. Eventually, the ascent leads to JO Pass (9444′) and a junction, 2.6 miles from the Rowell Meadows junction.

Turn right (west) and follow the crest of a gradually undulating ridge until switchbacks lead northwest down the hillside, from which you have momentary views of Jennie Lake through the trees. At 1.4 miles from JO Pass, find a junction with the very short lateral to the lake; turn left (south) on it. Like Weaver Lake, Jennie Lake (9012′; 11S 342382 4060976) is backdropped by impressive granite cliffs and rimmed by a light forest of red firs and lodgepole pines. Jennie Lake is larger than Weaver Lake. Overnighters can locate decent campsites on either side of the driftwood-choked outlet. Anglers may have better luck here than at Weaver, since Jennie is twice as far from the nearest trailhead and fishing pressure should be quite a bit less.

DAY 3 (Jennie Lake to Big Meadows Trailhead, 6.3 miles): Retrace your steps along the lateral to the main trail, turn left (northwest), and follow a gentle decline before making an ascending westward traverse across exfoliated granodiorite slopes and scattered forest, with fine views of the Monarch Divide along the way. Following the traverse, a steep, winding climb concludes at Poop Out Pass (9140′). A short descent from the pass brings you to a junction with the Stony Creek Trail.

Turn right (west) at the junction and make a moderate descent across the southern slopes of Shell Mountain to a crossing of a nascent, twin-channeled tributary of Stony Creek. From the creek, a gradual ascent around the nose of a ridge leads to a traverse across the west slope of Shell Mountain. Mostly open terrain allows excellent views of Big Baldy, Chimney Rock, and, if the ubiquitous haze abates, the San Joaquin Valley.

Return to forest cover as the track curves north-northwest, crosses a lushly lined, spring-fed brook, and follows a moderate descent across a second rivulet to Poison Meadow. Past the meadow, cross a third little stream, exit the signed Jennie Lakes Wilderness, and soon arrive at the junction where you close the loop. Turn left (south) and retrace your steps 2 miles to the trailhead.

Lodgepole Campground Trailhead

6771′; 11S 345864 4052373

DESTINATION/ UTM COORDINATES	TRIP TYPE	BEST SEASON	PACE (HIKING/ LAYOVER DAYS)	TOTAL MILEAGE
28 Ranger Lake 11S 348551 4059192	Out & back	Mid to late	2/1 Moderate	20
29 Deadman and Cloud Canyons 11S 364491 4055150 (at Colby Lake)	Semiloop	Mid to late	12/3 Strenuous	110.4

Information and Permits: This trailhead is in Sequoia National Park: 47050 Generals Hwy., Three Rivers, CA 93271, 559-565-3341, www.nps.gov/seki. Permits are required, there is a fee for them, and quotas apply. Some areas may have fire restrictions and bear-canister requirements. You may reserve a permit in advance for trips mid-May through September by mail or fax only, no earlier than March 1 and no later than three weeks before the start of your trip.

Driving Directions: Take the Generals Hwy. through the western edge of Sequoia National Park, north of the Giant Forest Museum, to the signed Lodgepole turnoff, where you head east into the Lodgepole complex. Continue east past the visitor center and ranger station (on-demand permits available here), as well as the store/snack bar/laundromat, to a parking area near the Lodgepole Nature Center. There are bear boxes where you can store any items you're not taking with you that might attract bears (food, cosmetics, etc.).

28 Ranger Lake

Trip Data: 11S 348551 4059192; 20 miles; 2/1 days

Topos: *Lodgepole, Mt. Silliman*

see map on p.114

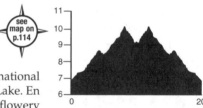

Highlights: Crossing the Silliman crest on the boundary between Sequoia and Kings Canyon national parks, this trip terminates at picturesque Ranger Lake. En route, the trail passes through fir forests, skirts flowery meadows, traces rambling brooks, and passes between a pair of shallow lakes whose inviting waters tempt dusty hikers.

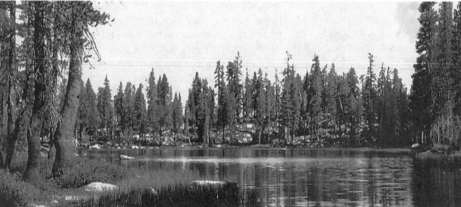

Ranger Lake, peaceful and lightly visited

GENERALS HWY

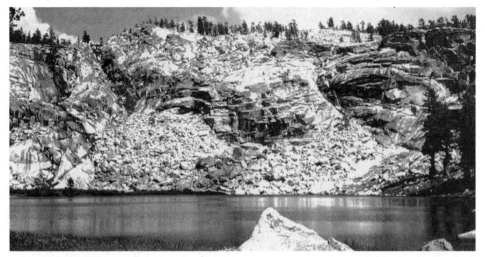

One of the Twin Lakes

DAY 1 (Lodgepole Campground Trailhead to Ranger Lake, 10 miles): From the parking lot, follow a dirt road northeast to a bridge over Marble Fork Kaweah River, cross the river, and pick up the trail. At a junction that comes up immediately, the track continues ahead (north) and curves west to skirt Lodgepole Campground on a moderate ascent through a dense forest cover of fir, pine, and cedar with a blooming understory. The path tops the moraine it's been climbing, turns north, and levels to ford Silliman Creek.

After passing shooting-star-fringed Cahoon Meadow, the trail continues its moderate ascent over duff-and-sand underfooting through stands of red and white fir and some meadows, crossing several streamlets, to Cahoon Gap. From here, the path descends moderately to ford the unnamed tributary just south of East Fork Clover Creek (campsite). A quarter mile beyond this ford, this trip turns right (northeast) at a junction where the trail to JO Pass goes north (ahead; campsite) and then fords East Fork Clover Creek.

Begin a moderate ascent in East Fork Clover Creek's drainage, which introduces lodgepole and western white pine into the forest cover. As the trail approaches Twin Lakes, open stretches between the trees are a high tide of floral colors. The last half mile to the timbered flats around Twin Lakes is a steep ascent. This area (9438´; 11S 346604 4058337) is heavily used, and there's even a pit toilet. However, by midsummer, this may be the last chance for a campsite with water before Ranger Lake.

Continuing toward Silliman Pass, the view of two large "pillars" of exfoliating granite (Twin Peaks) dominates the horizon during the steep progress to the pass. This ascent sees the end of fir and almost exclusive domination of lodgepole pine. At the unsigned pass (10,165´), there's a good view of flat-topped Mt. Silliman to the south, the heavily wooded Sugarloaf Creek drainage to the northeast, the Great Western Divide to the east, and the barren flats of the Tableland to the southeast.

From the pass, the trail drops steeply and then turns north to the nose of a granite ridge before switchbacking down. From the switchbacks, there are fine views of Ball Dome and much of the Kings River watershed, including the Monarch Divide. At the foot of the switchbacks, there's a junction where a trail leads right (southeast) to lovely but campsite-less Beville Lake. Continue ahead (east), and very shortly thereafter, a level duff trail leads left (north) to Ranger Lake, and to the excellent campsites on the southwest side of the lake (9212´; 11S 348551 4059192). Angling is good in the area, which also includes nearby Beville and Lost lakes.

DAY 2 (Ranger Lake to Lodgepole Campground Trailhead, 10 miles): Retrace your steps.

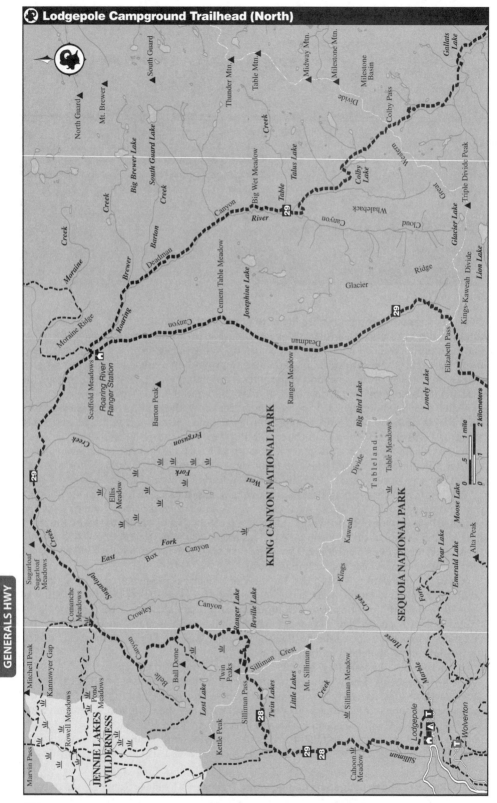

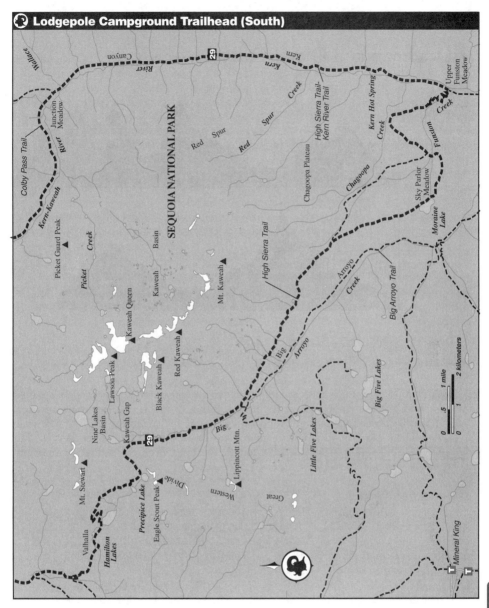

29 Deadman and Cloud Canyons

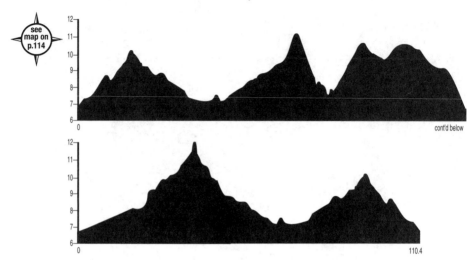

see map on p.114

cont'd below

Trip Data: 11S 364491 4055150 (at Colby Lake); 12/3; 110.4 miles

Topos: *Lodgepole, Mt. Silliman, Sphinx Lakes, Triple Divide Peak, Mount Kaweah, Chagoopa Falls*

Highlights: This is a long and unforgettable trip of stunning beauty and immense rewards—and one less traveled because of its length and the remoteness of its principal destinations: Deadman, Cloud, and Kern canyons, and the canyon of the Kern-Kaweah River. It will be the trip of a lifetime for many, so schedule as many layover days as your food-carrying ability allows. Because of its length, we don't recommend this trip for beginners.

SHORTENING TRIP 29

As an alternative for those with less experience or less time, go as far as Roaring River Ranger Station (Day 2, but can be done at a leisurely pace in 4 days with stops at Twin Lakes and Comanche Meadow) and take some layover days there to explore Deadman and Cloud canyons before retracing your steps. Another alternative is to make this a shuttle trip: From Roaring River Ranger Station, head to Deadman Canyon, over Elizabeth Pass to Bearpaw Meadow via the Over the Hill Trail to the High Sierra Trail, and take the High Sierra Trail west to its trailhead at Crescent Meadow, which is a few miles south of Lodgepole (see Trip 31 for directions for the shuttle car). You can do this in two more days from Lone Pine Creek with an overnight at Mehrten Creek (again, see Trip 31). A seasonal shuttlebus may be running to help you get back to Lodgepole. Or work out a return route on the trails linking Crescent Meadow and Lodgepole; some areas through which these trails pass are day-use only.

DAY 1 (Lodgepole Campground Trailhead to Ranger Lake, 10 miles): *(Recap: Trip 28, Day 1.)* Take a dirt road northeast to a bridge over Marble Fork Kaweah River and pick up the trail on the other side of the river. At a junction that comes up almost immediately, continue ahead (north) and curve west to skirt Lodgepole Campground while ascending. The path tops the moraine it's been climbing, turns north, and levels to ford Silliman Creek.

After passing Cahoon Meadow, continue the moderate ascent, crossing several streamlets, to Cahoon Gap. Descend moderately to ford the unnamed tributary just south of East Fork Clover Creek (campsite). A quarter mile beyond this ford, go right (east) at a junction where the trail to JO Pass goes north (ahead; campsite). Ford East Fork Clover Creek, and then turn northeast and ascend the creek's drainage toward Twin Lakes, climbing steeply in the last half mile. This area (9438´; 11S 346604 4058337 between the lakes) is heavily used but by midsummer may be the last chance for a campsite with water before Ranger Lake.

Continue toward Silliman Pass with Twin Peaks in view, topping out at the unsigned pass (10,165´), where there are fine views. From the pass, drop steeply and then turn north before switchbacking down. At the switchbacks' foot, there's a junction where a trail leads right (southeast) to campsite-less Beville Lake. Continue ahead (east) and, very shortly thereafter, follow a level duff trail leads left (north) to Ranger Lake and its excellent campsites on its southwest side (9212´; 11S 348551 4059192).

DAY 2 (Ranger Lake to Roaring River Ranger Station, 13 miles): Return to the junction with the main trail and turn left (east) on it, soon curving north. The track climbs a little ridge and passes the turnoff to Lost Lake; go ahead (generally north) on the main trail to circle Ball Dome. Passing through a moderate-to-heavy forest cover, the path emerges at a meadowed crossing of the outlet stream from Seville Lake.

Beyond this crossing is the signed Seville Lake/Rowell Meadow/Comanche Meadow junction. Turn right (northeast) toward Comanche Meadow on the northwest side of Sugarloaf Creek, descending, sometimes steadily and sometimes moderately, over duff-and-sand underfooting. This descent crosses an unnamed tributary and, a short distance beyond, reaches a junction with a trail to Marvin Pass. Go ahead (right, briefly north) here.

About 100 yards farther on, the trail passes the Kanawyer (k'n-OY-yer) Gap Trail to Marvin Pass and reaches Comanche Meadow in 5.5 miles, where there are fair campsites on Sugarloaf Creek (fair angling for brook) before the ford of the creek draining the meadow. Continuing toward Roaring River, ford the creek draining the meadow. Beginning a quarter mile after the ford, the hot, dusty trail drops moderately on sandy underfooting over a heavily forested slope that still shows some effects of a 1974 fire. Presently, as the trail levels out on the floor of Sugarloaf Valley, it follows the course of an old glacier.

Through the trees, hikers can see round, smooth, 1000-foot Sugarloaf Dome. More resistant than the surrounding rock, this granite island withstood the onslaught of the ice. The trail passes Sugarloaf Meadow (fair campsites) and parallels and then fords Sugarloaf Creek.

GENERALS HWY

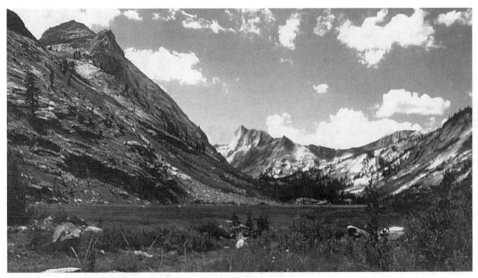

Looking up sublime Deadman Canyon toward Big Bird Peak

On the south side of this wide, shallow ford, the tread passes more campsites before crossing a series of sharp wrinkles in the terrain to reach Ferguson Creek and still more campsites. After fording this creek, the trail rounds a long, dry, timbered ridge nose before dropping down a steady slope to Roaring River, where the trail is briefly hemmed in on the river side by a cement-and-rock wall. At last, the track skirts Scaffold Meadows, reserved for NPS grazing. Signed SCAFFOLD MEADOWS TOURIST PASTURE across the river is also reserved for grazing and is open to the public.

Living up to its name, Roaring River can be heard a few yards to the left, and with this pleasant accompaniment, the trail ascends the last, gentle mile to good campsites near Roaring River Ranger Station (7415´; 11S 358361 4064111; toilet), fording the Barton Peak stream on the way. Fishing for rainbow and some golden trout is fair to good. Emergency services may be available from the resident summer ranger, whose cabin is nearby.

DAY 3 (Roaring River to Upper Ranger Meadow, 7 miles): There's a major junction near Roaring River Ranger Station; at this junction, begin the loop part of this trip by taking the Elizabeth Pass Trail right (south) toward Deadman Canyon and Elizabeth Pass.

Leaving Roaring River, the Elizabeth Pass Trail veers away from the river on a gentle-to-moderate ascent past well-charred Jeffrey pines. About 1.5 miles above the Roaring River bridge, your route ascends past several campsites; at the right time of summer, this short stretch has a wonderful display of wildflowers. The trail fords Deadman Canyon creek and, in 1.5 more miles, reaches a campsite. About 50 yards southeast of the campsite at the north end of a large, wet meadow lies the gravesite from which Deadman Canyon got its name.

THE GRAVE IN DEADMAN CANYON

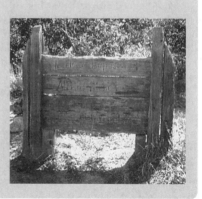

The citation on the grave reads: HERE REPOSES ALFRED MONIERE, SHEEPHERDER, MOUNTAIN MAN, 18– TO 1887. But it's a mystery now. Nobody knows who or what, if anything, is really in the grave or how it got there. At least two major versions of the story exist: The occupant was murdered nearby, or he died of illness before his partner could complete the two-week round trip to and from Fresno to bring back a doctor. Still, as Wilderness Press author Jeff Schaffer put it, no pharaoh in all his power and glory ever enjoyed a more magnificent setting for his tomb than this unknown soul does.

From this grave, the ascent continues, offering good views up the canyon of the spectacularly smoothed, unjointed, barren walls. Soon, the trail refords the creek and then climbs alongside a dramatic, green-water, granite-slab chute. The trail levels out in a dense stand of lodgepole and fir, and, passing a campsite, emerges at the north end of the open grasslands of Ranger Meadow. The precipitous canyon walls dominate the views from the meadow, and the cirque holding Big Bird Lake is clear on the west wall. By midsummer, this meadow is a colorful carpet of purple and red wildflowers.

At Ranger Meadow, the trail resumes its steady ascent over duff and sand, through stands of lodgepole and clumps of aspen. Below a forested bench, the creek streams down broad granite slabs. Just before the Upper Ranger Meadow flat, the route fords the creek to the east side. Here there are awesome glimpses of the headwall of the Deadman Canyon cirque, and this view continues to rule the skyline from the good campsites just beyond the drift fence at the north end of Upper Ranger Meadow (9200´; 11S 358329 4055282). Fishing for rainbow, brook, and hybrids is good. A cross-county route to Big Bird Lake takes off west across the creek here, becoming a well-worn tread as it ascends the slope south of the lake's outlet.

DAY 4 (Upper Ranger Meadow to Lone Pine Creek, 6.6 miles): This day's hike is a tough one: Though relatively short in total miles, it begins with a 2200-foot ascent to Elizabeth Pass that's followed by a 3200-foot descent from the pass. Get an early start. The Elizabeth Pass Trail is irregularly maintained and may be faint in places.

Leaving Upper Ranger Meadow, the exposed trail ascends gently through boulders, with Upper Ranger Meadow to the west. Low-growing willows line the stream, and clumps of wildflowers dot the green expanse. The ascent steepens to a moderate grade and then makes a very steep ascent of the headwall, paralleling a dramatic series of cascades and falls. Near the top of the falls is a bench. From here, note the sharp, gray, granite peak, shaped very like a ship's prow, high to the southwest. It's a helpful landmark.

Cross the stream above a long, dashing granite chute. Ignore the obvious, worn slot on the left (a remnant of an older trail) and instead bear slightly right to begin climbing gradually to moderately up the southwest side of the cirque on a newer trail made mostly of riprap (broken, fist-sized rocks) laid through a talus field. Where there are occasional gaps in the riprap, just look around for the next section of it. The ship's prow peak becomes increasingly visible near the top, as does another gray peak to its left and some red-and-gray peaklets still farther left. A crescent dip between the peaklets is Elizabeth Pass, and the steep switchbacks up it become easier to see as the trail approaches it.

The riprap finally turns to dirt for good just below the pass, where there is a Spartan campsite or two, as long the snowmelt holds out. The light-colored granite slabs contrast with the darker metamorphic rocks (around an old copper mine site) seen to the east, and this contrast is even more marked from the tiny saddle of Elizabeth Pass (11,380'). Views to the southwest from the pass include parts of the Middle Fork Kaweah River watershed, Moose Lake, and the jumbled peaks of the southernmost prominences of the Tableland Divide.

REVERSING THE STEPS OVER ELIZABETH PASS

If you are reversing these steps and coming over Elizabeth Pass from the High Sierra Trail side, you've been following a faint, ducked track. Once you've descended the dirt switchbacks on the Deadman Canyon side of the pass, look not for ducks but for the riprap trail. Hikers who miss the riprap track sentence themselves to a needlessly difficult, confusing, and exhausting descent.

From the pass, the trail initially descends steeply by switchbacks, then by a long but moderate traverse that crosses the outlet of Lonely Lake, and then again by a series of rocky switchbacks. Ducks are helpful in keeping to the route. At the foot of these zigzags, the path reaches a junction with a spur trail through Lone Pine Creek's canyon to Tamarack Lake. Turn left (east) toward Tamarack Lake and take the spur trail about a half mile up Lone Pine Creek to the first wooded area near the creek. There are sandy campsites near swimming holes on pleasant Lone Pine Creek here (about 8232'; 11S 357665 4049999). Ambitious hikers can continue to Tamarack Lake, finding campsites along the way and at the lake.

DAY 5 (Lone Pine Creek to Big Arroyo Trail Junction, 9 miles): Return to the Elizabeth Pass Trail junction and turn left (south) to descend another quarter mile to a junction.

Hikers continuing on this semiloop trip take the left fork south along Lone Pine Creek here toward a junction with the High Sierra Trail that's well east of Bearpaw Meadow: just east of a footbridge over Lone Pine Creek and near a bench with a campsite. Turn left (generally east) on the High Sierra Trail toward Hamilton Lakes. Make a steep, steady climb on

SHUTTLE OPTION: TO CRESCENT MEADOW

For hikers who wish to cut this trip short by taking the High Sierra Trail to Crescent Meadow (shuttle trip), take the right fork southwest at the Elizabeth Pass Trail junction; this is the 2.1-mile Over the Hill Trail, which meets the High Sierra Trail at Bearpaw Meadow. Follow this hot, exposed trail up over a hill and then down into forest near Bearpaw Meadow. Around this trail's high point, there are outstanding eastward views up Lone Pine Creek to Triple Divide Peak and, farther on, up toward Kaweah Gap. Upon reaching the High Sierra Trail, turn left (west) on it, and, in about 0.3 mile, find a turnoff left (south) for a spur trail going 200 yards down to overused Bearpaw Meadow Campground (poor campsites). From this junction, the High Sierra Trail continues generally west for 11 miles to the trailhead at Crescent Meadow. There are a few camping areas along the way, notably west of Buck Creek and at Mehrten Creek; the last legal one is 4 miles west of Crescent Meadow, near the westernmost tributary of Panther Creek. See Trip 31, days 1 and 2, for this part of the High Sierra Trail.

switchbacks into the awe-inspiring, polished-granite canyon of Hamilton Creek. The final climb to a ford of Hamilton Creek is overshadowed by the mighty rock on all sides: the sheer granite wall to the north called Angel Wings, the sharply pointed granite sentinels atop the south wall, and the wall's avalanche-chuted sides.

Under these heights, ford the stream a few hundred yards below the lowest of the Hamilton Lakes chain. From this ford, the trail climbs steeply over shattered rock to good campsites at the northwest end of Lake 8235 (Upper Hamilton Lake). Views from the campsites, including the silver waterfall ribbon at the east end, are superlative, and fishing for brook, rainbow, and golden is fair to good.

But the area is highly overused, so begin the steep 2500-foot climb to Kaweah Gap. The ascent is an engineering marvel of trail construction, which has literally blasted the way across vertical cliff sections. Beginning at the northwest end of Lake 8235, the trail ascends steadily up the juniper-and-red-fir-dotted slope with constant views of the lake and its dramatic walls and with seasonal wildflowers providing vivid touches of color.

After some doubling back, the trail turns south on a steep ascent to a point just above the north shore of Precipice Lake (10,200´), at the foot of the near-vertical north face of Eagle Scout Peak. The jagged summits of the peaks of the Great Western Divide dominate the skyline to the east during the final, tarn-dotted ascent to U-shaped Kaweah Gap. Approaching the gap, the equally spectacular summits of the Kaweah Peaks Ridge beyond pop into view. This colorful ridge dominates the views from Kaweah Gap (10,700´); below is Nine Lake Basin watershed to the north. Hikers with a penchant for exploring barren high country, or those interested in the good brook trout fishing, can detour across granite slab-and-ledge routes north to Nine Lake Basin and its good but exposed campsites.

The trail begins its steady-to-moderate southward descent along the west side of the headwaters of Big Arroyo Creek, fording over to the east side midway down. This descent crosses unjointed granite broken by substantial packets of grass and numerous runoff streams even in late season. Open stretches afford fine views of the U-shaped, glacially wrought Big Arroyo below, and the white, red, and black rocks of Black Kaweah and Red Kaweah peaks to the east.

The trail then reenters timber cover and arrives at some good campsites along the stream (9600´; 11S 362565 4043043). These campsites and an abandoned trail-crew cabin are about a quarter mile above the Little Five Lakes/Black Rock Pass Trail junction. Fishing for brook trout is fair to good. For anglers with extra time, the 2-mile side trip to Little Five Lakes offers fine angling for golden trout.

DAY 6 (Big Arroyo Trail Junction to Moraine Lake, 8 miles): *(Recap: Trip 31, Day 4.)* Continue ahead (south) to the Little Five Lakes junction and take the left fork southeast. The High

Sierra Trail begins a long, moderate ascent along the north canyon wall of Big Arroyo. The grade eases near a tarn, and then, swinging away from the lip of Big Arroyo, the trail begins a gradual descent to a junction in a meadow on the south side of a tributary of Chagoopa Creek.

Leave the official High Sierra Trail route at this junction and turn right (south) to descend through meadows and then more steeply over coarse granite sand to the Moraine Lake (9290´; 11S 369732 4036003). Good campsites on the south side of the lake provide views across the water of the Kaweah Peaks.

DAY 7 (Moraine Lake to Kern Hot Spring, 7 miles): *(Recap: Trip 31, Day 5.)* After traversing a moraine just east of Moraine Lake, the trail descends past an old stockman's cabin to superb Sky Parlor Meadow. Shortly beyond the ford of Funston Creek, at the east end of the meadow, this trip's route rejoins the official High Sierra Trail route. Turn right (northeast) toward Chagoopa Creek, where the track curves east and then southeast as it drops through changing life zones toward the bottom of Kern Canyon. After the trail re-fords Funston Creek, its final descent to the valley floor is on a series of steep, rocky switchbacks generally paralleling Funston Creek.

Now on the floor of Kern Canyon, the route turns left (north, upstream) on the Kern River Trail, drops into a marshy area, and then crosses a pair of meadows on wooden walkways. Then the trail leads gently upward through a forest of Jeffrey pine and incense-cedar. High on the western rim of the canyon, look for Chagoopa Falls. Past a manzanita-carpeted opening, the trail crosses the Kern River on a fine bridge and arrives at the south fork of Rock Creek. Then, around a point, the path leads to Kern Hot Spring (6880´; 11S 374055 4038030) and its very overused campsites. (Before continuing, see the sidebar on page 133 for warnings about Kern Hot Spring.)

DAY 8 (Kern Hot Spring to Junction Meadow, 8 miles): *(Recap: Trip 31, Day 6.)* Continuing north, the High Sierra Trail-Kern River Trail fords the upper fork of Rock Creek and traverses the gravelly canyon floor below the immense granite cliffs of the canyon's east wall. Past the confluence of Red Spur Creek, this route ascends beside the Kern River. The fords of the stream draining Guyot Flat, of Whitney Creek, and of Wallace Creek can be difficult in early season.

Beyond the ford of Wallace Creek, the trail reaches the overused campsites at Junction Meadow (8036´; 11S 373505 4048976) on the Kern River and a junction with the trail up the Kern-Kaweah River.

DAY 9 (Junction Meadow to Kern-Kaweah River, 6 miles): This day's route is irregularly maintained, but a backpacker with experience should have no trouble staying on it.

From the junction, leave the High Sierra Trail-Kern River Trail and take the left fork northwest 0.4 mile to a ford of the Kern River (very difficult in early season, but by late season, the river may be just a series of channels through a gravelly bed). Beyond the ford, the trail begins the steep ascent up the west Kern Canyon wall to the hanging valley above, the canyon of the Kern-Kaweah River. (Misnamed before it was fully explored, people once thought this stream might somehow link the Kern and Kaweah drainages. It doesn't.) Veering away from the Kern-Kaweah River, the path ascends to the north side of a granite knob, or spine, and passes through what has been called Kern-Kaweah Pass.

This difficult climb is repaid by the delightful valley above it, one of the finest in the Sierra. From the "pass," the trail makes a very steep, loose, and rocky (but mercifully short) descent, a moderate ascent, and, finally, a slight descent to what is left of Rockslide Lake (9040´)—two wide pools of crystal-clear, emerald-green water in the river. Utterly remote Kaweah Basin lies southwest of this region, possibly accessible cross-country.

Beyond the lake, the canyon widens into a granite amphitheater, where two tributary streams merge and dash into the main canyon over a rocky ledge to meet the main river below the fall, by which the river arrives at the bowl. From here, the ascent through a sparse-to-moderate lodgepole cover is moderate as the route threads the deep canyon lying between Kern Point and Picket Guard Peak.

One more steep ascent is required to reach the bowl that contains what is left of Gallats Lake (10,000´), a lovely oxbow in a large, wet meadow (fishing is good for golden). Fair campsites are here, but better ones lie a little less than 1 mile ahead, where the trail turns away from the river northwest toward Colby Pass. These campsites (10,170´; 11S 367129 4051182), perhaps the most remote on this trip, are a good explorer's base for excursions into the lightly visited headwaters of the Kern-Kaweah River and into Milestone Basin. Fishing is excellent for golden.

DAY 10 (Kern-Kaweah River to Roaring River Ranger Station, 12.8 miles): This is another long, tough day, so get an early start. The trail turns away from the Kern-Kaweah River to make a climbing traverse, at first moderate and then steep, west-northwest toward a tributary stream from Colby Pass. Ford the tributary twice and enjoy an easing of the grade as the route curves decidedly northward after the second ford, passing a meadow.

The slog to the pass soon begins as the trail fords the stream from lakes in Milestone Bowl to the northeast. Forest cover thins as the track winds through a series of bowls and then climbs steep, sandy-rocky switchbacks to reach the pass in 2.5 miles from last night's campsite. Over-the-shoulder views on the climb take in the Kern-Kaweah's canyon as well as Kaweah Peaks Ridge.

At the pass (12,000´), there are excellent views back (south) toward Kaweah Peaks Ridge and north over Cloud Canyon to Palmer Mountain, seemingly framed by the canyon's walls. Begin the steep, zigzagging descent of a narrow, rocky chute toward Colby Lake (10,584´), a scenic gem with exposed campsites in a cirque high above Cloud Canyon's floor. Cross the lake's inlet as the trail traverses the lake's east side at a little under 4 miles. For those who love alpine conditions, the temptation to stop here is almost irresistible, especially because fishing for rainbow and brook is good.

Leaving Colby Lake, ford its outlet and curve west into the upper reaches of the cirque east of the striking Whaleback, which separates Cloud Canyon from this cirque. Switchback steeply down the cirque's eastern wall before making a descending traverse northwest to the cirque floor and its creek. The trail fords the creek several times on its way north and then northwest to the northern tip of the Whaleback.

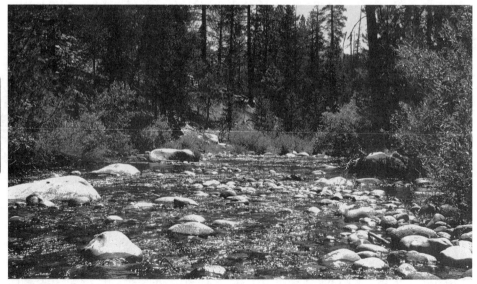

Roaring River bubbles along next to the trail.

Begin a steep descent of the Whaleback that finally eases on a long, moderate-to-gradual switchback to the bottom of Cloud Canyon. Ford the stream draining Cloud Canyon, which becomes Roaring River, for the first time. There are good campsites near this ford. But heading north, leave trailless upper Cloud Canyon behind (there used to be a trail, but it's long since disappeared from neglect). Pass over a wood platform above a spring-fed pool and descend past one of trapper Shorty Lovelace's small line cabins, a few yards off the trail and worth a peek (don't harm it; see Trip 26, Day 3, for more on Shorty).

Beyond Shorty's cabin, ford the stream again and then ford Table Creek. Just beyond, drop steeply to ford Roaring River (ford not shown on the topo) and climb away from the crossing. The trail wanders north toward Big Wet Meadow; pause to enjoy the incredible scenery here, especially upstream toward the Whaleback. From Big Wet Meadow, descend through forest and meadows to ford Cunningham Creek, pass campsites and a hitching post, and reach Cement Table Meadow.

From Cement Table Meadow, the trail angles northwest through Jeffrey pines as it descends gradually near the tumbling river. Presently, the track fords the two channels of Barton Creek and soon after fords Brewer Creek. Two more miles of pleasant, scenic descent bring hikers to a footbridge over Roaring River.

Cross to the river's west side, veer south, and shortly find the junction and nearby campsites at Roaring River Ranger Station, closing the loop part of this trip.

Days 11–12 (Roaring River Ranger Station to Lodgepole Campground Trailhead, 23 miles):
Retrace your steps of Day 1 and Day 2 to the trailhead.

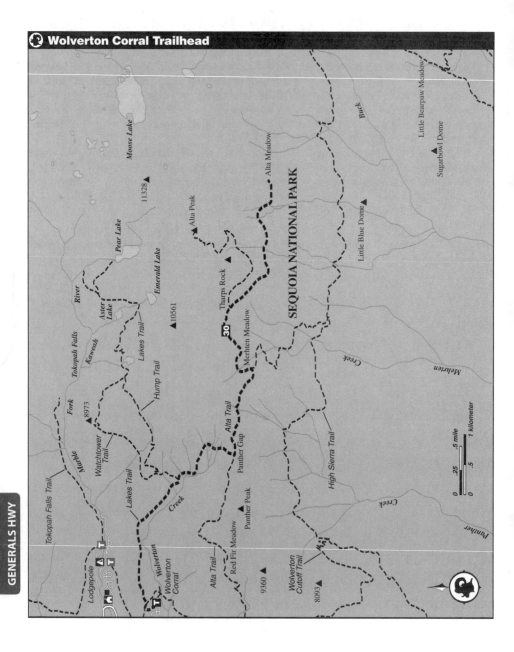

Wolverton Corral Trailhead

Wolverton Corral Trailhead   7325'; 11S 342917 4053326

DESTINATION/ UTM COORDINATES	TRIP TYPE	BEST SEASON	PACE (HIKING/ LAYOVER DAYS)	TOTAL MILEAGE
30 Alta Meadow 11S 350980 4049489	Out & back	Mid to late	2/1 Leisurely	13

Information and Permits: This trailhead is in Sequoia National Park: 47050 Generals Hwy., Three Rivers, CA 93271, 559-565-3341, www.nps.gov/seki. Permits are required, there is a fee for them, and quotas apply. Some areas may have fire restrictions and bear-canister requirements. You may reserve a permit in advance for trips mid-May through September by mail or fax only, no earlier than March 1 and no later than three weeks before the start of your trip.

Driving Directions: From Visalia, drive east on State Hwy. 198 for 40 miles through Woodlake village, around Lake Kaweah, and through Lemon Cove, Three Rivers, and Hammond villages. Continue 17 more miles to Giant Forest and then about another 2.25 miles to the turnoff right (east) to the General Sherman Tree and to Wolverton. Turn toward Wolverton, avoid the General Sherman Tree turnoff, and follow this road to the parking loop at its end, 1.5 miles from the Generals Hwy. The trailhead is on the upper side of the loop, easily distinguished by a large sign and a set of concrete stairs. There are bear boxes where you can store any bear-attracting items you're not taking with you.

30 Alta Meadow

Trip Data: 11S 350980 4049489; 13 miles; 2/1 days

Topos: *Lodgepole*

Highlights: Natural gardens and wonderful panoramas make the hike to Alta Meadow a treat, while the huge meadow itself—seasonally carpeted in wildflowers—is a delight to visit. Taking the trail to Alta Peak is a popular dayhike from here.

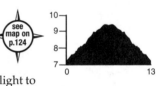

HEADS UP! The exposure on the Alta Trail may trouble acrophobics. Also, a trail that once went across Alta Meadow to Moose Lake no longer exists—even across the meadow, it is barely a use trail—and trying to follow its route is a frustrating exercise in bashing through deadfall and over animal trails. A better route to Moose Lake may be to go cross-country at or above treeline—a rough route for hardier hikers, especially for those who wish to loop over to Pear Lake.

DAY 1 (Wolverton Corral Trailhead to Alta Meadow, 6.5 miles): Begin your hike on the Lakes Trail (7283'; 11S 344858 4051524 (field)) with a moderate-to-steep climb northward, first up the stairs and then up the duff trail under a dense fir forest, shortly passing a spur left (west) to the Long Meadow Loop. Continue ahead (north) to another junction, this one on the right (south-southeast). Stay on the Lakes Trail (now eastward) as it travels this forested ridge. After about 0.75 mile, the path traverses above musical Wolverton Creek before descending into the meadow along the creek for a welcome and flowery break from the dense forest.

At 1 mile, the trail hooks right (southeast), and hereafter openings in the forest provide displays of abundant wildflowers. The grade steepens around 1.5 miles, and the path soon fords a stream. Around 1.6 miles, there's a major junction (8102'; 11S 347038 4051071): The Lakes Trail turns left (north) toward Heather and its sister lakes, while this trip continues ahead (east-southeast) toward Panther Gap. On its way to Panther Gap, the trail crosses numerous small streams that nourish hillside meadows and one glorious flower garden after another.

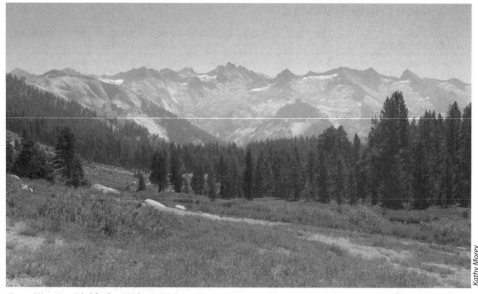

Kathy Morey

Great Western Divide from Alta Meadow

Beyond the last stream at 2.3 miles, the trail climbs a steep switchback to Panther Gap (8520´; 11S 347334 4050181 (field)). Be sure to take in the sublime views from the south edge of Panther Gap over unseen Middle Fork Kaweah River to Castle Rocks and the jagged peaks of the Great Western Divide. The gap also offers a couple of dry bivouac sites. A junction at the gap gives a choice between a faint route to Giant Forest (right/west); this trip turns left (east) on the Alta Trail toward Alta Meadow.

After wandering first to one side of the gap and then to the other, the trail settles down for a gradual, ascending, eastward traverse of the south side of this ridge, which separates the Kaweah River's Middle and Marble forks. While the Lakes Trail continues up the Marble Fork, the Alta Trail is a narrow, sandy, mostly exposed track as much as 5000 feet above the Middle Fork, almost paralleling the famed High Sierra Trail (about 1500 feet below on the same slopes). Chinquapin, manzanita, and a few red and white firs clothe the slopes around you but hardly interfere with the panoramic views.

Beyond a spring-fed garden, the path switchbacks up and then resumes its traverse, soon crossing a tiny meadow. At a signed but faint junction (8990´; 11S 348794 4049788 (field)) with a connector right (east-southeast) down to the High Sierra Trail, the Alta Trail bears left (north), curves up, and soon reaches Mehrten Meadow, with its welcome creek, shade, and a few campsites. Ignore a use trail that darts right and steeply down to a creek crossing and eventually a tent spot; continue ahead (north and then east) to ford two forks of the creek and perhaps take a well-earned rest.

From Mehrten Meadow onward, the Alta Trail is better shaded than before, the downhill slopes seem less precipitous, and the views are less frequent. The trail soon passes above a vigorous spring and then a hillside meadow. Nearing Tharps Rock, the track crosses a trio of seasonal streams and soon meets the trail to Alta Peak (9330´; 11S 349862 4050173 (field)) in an open area with good views upslope to the peak. Left (north) goes to the peak; this trip continues ahead (east) to Alta Meadow, now about a mile away. There are bivouac sites near this junction.

A hundred yards farther east, on the edge of the open area, the trail fords a stream and shortly passes a campsite just downhill. Beyond the previous junction, the path seems to deteriorate somewhat and crosses a runoff channel. Still, at open areas, the views are splendid down to Little Blue Dome and east toward the Great Western Divide.

Presently, the trail traverses above a great downslope sweep of granite (superb views!) and then fords a year-round stream that nourishes a very steep meadow. Just beyond, the maintained trail peters out at a sandy spot on a south-trending ridge on huge Alta Meadow's west side (9356´; 11S 350980 4049489 (field)). This ridge has moderate forest cover and offers the best campsites at Alta Meadow. The best water source is the stream just forded; water on this side of the meadow consists of inadequate seeps and scummy pools. Nevertheless, it's hard to beat a perch in Alta Meadow, where you can enjoy the flowers and the stirring spectacle of the Great Western Divide.

Beyond here, the topo is badly out of date: The route across the meadow barely qualifies as a use trail and ends altogether a few yards into the trees on the meadow's east side. Campsites on that side virtually have been wiped out by deadfall, runoff, and overgrowth.

DAY 2 (Alta Meadow to Wolverton Corral Trailhead, 6.5 miles): Retrace your steps to the trailhead.

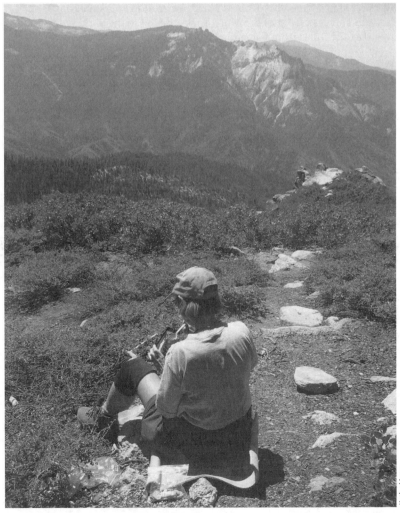

Castle Crags from a rest stop at Panther Gap

Crescent Meadow Trailhead

DESTINATION/ UTM COORDINATES	TRIP TYPE	BEST SEASON	PACE (HIKING/ LAYOVER DAYS)	TOTAL MILEAGE
31 High Sierra Trail 11S 358453 4039042 (trans-Sierra)	Shuttle	Mid to late	9/3 Moderate	67

Information and Permits: This trailhead is in Sequoia National Park: 47050 Generals Hwy., Three Rivers, CA 93271, 559-565-3341, www.nps.gov/seki. Permits are required, there is a fee for them, and quotas apply. Some areas may have fire restrictions and bear-canister requirements. You may reserve a permit in advance for trips mid-May through September by mail or fax only, no earlier than March 1 and no later than three weeks before the start of your trip.

Driving Directions: From Fresno, take Hwy. 180 east approximately 50 miles into Kings Canyon National Park and a junction with the Generals Hwy. Turn south on the Generals Hwy., toward Giant Forest. Near the Giant Forest Museum, turn west toward Crescent Meadow onto narrow Crescent Meadow Road, a circuitous ribbon of old asphalt that then wanders south and east. Go past the Moro Rock junction to the parking lot and toilet at the end of the road, 2.5 miles from Generals Hwy.

31 High Sierra Trail

Trip Data: 11S 358453 4039042; 67 miles; 9/3 days

Topos: *Lodgepole, Triple Divide Peak, Mt. Kaweah, Chagoopa Falls, Mt. Whitney, Mt. Langley*

Highlights: This dramatic trans-Sierra route follows the renowned High Sierra Trail from Crescent Meadow to Whitney Portal, visiting many classic Sierra points and crossing the Great Western Divide at Kaweah Gap and the Sierra Crest at Trail Crest, the Sierra's highest on-trail pass. From a junction near there, bagging Mt. Whitney's summit is an integral part of this trip along the way. The High Sierra Trail is the quintessential Sierra crossing—and there's plenty of fine fishing along the way.

HEADS UP! *This trip enters the Mt. Whitney Zone, which requires an additional permit reservation and per-person fee. Apply for it at the same time you apply for your trailhead permit reservation. For details, see www.fs.fed.us/r5/inyo/recreation/wild/mtwhitney.shtml. Bear canisters are required on the Mt. Whitney Trail.*

The Forest Service asks that hikers on Mt. Whitney pack out their solid wastes. See www.fs.fed.us/r5/inyo/recreation/wild/packitout.shtml for how to get the ingenious pack-out kits, use them, and dispose of them.

Shuttle Directions: From Hwy. 395 in Lone Pine, at its only stoplight, head west on Whitney Portal Road for 13 miles to the large overnight parking lot near the end of the road (toilet, water, store, nearby campground).

DAY 1 (Crescent Meadow Trailhead to Merhten Creek Camp, 5.5 miles): From the parking loop, circumvent the meadow on an asphalt path and begin climbing steadily and generally eastward through a forest of giant sequoias, sugar pines, and white firs. Soon after passing a junction on the left on a forested saddle with a trail to Giant Forest, continue ahead (generally eastward) on the High Sierra Trail and break out of the trees into the open above the Middle Fork Kaweah River. Soon, the trail reaches Eagle View overlook, where the view is indeed stunning: Moro Rock pops up in the west, far below is the churning river, and to the east are the heavily glaciated peaks of the Great Western Divide.

The course of the trail does not follow a "natural" route, but instead makes a high traverse across the north wall of the Middle Fork Kaweah River's canyon. However, the traverse is not level: Frequently, the trail undulates over 400-foot rises, only to dip down into a secondary tributary canyon, and then emerge to climb again.

The trail, for now shady and nearly level, continues generally northeastward in a forest of ponderosa and sugar pine, black oak, incense-cedar, and white fir, mixed with manzanita, whitethorn scrub, and much fragrant kit-kit-dizze. Across the canyon, those impressive sentinels of the valley, Castle Rocks, fall slowly behind as the path marches up the canyon.

After negotiating three switchbacks, resume the stroll and soon pass a junction with the Wolverton Cutoff, used mainly by stock. Go ahead (north here). Legal camping begins just past this junction, at the point where a tributary of Panther Creek splashes steeply down granite—not that any campsites are yet apparent. Where another tributary of Panther Creek descends a loose slot to cross the trail at about 7080 feet, look for campsites some 150 yards farther east in a shallow, forested draw below the trail. Spring-fed streams cross the trail in this vicinity late into the season.

Yellow-throated gilia and mustang clover are abundant along the trail until late in the season. Climb over Sevenmile Hill and continue to the crossing of Mehrten Creek (7685´; 11S 349362 4048752), 5.5 miles from the trailhead. On the west side of the creek, a use trail leads steeply up the hillside to campsites with a bear box.

DAY 2 (Merhten Creek Camp to Upper Hamilton Lake, 8.5 miles): Beyond Mehrten Creek, pass a junction with the Sevenmile Trail, which provides a 2.2-mile connection to the Alta Trail, 1300 feet above. Continue ahead, generally eastward.

From that junction, descend to a ford of an unnamed tributary and then climb steeply. Views to the south and southeast include the spectacular granite-dome formations of Sugarbowl Dome and Castle Rocks above the timbered valley floor. At each ford of the unnamed tributaries draining the slopes of Alta Peak, the trail passes precariously perched campsites. The next developed campsite with a bear box is 8.5 miles from Crescent Meadow, near the first branch of the twin-channeled tributary before to the main branch of Buck Creek. Beyond the streams, the trail bends around the mostly open slopes of Buck Canyon and then descends to a bridge over Buck Creek.

A switchbacking climb leads up the forested east wall of Buck Canyon to the top of a low ridge and the signed 200-yard lateral south to Bearpaw Meadow Campground (7650´; 11S 354657 4047140). There, viewless, very overused, designated campsites sheltered by dense timber have bear boxes, pit toilets, and piped water. Open fires are not allowed. In about 0.3 mile, reach a junction with the northeast-bound Over the Hill Trail; stay on the High Sierra Trail as it curves south for a bit. Emergency services are usually available from the nearby A-framed ranger station. Near the ranger station is Bearpaw High Sierra Camp.

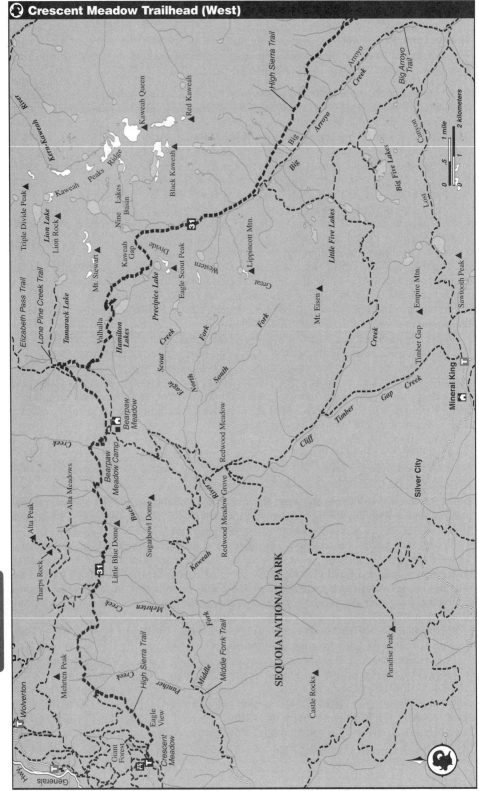

SEQUOIA NATIONAL PARK

GENERALS HWY

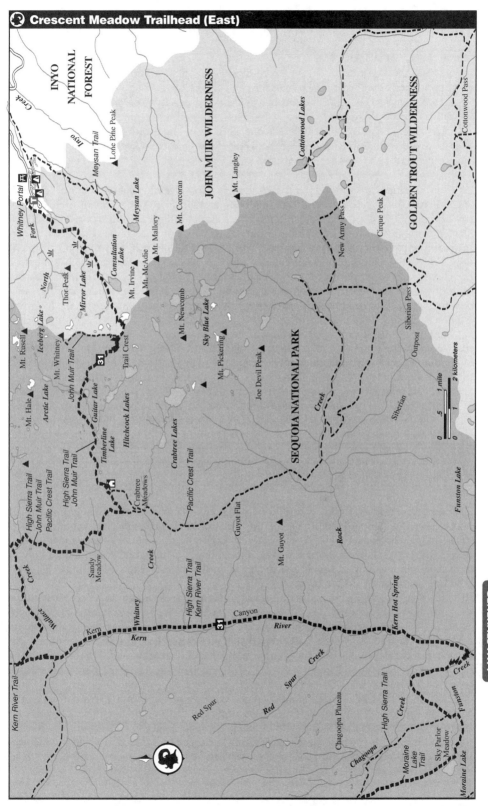

INYO NATIONAL FOREST

JOHN MUIR WILDERNESS

GOLDEN TROUT WILDERNESS

SEQUOIA NATIONAL PARK

Inyo Creek

Lone Pine Peak

Meysan Trail

Whitney Portal

North Fork

Meysan Lake

Mt. Corcoran

Mt. Langley

Cottonwood Lakes

Cottonwood Pass

Consultation Lake

Mt. Mallory

Mt. McAdie

Mt. Irvine

Thor Peak

Mirror Lake

Iceberg Lake

New Army Pass

Cirque Peak

Mt. Russell

Mt. Whitney

Mt. Hale

Arctic Lake

John Muir Trail

Trail Crest

Guitar Lake

Mt. Newcomb

Sky Blue Lake

Mt. Pickering

Joe Devil Peak

Siberian Pass

Outpost

Siberian

Creek

Hitchcock Lakes

Timberline Lake

High Sierra Trail
John Muir Trail
Pacific Crest Trail

Crabtree Lakes

Pacific Crest Trail

Crabtree Meadows

Guyot Flat

Funston Lake

1 mile
1 kilometer
2 kilometers
.5
0
1
0

High Sierra Trail
John Muir Trail
Pacific Crest Trail

Sandy Meadow

Whitney Creek

Mt. Guyot

Rock Creek

Kern Hot Spring

Kern River Trail

Wallace Creek

Kern

Whitney

Kern

High Sierra Trail
Kern River Trail

Canyon

River

Red Spur Creek

Red Spur

Red

Chagoopa Plateau

Spur Creek

Funston Creek

Creek

High Sierra Trail

Moraine Lake Trail

Sky Parlor Meadow

Chagoopa Creek

Moraine Lake

GENERALS HWY

131

BEARPAW HIGH SIERRA CAMP

At this backcountry lodge, like the famed High Sierra Camps of Yosemite, guests sleep in tent cabins and enjoy hot meals for breakfast and dinner (by reservation only). Unlike the claustrophobic backpackers' camp, Bearpaw's location on the edge of Middle Fork Kaweah River's canyon offers expansive views of the glacier-scoured surroundings, including such notable landmarks as Eagle Scout Peak and Mt. Stewart on the Great Western Divide, the Yosemite-esque cleft of Hamilton Creek, and Black Kaweah above Kaweah Gap. A tiny "store" may offer snacks, batteries, and other supplies.

Continue the eastward trek on the High Sierra Trail, leaving the backcountry hubbub around Bearpaw Meadow and descending moderately through sparse stands of mixed forest. Rounding the slope and descending toward River Valley, the trail traverses a section blasted from an immense exfoliating granite slab. Views of clearcut avalanche chutes on the south wall of the canyon accompany the descent to the bridge over wild, turbulent Lone Pine Creek. This stream cascades and plunges down a narrow, granite chasm below the culvert; the torrential force down the slender, V-shaped slot is clear evidence of the sculpting power of water. From the creek, the trail ascends an exposed slope, passing a side trail to Tamarack Lake and Elizabeth Pass (good campsites near the junction). Go ahead (southeast) here.

Continuing the steady ascent, you will be overwhelmed by the gigantic scale of the rock sculpting by ice, rock, and snow to the east and southeast. The final climb to the ford of Hamilton Creek is overshadowed by the mighty rock on all sides: the sheer granite wall to the north called Angels Wings, the sharply pointed granite sentinels atop the south wall, and its avalanche chutes—all are constant sources of awe.

Under these heights, ford the creek a few hundred yards below the lowest Hamilton Lake and then climb steeply over shattered rock to good campsites at the northwest end of Upper Hamilton Lake (8235; 11S 358787 4047703; two-night limit at this overused lake). Views from the campsites, including the silver waterfall ribbon at the east end, are superlative, and fishing for brook, rainbow, and golden is fair to good.

DAY 3 (Upper Hamilton Lake to Big Arroyo Trail Junction, 8 miles): Regain the High Sierra Trail and go generally east toward Kaweah Gap on a 2500-foot climb that is something of an engineering marvel, with sections literally blasted out of a vertical cliff. Beginning at the northwest end of Upper Hamilton Lake, the trail ascends steadily up a juniper-and-red-fir-dotted slope with constant views of the lake and its dramatic cirque wall. Despite the rocky terrain, many wildflowers line this ascent, and among the manzanita and chinquapin, you may see lupine, yellow columbine, penstemon, Indian paintbrush, white cinquefoil, false Solomon's seal, and Douglas phlox.

After some doubling back, the trail turns south on a steep ascent to a point just above the north shore of Precipice Lake (10,200´) at the foot of the near-vertical north face of Eagle Scout Peak. The jagged summits of the Great Western Divide dominate the skyline to the east during the final, tarn-dotted ascent to U-shaped Kaweah Gap, but on the approach, the equally spectacular ridges of the Kaweah Peaks come into view beyond. This colorful ridge dominates the view from Kaweah Gap (10,700´), which also includes the Nine Lakes Basin watershed to the north.

From the gap, hikers ready to stop for the day can turn left (north), find a very easy cross-country into Nine Lakes Basin, and soon arrive at the roughly horseshoe-shaped first lake (10,450´; 11S 361539 4074018), with numerous fair-to-good campsites and good fishing for brook trout. A base camp here makes a fine springboard for excursions to the increasingly secluded and dramatic lakes to the north and east. Climbers will find a wealth of steep faces west and east of this fine base camp.

For this trip, the trail continues a steady, moderate southward descent along the west side of Big Arroyo Creek, fording to the east side midway down. Descend over unjointed granite broken by substantial pockets of grass and numerous runoff streams that continue to flow even late into the season. Open stretches afford fine views of U-shaped, glacially wrought Big Arroyo below, and the white, red, and black rocks of Black Kaweah and Red Kaweah peaks to the east.

The route then reenters timber cover and arrives at some good campsites (9600′; 11S 362446 4043234) along the stream, about a quarter mile above the Little Five Lakes/Black Rock Pass junction. Fishing in the creek for brook trout should be fair to good, but anglers with extra time should take the 2-mile side trip to Little Five Lakes to enjoy the fine angling for golden trout.

DAY 4 (Big Arroyo Trail Junction to Moraine Lake, 8 miles): Continue ahead (southeast) past the Little Five Lakes junction. The High Sierra Trail begins a long, moderate ascent along the north canyon wall of Big Arroyo. This route parallels the course of a trunk glacier that once filled Big Arroyo, overflowed the benches on either side, and contributed to the main glacier of Kern Canyon. The track climbs the wall of this trough amid sparse timber and a bounty of wildflowers tucked between sagebrush, manzanita, and chinquapin; the most colorful flowers include columbine, bright Indian paintbrush, and purple lupine.

The grade eases near the mirrored surface of a tarn, and then, swinging away from the lip of Big Arroyo, the trail begins a gradual descent through alternating stretches of timber and meadow. Tree-interrupted views of the jagged skyline of the Great Western Divide accompany the descent on the way to a trail junction in a meadow on the south side of a tributary of Chagoopa Creek.

Leave the official High Sierra Trail route at this junction and turn right (south) through meadows filled with clumps of shooting stars. This descent grows steeper over coarse granite sand amid dense stands of lodgepole and foxtail pine, with superlative views down into Big Arroyo to the drainages of Soda and Lost Canyon creeks. This steadily down-winding trail leads to the wooded shores of Moraine Lake (9290′; 11S 369732 4036003). Good campsites on the south side of the lake provide views across the water of the Kaweah Peaks, along with nearby gardens of wild azalea.

CROWDS AT KERN HOT SPRING

Before resuming the trip, be advised of the terrible overcrowding at Kern Hot Spring, tomorrow's destination. This overcrowding has resulted in great disappointment for those expecting wilderness solitude at this remote hot spring. Consider an alternative to camping at Kern Hot Spring, where campers are required to stay in the adjacent, badly overused campground. Campsites may be available on the west side of the river, before crossing to the spring on the east side, and also a few hundred yards to a quarter mile away from the spring on the east side of the river. Consider taking a dip around midday on the way to campsites either well below or well above the hot spring: Crowds might be lower then, when backpackers taking a layover day or week or a month or the whole summer at the hot spring could be out dayhiking and the evening's horde of newcomers have yet to arrive.

DAY 5 (Moraine Lake to Kern Hot Spring, 7 miles): After traversing a moraine just east of Moraine Lake, the trail descends moderately, then gently, passing an old stockman's cabin before reaching superb Sky Parlor Meadow, with excellent views back across this flower-filled grassland to the Great Western Divide and Kaweah Peaks. Shortly beyond the ford of Funston Creek, at the east end of the meadow, this trip's route rejoins the official High Sierra Trail route and begins the moderate, then steep, descent to the bottom of Kern Canyon.

Along the initial descent, lodgepole pine is replaced by lower-altitude white fir and Jeffrey pine; farther down, the trail descends steeply through manzanita and snowbush beneath an occasional juniper or oak. The unmistakably U-shaped Kern Canyon is typical of glacially modified valleys. The final descent to the valley floor is accomplished via a series of steep, rocky switchbacks generally paralleling the plunge of Funston Creek.

Now on the floor of Kern Canyon, the route turns north, upstream, on the Kern River Trail, drops into a marshy area, and then crosses a pair of meadows on wooden walkways. Then the trail leads gently upward through a forest of Jeffrey pine and incense-cedar. High on the western rim of the canyon, look for Chagoopa Falls, a fury of plunging whitewater when the stream is full.

Past a manzanita-carpeted opening, the trail crosses the Kern River on a fine bridge and arrives at the south fork of Rock Creek. Then, around a point, the path leads to Kern Hot Spring (6880'; 11S 374055 4038030)—a therapeutic treat for the tired and dusty hiker. Although the cement tub screened by wood planks would appear crude by suburban backyard standards, here in the midst of the backcountry, Kern Hot Spring is a regal, heated paradise. Just a dozen yards away from the 115°F pool, the great Kern River rushes past. Campers must stay near the spring in the aforementioned designated campground, which has bear boxes and a pit toilet. Fishing in the Kern is good for rainbow and golden-rainbow hybrids.

DAY 6 (Kern Hot Spring to Junction Meadow, 8 miles): Continuing north, the route fords the upper fork of Rock Creek and traverses the gravelly canyon floor below the immense granite cliffs of the canyon's east wall. Past the confluence of Red Spur Creek, this route ascends gradually, sometimes a bit steeply, beside the Kern River, heading almost due north.

KERN TRENCH

The U-shaped trough of the Kern River, known as the Kern Trench, is remarkably straight for about 25 miles along the course of the Kern Canyon fault. The fault, a zone of structural weakness in the Sierra batholith, is more susceptible to erosion than the surrounding rock, and this deep canyon has been carved by both glacial and stream action. Many times, glaciers advanced down the canyon, shearing off spurs created by stream erosion and leaving some tributary valleys hanging above the main valley. The glaciers also scooped and plucked at the bedrock, creating basins in the granite, which later became lakes when the glaciers melted and retreated.

The walls of this deep canyon, from 2000 to 5000 feet high, are spectacular, with a number of streams cascading and falling down granite faces. (The fords of the stream draining Guyot Flat, of Whitney Creek, and of Wallace Creek can be difficult in early season.) Beyond the ford of Wallace Creek, the trail enters a park-like grove of stalwart Jeffery pines, providing a noble setting for the overused campsites at Junction Meadow (8036'; 11S 373505 4048976) on the Kern River, where fishing should be good for rainbow and some brook trout.

DAY 7 (Junction Meadow to Crabtree Ranger Station, 8.5 miles): The trail leaves the park-like Jeffrey pines of Junction Meadow and heads north to ascend steeply on rocky underfooting over a slope covered by manzanita and currant. Over-the-shoulder views down Kern Canyon improve continuously, as the occasional Jeffrey, lodgepole, and aspen offer frames for the photographer composing a shot of the great cleft.

After a mile, reach a junction of the Kern River Trail and the High Sierra Trail, where your route turns right (southeast), back toward Wallace Creek's canyon. At 10,400 feet is another junction, this one with PCT/JMT. Turn right (south) onto the PCT/JMT, which, in this area, is also the route of the High Sierra Trail. Immediately ford Wallace Creek (difficult in early season), pass some campsites, and then continue southward on generally gentle gradients through sporadic stands of lodgepole and foxtail pine.

At approximately 10,800 feet, reach a junction (campsites) between the PCT, which continues south, and the JMT and High Sierra Trail, which both turn east here. Take the left fork east and follow the JMT/High Sierra Trail on a climb over a bench through lodgepole and foxtail pines, staying well above the north bank of Whitney Creek. About a mile from the PCT junction, come to a junction (campsites) with a lateral that drops to a ford of Whitney Creek and continues south through upper and lower Crabtree Meadows, eventually joining the PCT south of here.

On the far side of Whitney Creek are a bear box and a junction with a lateral to Crabtree Ranger Station and the fair campsites nearby (10,700´; 11S 379376 4047420). Emergency services are sometimes available at the ranger station. Fishing in Whitney Creek is fair for golden trout.

DAY 8 (Crabtree Ranger Station to Trail Camp, 7 miles): From the vicinity of the ranger station, return to the JMT/High Sierra Trail and climb east along the north side of Whitney Creek to Timberline Lake, a small, irregular-shaped body of water most noted for reflecting the west face of Mt. Whitney—a favorite subject of both amateur and professional photographers. The lake is closed to camping, and the Mt. Whitney Zone begins around here.

Skirt the north side of the lake and continue a gentle ascent past timberline into an alpine meadow on the way around Guitar Lake. Backpackers in search of overnight accommodations may find decent campsites near the "guitar's neck" and near the crossing of Arctic Lake's outlet.

Away from Guitar Lake, the trail climbs to a bench with some tiny ponds and poor campsites. Traverse an alpine meadow and then start climbing on long, rocky switchbacks across the west face of Mt. Whitney to a junction of the JMT/High Sierra Trail heading to the summit of Mt. Whitney and the Mt. Whitney Trail from Whitney Portal.

SIDE TRIP TO MT. WHITNEY

To come all this way and not take the 2-mile trail to the summit of the highest peak in the lower 48 would be unforgivable. It's an integral part of the High Sierra Trail.

First, stash your heavy backpack into clefts of rock near the junction and don a daypack with the usual essentials. Then follow a steady climb along the west side of Whitney's south ridge, where the trail periodically enters notches with acrophobic vistas straight down the east face. As you ascend the rocky trail, sharp eyes will soon spy the summit hut, built for research purposes by the Smithsonian Institute in 1909. Nearing the final slope, the grade increases, as multiple paths lead toward the top. Cairns may aid in finding a route to the summit, but the way from here is unmistakable—simply head for the top.

Cresting the broad summit plateau of jumbled slabs and boulders, the roof of the hut comes into view, and soon you find yourself at 14,491 feet, the top of the continental US. Toward the edge of the plateau is a pit toilet, not only the highest waste receptacle in the lower 48, but perhaps the one with the grandest view as well. Any adjective used to describe the incredible summit vista is grossly inadequate. Suffice to say, the view from the highest point in the lower 48 is a complete, 360-degree panorama, with each bearing of the compass holding something extraordinary to discover—a just reward for the toil necessary to reach such a lofty goal. Be sure to record your name in the summit register near the hut before backtracking the 2 miles to the trail junction. Officially, the JMT ends (or begins) at the summit, but the High Sierra Trail continues. Alas, there is no solitude here: Any halfway decent day sees dozens of hikers milling around the summit plateau.

If you took the side trip up Mt. Whitney, retrace your steps to the junction with the main trail. From the junction, make a short climb up to Trail Crest (13,620´) along the spine of the Sierra and on the boundary between Sequoia National Park to the west and John Muir Wilderness to the east. From Trail Crest, the Mt. Whitney Trail angles east around the top of a steep chute before embarking on a seemingly interminable descent down about a hundred tight switchbacks. Midway down is a stretch of trail that routinely ices up, providing tenuous footing; a steel cable is usually in place to aid in negotiating this sometimes tricky section. The demanding, 1600-foot descent finally eases on the approach to the seemingly barren terrain of Trail Camp, the highest legal camping area along the Mt. Whitney Trail.

Hordes of expectant peakbaggers may be camped in sandy sites between boulders at Trail Camp (12,035′; 11S 385533 4047132), which lends a somewhat circus-like atmosphere to the surroundings on a typical summer day. Despite the crowd, the alpine setting below the east face of the Whitney massif is spectacular. To the north is Wotan's Throne, with Pinnacle Ridge behind, and, to the south, 13,680-foot Mt. McAdie and 13,770-foot Mt. Irvine form a striking amphitheater for the icy waters of Consultation Lake. Water is readily available from nearby streams and tarns.

DAY 9 (Trail Camp to Whitney Portal, 6.5 miles): Beyond Trail Camp, head east-northeast to descend some poured concrete steps and continue steeply down a granite trail, witnessing ivesia, currant, creambush, and gooseberry growing in between the boulders. The outlet of Consultation Lake cascades down a ravine southeast of the trail. Ford Lone Pine Creek and pass tiny Trailside Meadows (no camping), carpeted with lush grasses and brightened by shooting stars, paintbrush, and columbine. Beyond the meadows, the trail refords Lone Pine Creek and then switchbacks down to sparse timber, finally leveling out near Mirror Lake (10,650′; no camping), cradled in a cirque beneath the south face of Thor Peak.

After fording Mirror Lake's outlet, the descent continues down a slope blooming with senecio, fireweed, pennyroyal, currant, Newberry's penstemon, Sierra chinquapin, Indian paintbrush, and creambush. Upon leveling out, the trail crosses Lone Pine Creek and enters a large meadow on the way to Outpost Camp (10,367′), which has several campsites.

From Outpost Camp, the trail crosses Lone Pine Creek, skirts a willow-lined meadow dotted with wildflowers, and then switchbacks down to a junction with a lateral to Lone Pine Lake (campsites). Ford Lone Pine Creek again and begin a final set of long, dusty, switchbacks that pass through open areas of sagebrush, chinquapin, mountain mahogany, and other members of the chaparral community common to the east side of the Sierra.

Two more fords of Lone Pine Creek provide cool nooks on the hot descent. Views down the V-shaped canyon of the Alabama Hills provide a fine diversion along the drop toward the trailhead. Exit John Muir Wilderness and soon reach the paved road loop at shady Whitney Portal (8361′; 11S 389060 4049762), where a hamburger and milkshake from the café should be a rewarding temptation after more than a week dining on trail food. In addition to the café, Whitney Portal offers campgrounds, restrooms, water, and a small store.

Sawtooth-Monarch Trailhead

7800'; 11S 356884 4035385

DESTINATION/ UTM COORDINATES	TRIP TYPE	BEST SEASON	PACE (HIKING/ LAYOVER DAYS)	TOTAL MILEAGE
32 Pinto Lake 11S 358453 4039042	Out & back	Mid to late	2/1 Moderate	17
33 Nine Lakes Basin 11S 361539 4074018	Out & back	Mid to late	6/3 Moderate, part cross-country	44
34 Big and Little Five Lakes 11S 358453 4039042	Loop	Mid to late	6/2 Moderate	40.5

Information and Permits: This trailhead is in Sequoia National Park: 47050 Generals Hwy., Three Rivers, CA 93271, 559-565-3341, www.nps.gov/seki. Permits are required, there is a fee for them, and quotas apply. Some areas may have fire restrictions and bear-canister requirements. You may reserve a permit in advance for trips mid-May through September by mail or fax only, no earlier than March 1 and no later than three weeks before the start of your trip.

Driving Directions: From Visalia, drive east on State Hwy. 198 for 40 miles through Woodlake village, around Lake Kaweah, and through Lemon Cove and Three Rivers villages. Continue about 6 more miles to Hammond village to a junction with the infamous Mineral King Road. Turn right onto it and follow the narrow, twisting road 23 miles through Silver City to the Sawtooth-Monarch Trailhead on the left, 0.8 mile past the ranger station. Parking is across the road.

32 Pinto Lake

Trip Data: 11S 358453 4039042; 17 miles; 2/1 days

Topos: *Mineral King*

Highlights: The fine scenery of the Cliff Creek drainage, the good camping, and the relatively warm swimming in Pinto Lake make this trip worthwhile in spite of the tough hike.

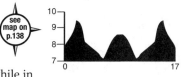

see map on p.138

DAY 1 (Sawtooth-Monarch Trailhead to Pinto Lake, 8.5 miles): From the trailhead, the route climbs north-northwest on manzanita-and-sagebrush-flanked trail to a junction. Turn left (north) and begin a relentless 1600-foot climb up a southwest-facing slope that can be quite hot in midsummer. Fortunately, a good part of the climb is under red fir forest. At the top of some switchbacks, the trail leaves the trees and makes a long, ascending traverse toward Timber Gap. Before heading back into the trees just below the gap, turn around and take in the fine view down toward Mineral King Valley, and then conclude the ascent at the forested saddle of Timber Gap (9511').

From the gap, the trail drops steeply on switchbacks through red fir forest toward a crossing of Timber Gap Creek, where a long swath of flower-filled meadow supplants the forest. The delightful garden is one of the largest and most vibrant in the Sierra. Soon, cross back over the creek and then hop over a number of lush, spring-fed rivulets on the way down the drainage. Eventually, the trail leaves Timber Gap Creek, rounds the nose of a

HWY 198

137

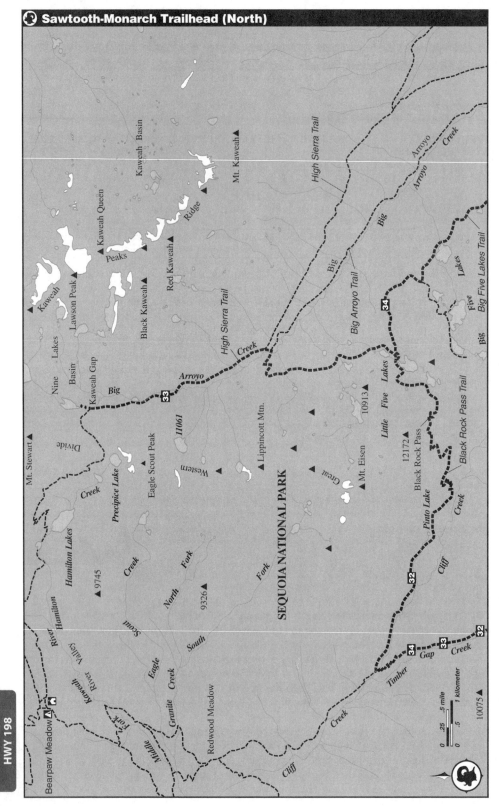

SEQUOIA NATIONAL PARK

Mt. Stewart ▲

Divide

Precipice Lake

Eagle Scout Peak ▲

11061

Western

Lippincott Mtn. ▲

Great

Mt. Eisen ▲

10913 ▲

Little Five Lakes

12172 ▲

Black Rock Pass

Black Rock Pass Trail

Pinto Lake

Cliff

Creek

Big Five Lakes Trail

Big   Five   Lakes

Arroyo   Creek

Arroyo

Big

Big

Big Arroyo Trail

High Sierra Trail

Mt. Kaweah ▲

Kaweah Basin

Kaweah Queen ▲

Peaks

Red Kaweah ▲

Ridge

Black Kaweah ▲

Lawson Peak ▲

Kaweah ▲

Nine   Lakes

Basin

Kaweah Gap

Big

Arroyo

33

High Sierra Trail

Creek

34

Hamilton Lakes

Creek

9745 ▲

North   Fork

9326 ▲

Hamilton

River

Kaweah River Valley

Eagle

Granite Creek

Middle   Fork

Redwood Meadow

South

Scout

Fork

Cliff

Creek

Bearpaw Meadow ▲ ⛺

Timber   Gap   Creek

34

33

32

32

10075 ▲

0   .25   .5   1 kilometer
0   .5 mile

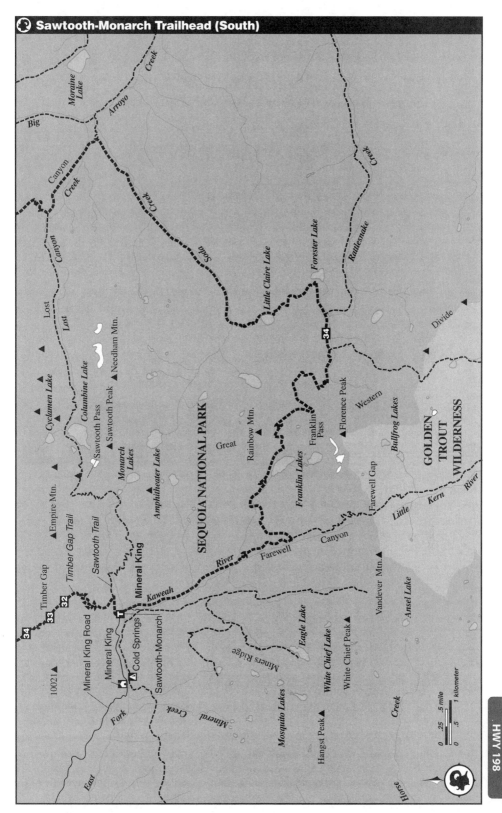

Moraine Lake

Big

Arroyo

Creek

Creek

Canyon Creek

Soda Creek

Forester Lake

Little Claire Lake

Rattlesnake Creek

Lost Creek

Lost

Divide

Cyclamen Lake

Columbine Lake

▲ Needham Mtn.

Sawtooth Pass

▲ Sawtooth Peak

Monarch Lakes

SEQUOIA NATIONAL PARK

Great

▲ Rainbow Mtn.

Franklin Lakes

Franklin Pass

▲ Florence Peak

Western

Bullfrog Lakes

34

GOLDEN TROUT WILDERNESS

▲ Empire Mtn.

Amphitheater Lake

Farewell Gap

Little Kern River

Timber Gap

Sawtooth Trail

Sawtooth Gap Trail

Mineral King

River

Farewell

Canyon

34 **33** **32**

Mineral King Road

Cold Springs

Kaweah

Sawtooth-Monarch

▲ Vandever Mtn.

Ansel Lake

10021 ▲

Mineral King

East Fork

Mineral

Creek Fork

Miners Ridge

Mosquito Lakes

▲ Hangst Peak

White Chief Lake

White Chief Peak ▲

Eagle Lake

Creek

Horse

0   .25   .5 mile
0   .5   1 kilometer

ridge, and then switchbacks down toward Cliff Creek through dense coniferous forest. Immediately after a ford of Cliff Creek (difficult in early season), find tiny Cliff Creek Camp (7125´), complete with bear box, and a signed junction with the Black Rock Pass Trail. There are no campsites between Cliff Creek Camp and the Pinto Lake area.

Turn right (southeast) and climb up Cliff Creek's canyon on the Black Rock Pass Trail through wildflowers, pockets of shrubs, and scattered firs, and across several meadow-lined creeklets. In early summer, the fine wildflower displays include mariposa lily, rein orchid, wild strawberry, monkeyflower, wallflower, corn lily, delphinium, yellow-throated gilia, and buckwheat.

Farther up the canyon, the trail emerges from the forest at an extensive boulder field, under which the creek temporarily flows. Ahead, the creek spills down a rock wall on the canyon's south side. Switchbacks lead up-canyon along the creek's north fork through dense willow, sagebrush, whitethorn, and bitter cherry, to a ford of Pinto Lake's outlet. Shortly after, reach an unmarked junction with a lateral on the right to well-used campsites on a forested bench south of Pinto Lake (bear box). Pinto Lake (8685´; 11S 358453 4039042) hides in a dense thicket of willows nearby, offering surprisingly pleasant swimming.

DAY 2 (Pinto Lake to Sawtooth-Monarch Trailhead, 8.5 miles): Retrace your steps to the trailhead.

33 Nine Lakes Basin

Trip Data: 11S 361539 4074018; 44 miles; 6/3 days

 see map on p.138

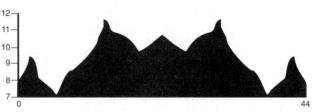

Topos: *Mineral King, Triple Divide Peak*

Highlights: Nine Lakes Basin offers seclusion that only cross-country destinations seem to possess. While hundreds tramp the High Sierra Trail, not more than a half mile away, and many throng to Little Five Lakes, through which this trip passes, few visit this wild basin, with its splendid lakes and majestic scenery.

HEADS UP! The trail is relatively easy, and the route to the lowest lake in Nine Lakes Basin is straight-forward but trackless: Just follow the outlet stream. Map-and-compass skills and some cross-country experience are prerequisites for exploring the basin's highest lakes.

DAY 1 (Sawtooth-Monarch Trailhead to Pinto Lake, 8.5 miles): *(Recap: Trip 32, Day 1.)* Ascend shrub-covered slopes north-northwestward to a junction with the Sawtooth Pass Trail, and turn left (north). Continue climbing to forested Timber Gap. Descend from the gap, following the course of Timber Gap Creek through flower-covered meadows and dense forest. Round the nose of a ridge, descend to a crossing of Cliff Creek, and immediately reach Cliff Creek Camp (bear box; last campsites before Pinto Lake area), near a junction with the Black Rock Pass Trail.

Turn right (southeast) and follow the Black Rock Pass Trail through a mixture of meadowlands and forest to a crossing of Pinto Lake's outlet. Just beyond, a lateral leads to campsites (bear box) south of nearby Pinto Lake (in dense willow thickets).

DAY 2 (Pinto Lake to Little Five Lakes, 7 miles): Head across the meadows southwest of Pinto Lake to find the Black Rock Pass Trail in talus on the cirque's north wall; don't take the well-trod use trail up the meadows. Start climbing across slopes covered with sagebrush, chinquapin, and willows. Early summer puts on quite a wildflower display, with forget-me-nots, paintbrush, lupine, phlox, wallflower, yampa, larkspur, senecio, and Bigelow sneezeweed. Soon, you encounter the first of many switchbacks that lead to Black Rock Pass.

The interminable slog is made more tolerable by the incredible scenery along the way, including the cascades below Spring Lake and the classic chain of cirque lakes consisting of Spring Lake itself, Cyclamen Lake, and Columbine Lake, often still icebound in early summer.

PATERNOSTER LAKES

When books on Sierra geology discuss "paternoster lakes," a series of lakes in glacier-carved basins, strung like rosary beads one after the other on the stream connecting them, they often choose a photo of these very lakes (Spring, Cyclamen, and Columbine) to illustrate the concept.

Finally, the rocky path attains Black Rock Pass (11,630'), where the views are vast. To the east and southeast, the companion basins of Little Five Lakes and Big Five Lakes drop off into Big Arroyo, and beyond this chasm rise the multicolored Kaweah Peaks. In the distant east is the 14,000-foot Whitney Crest, backbone of the Sierra.

From the pass, the zigzagging downgrade trends southeast and then angles northeast to pass above the highest of the Little Five Lakes, which actually comprise more than a dozen lakes. (When snow obscures the trail in early season, keep to the left so as not to end up off-route too far to the right and come out onto some cliffs.) A couple of Spartan campsites nestle in the rocks above the highest lake, which has a large tarn to the south. At the north end of the main (second) lake (10,476'; 11S 362402 4039601), overused campsites are huddled around a bear box, just east of a peninsula (no camping) and a bay. Stroll out onto the peninsula at sunset to catch the alpenglow on Kaweah Peaks Ridge. A summer ranger station across the bay may offer emergency services. The other lakes may offer more privacy.

DAY 3 (Little Five Lakes to Nine Lakes Basin, 6.5 miles, part cross-country): Just below the second of the Little Five Lakes, the trail fords the outlet and meets the trail to Big Five Lakes. Turn left (northeast) here and continue down the Little Five Lakes chain to another ford of the stream that links them. Soon, the trail crosses the outlet of the northern cluster of Little Five Lakes.

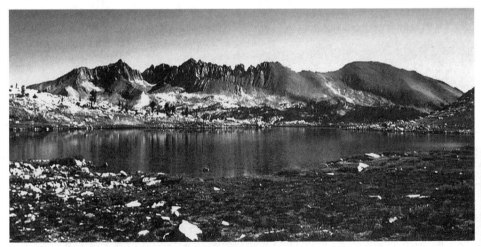

Kaweah Peaks Ridge from the highest of the Little Five Lakes

After an easy rise out of the basin, the trail descends into Big Arroyo, a large, west-bank canyon whose stream is a tributary of the Kern River. The route becomes increasingly steep as it turns northeast. Beyond a ford of Big Arroyo's stream, reach a junction with an unsigned trail heading down Big Arroyo. Head left (north), now on the High Sierra Trail, to ascend gently up this broad glacial valley past numerous potential campsites with great views of Lippincott Mountain and Eagle Scout Peak towering in the west, and metamorphic Black Kaweah and Red Kaweah piercing the eastern sky.

The trail fords Big Arroyo's creek again and then climbs over grassy pockets and granite slabs toward Kaweah Gap, a distinctive low spot on the Great Western Divide to the northwest. Where the High Sierra Trail swings west to Kaweah Gap, your cross-country route heads north into Nine Lakes Basin and soon arrives at the roughly horseshoe-shaped first lake (10,450´; 11S 361528 4046997), with numerous fair to good campsites, good fishing for brook trout, and fine opportunities to explore this fascinating basin.

DAYS 4–6 (Nine Lakes Basin to Sawtooth-Monarch Trailhead, 22 miles): Retrace your steps to the trailhead.

34 Big and Little Five Lakes

Trip Data: 11S 358453 4039042; 40.5 miles; 6/2 days

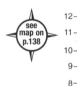

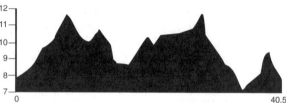

Topos: *Mineral King, Chagoopa Falls*

Highlights: This trip, which visits Big and Little Five Lakes, is perhaps the best backpackers' route for looping the dramatic alpine country east of Mineral King. Challenging passes and remote lakes reward the hiker, and fishing for golden and brook is good to excellent.

HEADS UP! *You'll need to be in excellent shape in order to enjoy this challenging trip.*

DAY 1 (Sawtooth-Monarch Trailhead to Franklin Lakes, 6 miles): From the parking lot, return to Mineral King Road. Walk east and then south up the road to the pack-station access road, and then follow that road south-southeast up the canyon past the pack station and a sign indicating that you're now on the Franklin Lakes/Farewell Gap Trail. Continue past corrals and through the open terrain of the East Fork Kaweah River's valley. Gazing southeast, spot the prominent, V-shaped notch of Farewell Gap at the head of the canyon. Just right (west) of the road, the hurried waters of the river are hidden by a screen of willows. On the approach to Crystal Creek, scattered clumps of juniper and red fir contrast vividly with the ghost-white trunks of some cottonwoods

Ford Crystal Creek and then branch left (south-southeast) onto an unsigned, single-track trail, as the road, closed to vehicles, veers right toward Soda Spring. Along the rocky trail, enjoy the fragrance of sagebrush, and between the sagebrush and gooseberry of these lower slopes, find spots of color provided by a variety of wildflowers, including paintbrush, fleabane, cow parsnip, and ipomopsis. A gradual-to-moderate climb leads to a ford of dashing Franklin Creek (difficult in early season) and the start of a steep, switchbacking, exposed climb, interrupted by an ascending traverse near the midpoint of the switchbacks. Above the switchbacks, reach a junction of the Franklin Lakes and Farewell Gap trails.

Turn left (northeast) at the junction and follow the Franklin Lakes Trail on a long, ascending traverse across the northwest slopes of Tulare Peak. Here you will enjoy fine views down the Kaweah River's canyon to Mineral King and up to Farewell Gap. The contrast between the green hillside and the red of Vandever Mountain in the south is especially striking in the morning light. Enter a sparse forest of mature foxtail pines and cross red-hued, rocky slopes dotted with spring flowers and laced with tiny snowmelt rills, as the trail turns northeast into Franklin Creek's upper canyon. Drop briefly to a ford of willow-lined Franklin Creek and resume a switchbacking climb toward the lakes. Pass the first campsites along the creek just below the rock-and-concrete dam across the outlet of the lower lake.

Continue climbing on the trail as it rises well above the shore of Lower Franklin Lake (10,300´; 11S 360092 4031802) to the first of a pair of paths that lead down to view-filled campsites (bear box) notched into sandy ledges on the sloping hillside above the lake. The second path accesses campsites (bear box, pit toilet) near the east inlet about 400 feet above the lake. The popularity of the lakes, combined with the limited number of viable campsites, may lend more of a feeling of a trailer park than remote backcountry on busy summer weekends; don't expect solitude.

Backpackers who haven't expended all their energy on reaching the first campsites may escape some of the crowd by continuing another half mile to a bench between the lower and upper lakes. Campsites on the bench are treeless and exposed but see far fewer visitors. A short romp from the bench over boulders leads to Upper Franklin Lake (10,578´), directly below the cirque wall between Florence and Tulare peaks.

VIEWS AND FISHING AT FRANKLIN LAKE

A bizarre conglomeration of colors appears in Upper Franklin Lake's dramatic cirque basin. To the northeast, the slopes of Rainbow Mountain are a study of gray-white marble whorls set in a sea of pink, red, and black metamorphic rocks. To the south, the slate ridge joining Tulare Peak and Florence Peak is a hue of chocolate red that sends photographers scrambling for viewpoints from which to foreground the contrasting blue of Lower Franklin Lake against this colorful headwall. Anglers should find the fishing for brook trout good at the lower lake and perhaps better at the upper lake.

DAY 2 (Franklin Lakes to Little Claire Lake, 7 miles): Away from Lower Franklin Lake, the trail rises steadily eastward and then climbs steep switchbacks. Views of the Franklin Lakes' cirque improve with elevation, with both lakes eventually coming into view. The ascent leaves forest cover behind as the trail crosses and recrosses a field of coarse granite granules dotted with bedrock outcropping. Despite the sieve-like drainage of this slope, wildflowers abound. High up on the slope, two adjacent, year-round rivulets nourish gardens of yellow mimulus and lavender shooting stars. At windy Franklin Pass (11,760´), views are panoramic.

VIEWS AT FRANKLIN PASS

Landmarks to the northwest include Castle Rocks and Paradise Peak; to the east is the immediate unglaciated plateau above the headwaters of Rattlesnake Creek, as well as Forester Lake on the wooded bench just north of the creek. East of the Kern Trench and plateaus is Mt. Whitney along the Sierra Crest.

The initial descent from the pass, unlike the west-side ascent, zigzags down a slope mostly covered with disintegrated quartz sand and, oddly, sprinkled with small, wind-sculpted granite domes. Eventually, very widely scattered stunted pines begin to reappear prior to some switchbacks that lead down to a small meadow in the Rattlesnake Creek drainage (campsites in the vicinity; fine fishing). On the way, pass a signed junction with the faint Shotgun Pass Trail on the right. Skirt the meadow and continue downstream to a junction of the Soda Creek and Rattlesnake Creek trails.

From the junction, go left (east-northeast) on the Soda Creek Trail. Walk through light, lodgepole pine forest on a gradual ascent to Forester Lake (10,190´), a little more than 3 miles from the pass. The lake is rimmed by grass and pine, with plenty of campsites spread around the shore. Fair-size brook trout should tempt the angler.

From the lake, head north for a moderate climb, interrupted briefly by a short stroll across a meadow-covered bench, leading to the top of a rise. From there, follow a moderate ascent to the sandy crown of a ridge dividing the Rattlesnake Creek and Soda Creek drainages. At this rounded summit, the crests of Sawtooth Ridge and Needham Mountain are easily visible to the north, and they remain in view as the trail descends moderately to the south end of Little Claire Lake. You may hear the effervescent burble of the Brewer blackbird and the raucous call of the Clark nutcracker as you skirt the east side of the lake to the good campsites on a sandy slope dotted with foxtail pines at the north end of Little Claire Lake (10,450´; 11S 363656 40323021). Fishing for brook trout may be excellent.

DAY 3 (Little Claire Lake to Big Five Lakes, 8 miles): The trail west of the outlet stream from Little Claire Lake follows well-graded switchbacks northward down a steep, forested slope for more than a mile. At the bottom of this 900-foot, precipitous, duff-and-rock slope, the route fords Soda Creek, descends gently over duff and sand through a moderate forest cover, and then becomes steeper. (Contrary to the 7.5´ topo, the trail doesn't ford the creek again.) Marmots on the rocky slope south of the creek whistle excitedly as unexpected visitors pass by, but they usually fail to stir from their lookout posts unless travelers show more than passing interest.

During the next several miles of undulating descent through lodgepole forest and across dry slopes, usually well away from Soda Creek, the trail leads across occasional refreshing tributaries, one of which is spanned by a boardwalk, and passes a half-dozen campsites of uneven quality. Among the lodgepoles, notice an occasional whitebark pine and then red fir. Clumps of sagebrush fill gaps between the stands of timber, and nestled next to their aromatic branches are healthy patches of Douglas phlox and Indian paintbrush.

The appearance of Jeffrey pine heralds the approach to a signed junction with the route along the Sawtooth Pass Trail to the left (northwest) and a trail branching right down into Big Arroyo. Turn left on the Sawtooth Pass Trail. (Fortunately, the Park Service has rerouted what was once a steep, rocky, loose, hot, exposed ascent to the foot of Lost Canyon.)

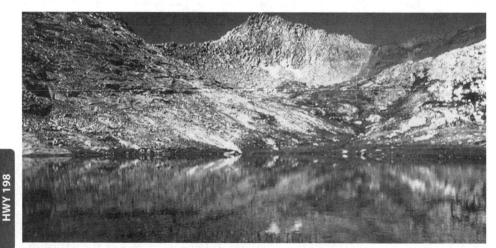

The highest of the Little Five Lakes, looking south to an unnamed peak

Beyond a crossing of Lost Creek, the trail follows a zigzagging climb through light forest to a meadow with a nearby campsite. Past the meadow, a more moderate ascent continues up Lost Canyon to a junction with the trail to Big Five Lakes. From here, campsites with a bear box are a short distance farther up the Sawtooth Pass Trail near another crossing of Lost Creek.

However, today's route turns right (north) at the junction and follows switchbacks up a hillside covered with lodgepole pines and chinquapin. Reach a bench where a tepid tarn at 10,084 feet offers the possibility of a fine swim and secluded camping above the heather-lined shore. Beyond the bench, resume a moderate climb amid boulders and slabs to the apex of a ridge overlooking the Big Five Lakes' basin. A rocky, steep descent leads to the first of the lakes (9830'; 11S 365026 4038630), where backpackers can overnight at good campsites near the log-jammed outlet or along the north shore.

DAY 4 (Big Five Lakes to Little Five Lakes, 4 miles): From the outlet of the lowest Big Five Lake, Lake 9830, follow the trail around the north shore to an informal junction with a use trail to campsites and ahead to the next lake. Take the right-hand fork northwest and make a steep, zigzagging, milelong climb to a T-junction with the trail to the upper Big Five Lakes (very beautiful, campsites) and the path to Little Five Lakes.

Turn right (north) and follow the Little Five Lakes Trail to the top of a ridge. The trail undulates for a dry mile, with periodic great views of Mt. Kaweah, the Kaweah Peaks Ridge, and, at the ridge's west end, Red Kaweah and Black Kaweah.

The dry stretch ends when the trail dips to traverse a boardwalk over a small, intimate valley, where a stream flows at least until late summer. From this brook, climb for several hundred vertical feet through a moderate lodgepole forest, level off, and then gain sight of the main Little Five Lake, Lake 10476, bordered by a large meadow. Soon, the trail reaches the north end of the lake (10,476'; 11S 362026 4038630), where overused campsites are huddled around a bear box. A summer ranger station may offer emergency services.

DAY 5 (Little Five Lakes to Pinto Lake, 7 miles): *(Recap in Reverse: Trip 33, Day 2.)* From the north end of Lake 10476, follow the trail around the west shore and then climb moderately above the lake to the north before angling south to pass above the highest of the Little Five Lakes. Leaving the lakes behind, a zigzagging climb leads to 11,630-foot Black Rock Pass on the Great Western Divide.

Rocky switchbacks lead from the austere surroundings of the pass down into the more hospitable surroundings of some subalpine meadows near Cliff Creek. Find an unsigned junction with a use trail on the left that leads roughly south to shady campsites with bear box. Nearby, Pinto Lake (8685'; 11S 358453 4039042) hides in a pocket of thick willows, offering surprisingly pleasant swimming.

DAY 6 (Pinto Lake to Sawtooth-Monarch Trailhead, 8.5 miles): *(Recap in Reverse: Trip 32, Day 1.)* From the vicinity of Pinto Lake, the trail heads generally west-northwest down the canyon, crosses the lake's outlet, and then switchbacks down the north wall of the canyon, well above the course of Cliff Creek. At the bottom of this descent, reach a signed junction with the Timber Gap Trail near Cliff Creek Camp (campsites, bear box).

Turn left (southwest), immediately ford Cliff Creek (difficult in early season), and make a switchbacking climb up a hillside. Above the switchbacks, climb around the nose of a ridge into the drainage of Timber Gap Creek. Ascend the canyon; farther upstream, the trail crosses the main creek a couple of times in a splendid, flowery meadow. A final, switchbacking climb through red firs leads to aptly named Timber Gap (9511').

Drop southeast away from Timber Gap, eventually breaking out of the trees to a tremendous view down into Mineral King's subalpine valley. After a while, a series of switchbacks descends through red firs before traversing open slopes to a junction with the Monarch Lakes-Sawtooth Pass Trail. Take the right fork southeast here. A steeper descent from there leads down to the Sawtooth-Monarch Trailhead.

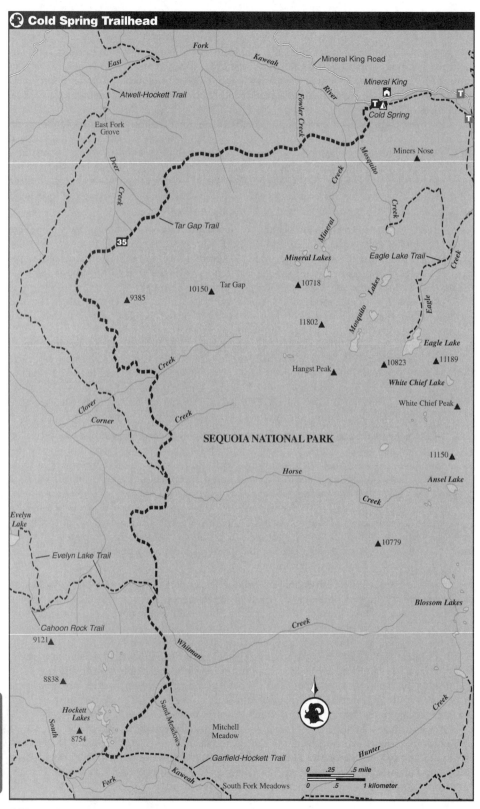

East Fork

Kaweah

Fork

Mineral King Road

Atwell-Hockett Trail

Mineral King

Fowler Creek

River

T

🏠

Cold Spring

T

T

East Fork Grove

Miners Nose ▲

Deer

Creek

Tar Gap Trail

Mineral

Creek

35

Mineral Lakes

Eagle Lake Trail

Creek

10150▲   Tar Gap

▲10718

Mosquito Lakes

Eagle

9385▲

11802▲

Eagle Lake

Hangst Peak▲

▲10823

▲11189

White Chief Lake

White Chief Peak ▲

Creek

Clover

SEQUOIA NATIONAL PARK

11150▲

Corner

Creek

Horse

Ansel Lake

Creek

Evelyn Lake

▲10779

Evelyn Lake Trail

Blossom Lakes

Cahoon Rock Trail

9121▲

Creek

Whitman

8838▲

Hockett Lakes

Sand Meadows

Mitchell Meadow

Hunter

▲ 8754

South

Garfield-Hockett Trail

Creek

Kaweah

South Fork Meadows

Fork

0   .25   .5 mile

0   .5   1 kilometer

Cold Spring Trailhead

7452'; 11S 355367 4035231

DESTINATION/ UTM COORDINATES	TRIP TYPE	BEST SEASON	PACE (HIKING/ LAYOVER DAYS)	TOTAL MILEAGE
35 Hockett Lakes 11S 350479 4124418	Out & back	Mid to late	6/1 Leisurely	28

Information and Permits: This trailhead is in Sequoia National Park: 47050 Generals Hwy., Three Rivers, CA 93271, 559-565-3341, www.nps.gov/seki. Permits are required, there is a fee for them, and quotas apply. Some areas may have fire restrictions and bear-canister requirements. You may reserve a permit in advance for trips mid-May through September by mail or fax only, no earlier than March 1 and no later than three weeks before the start of your trip.

Driving Directions: From Visalia, take Hwy. 198 east for 37 miles to the signed Mineral King junction with eastbound Mineral King Road. Turn onto Mineral King Road and follow the narrow, winding road 23 miles to the Mineral King Ranger Station. Almost all of this road is paved, but it nonetheless takes more than an hour to drive. The Cold Spring Campground is a half mile before the ranger station. Look for parking along Mineral King Road before entering the campground. Marmots can pose a threat to parked cars in the early season; check with the ranger station for the current situation.

35 Hockett Lakes

Trip Data: 11S 350479 4124418; 28 miles; 6/1 days

Topos: *Mineral King, Silver City, Moses Mtn.*

see map on p.146

Highlights: This enjoyable hike takes travelers south to the striking Hockett Plateau; touring stands of pine interspersed with giant sequoia trees and several luxuriant subalpine meadows line the way to quiet and solitude at Hockett Lakes.

DAY 1 (Cold Spring Trailhead to Deer Creek, 4.5 miles): The route leaves the southwest end of Cold Spring Campground following signs for Tar Gap to the obvious trail heading south up the hill. (There is drinking water available at several taps in the campground until the middle of October.) Immediately after leaving the campground, the route climbs moderate switchbacks for about a mile.

After about 500 feet of elevation gain, the trail levels out, heading west, and begins to traverse granite boulders, fording several small branches of Mosquito Creek. In another half mile, the trail fords Mineral Creek and begins a gentle ascent through juniper and red fir trees. Here, dappled sunlight filters through the tall boughs of pine, illuminating brightly colored patches of fern and heather on the forest floor. Shortly thereafter, the forest opens to the north, and expansive vistas of Conifer Ridge and Paradise Peak appear across the valley.

After fording Fowler Creek, the trail again climbs gently and begins to turn toward the southwest. The path continues to climb at intervals over the next 2 miles, lazily angling toward the southwest. There is an obvious point where the trail leaves a dense stand of pine, jogs briefly to the south, and then turns back toward the southwest. Shortly after this jog in the path, and a quarter mile before fording Deer Creek, you'll reach a few fine campsites on the northwest side of the trail under tree cover (8240'; 11S 351240 4033360). Get water from Deer Creek, a quarter mile farther along the trail.

DAY 2 (Deer Creek to Horse Creek, 5.5 miles): After leaving the peaceful campsites behind, the trail comes to fields of tall ferns. A little bushwacking may be required here, but the trail remains plain underfoot. Deer Creek is a welcome sight ahead, cheerily tinkling over boulders as it streams downhill to the north. Once past the ford, the trail continues southwest for another mile before rounding a sharp bend and making a permanent tack toward the south. A truck-sized boulder is an obvious landmark just west of the trail here, a sentinel for this trail section.

The well-defined track continues through stands of pine and fir, with majestic sequoias interspersed among the smaller conifers. There are many charred trunks along this section of trail, evidence of a fire that left remains of these giant trees scattered along the slopes. Clover Creek's ford appears about 1.5 miles after Deer Creek, and Corner Creek lies another half mile down the trail. Although both Clover and Corner creeks may be low in late season, they will provide adequate drinking water.

After fording Corner Creek, the trail descends a final 200 feet on gravel and dirt before reaching the signed junction with the Atwell Mill Trail. Now joined, the trails continue south and then southwest toward Horse Creek, a quarter mile ahead and heard before it can be seen. There are several well-used campsites on the banks of Horse Creek, the majority lying on the east side of the trail (8560´; 11S 351701 4028671). There is also a convenient food-storage system here, consisting of a wire-and-pulley arrangement suspended between two pines, allowing you to hang food in the evening.

DAY 3 (Horse Creek to Hockett Lakes, 4 miles): The ford of Horse Creek lies just south of the campsites (wet in early season). After the ford, the path ascends a gravel wash and then winds and rolls through 1.5 miles of open forest and brush before arriving at the foot of

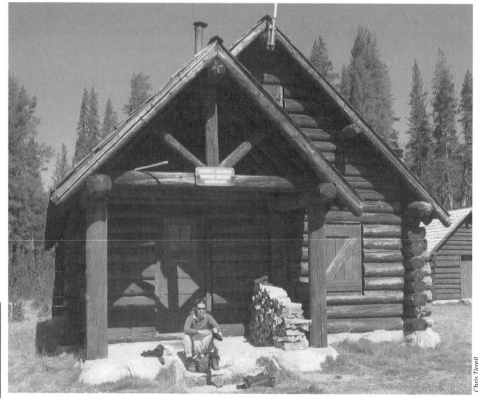

Hockett ranger station

HWY 198

Chris Tirrell

Hockett Meadow. Appearing suddenly from the trees, Hockett Meadow is a lush, open field ringed with pine and sprawling away to the south. Standing in the meadow, you'll enjoy sweeping views of Hengst and White Chief peaks to the northeast and Vandever Mountain to the east.

Whitman Creek enters at the foot of the meadow, and its picturesque banks are lined with colorful wildflowers and shade trees. Meet the trail to Evelyn Lake just before entering Hockett Meadow; continue ahead (south) here on the main trail. Or turn right (northwest) on the Evelyn Lake Trail to find several appealing campsites on Whitman Creek's north bank. There is also a seasonally occupied ranger station at Hockett Meadow.

The path crosses Whitman Creek on a small wooden bridge and ascends stairs to gain a bench just above the meadow. The route meanders through juniper and pine for a mile to reach the signed South Fork Meadow/Hockett Lakes junction. Go right (southwest) here.

Sand Meadows appears in the east, and its short meadow-grass rustles in the wind, giving an illusion of movement to this otherwise placid landscape. The trail reenters open forest and follows a drainage to the signed Sand Meadow/South Fork Crossing junction. Turn right (southwest) and follow this trail, glimpsing the Hockett Lakes through the trees to the north. A lateral heading right (north) to the southernmost Hockett Lake appears shortly. A few scattered campsites lie on the south bank, protected from the wind. It is also possible to find campsites on the east side of the lakes by skirting the southern shore through the dense cover (8574´; 11S 350479 4124418). A layover day here allows exploration of this remote corner of Sequoia National Park.

DAYS 4–6 (Hockett Lakes to Cold Spring Trailhead, 14 miles): Retrace your steps.

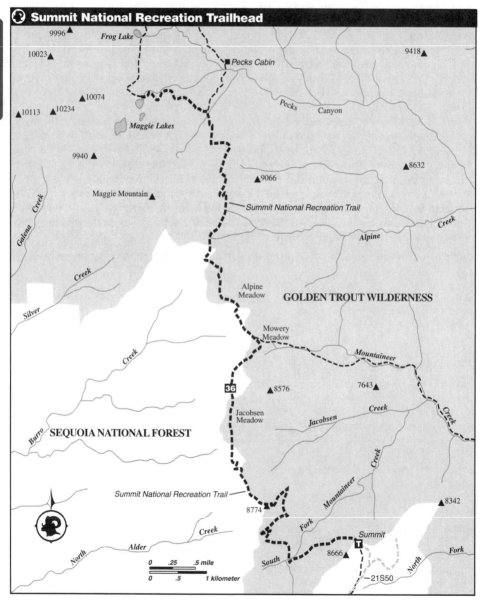

Summit National Recreation Trailhead

Summit National Recreation Trailhead

8296'; 11S 0358157 4008459 (field)

DESTINATION/ UTM COORDINATES	TRIP TYPE	BEST SEASON	PACE (HIKING/ LAYOVER DAYS)	TOTAL MILEAGE
36 Maggie Lakes 11S 358157 4008459	Out & back	Mid to late	4/1 Leisurely	19.8

Information and Permits: This trailhead is in Sequoia National Forest: 900 West Grand Avenue, Porterville, CA 93257, 559-784-1500, www.fs.fed.us/r5/sequoia/. Permits are required for overnight stays; there are no formal quotas, but offices may exercise discretion in issuing permits, refusing if they judge an area is overused at the time.

Driving Directions: From Porterville, go east on Hwy. 190 through Springville, winding slowly up into the southern Sierra almost 28 miles past Springville. Go past the turnoff to Camp Nelson (last chance for gas) and continue toward Quaking Aspen Campground. At 27.9 miles from Springville, or 0.1 mile before (just west of) Quaking Aspen Campground, turn left (northeast) on inconspicuously signed, initially paved Forest Road 21S50. Ignore dirt side roads, even when 21S50 turns to dirt, too. Summit National Recreation Trail crosses or grazes this road several times. Don't be fooled by signs into stopping too soon; your goal is the roadend. At a Y at 4.4 miles, turn left to Summit Trailhead; now the road, still 21S50, is dirt. At the next Y, at 5.5 miles, following signs, go right on 21S50. After a brief paved stretch at 6 miles, the road becomes narrow and rough. At a signed Y at 7.2 miles, go right. At another Y at 7.7 miles, go left on 21S50. At 7.9 miles, go right on 21S50. Soon, the road descends and becomes very rough. There's some improvement when the road levels out. At 9.6 miles at a Y, go left onto what's faintly signed as Forest Road 31F11 but, according to the map, is still 21S50; it's very rough. At 9.9 miles, at the end of the road, find parking and poor signage for Summit National Recreation Trail; the trailhead for Maggie Lakes is on the right (northwest) of the waterless parking lot.

36 Maggie Lakes

Trip Data: 11S 358157 4008459 (field); 19.8 miles; 4/1 days

Topos: *Camp Nelson, Quinn Peak*

Highlights: Cool, deep fir forest alternates with

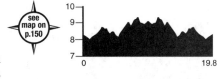

marvelous meadows on the way to the lovely, peaceful Maggie Lakes, a bit of High Sierra beauty in this largely lakeless southern Sierra landscape.

HEADS UP! *Maps show a number of trails intersecting Summit National Recreation Trail, but years of neglect has left many of them almost invisible or impassable or both. It's tempting to make this a loop trip, but that "loop" may be very hard to find and follow.*

DAY 1 (Summit National Recreation Trailhead to Mowery Meadow, 5 miles): Head north, briefly through scrub, soon curving west into moderate to dense fir forest on gradually descending, dusty trail. The trail becomes unpleasantly rocky just before it descends abruptly to South Fork Mountaineer Creek, just below two tributaries that nourish a wonderful hillside meadow just left (west) of the trail. Ford the creek and climb steeply away, leveling out and heading north near a lovely meadow on the east (right). Soon the track leaves the meadow behind and begins climbing gradually on long switchbacks up a densely forested ridge, just missing the ridge's high point but breaking into the clear shortly thereafter. Here, there are marvelous views west down the mountains' intricately folded slopes to the Central Valley and north toward the true High Sierra.

Leaving the viewpoint, descend across a long, open saddle before veering back into dense forest and dropping on long, gradual, sometimes rocky switchbacks to a junction with largely vanished Jacobsen Trail. Continue ahead (north) here to skirt large, flowery Jacobsen Meadow, where there's a signed "fire safe" campsite just off the trail. This is Sequoia National Forest's way of showing that with a California Campfire Permit, a campfire is legal here. As with other meadowside campsites in this area, search for water in the meadow, possibly downstream along the creek that flows out of it.

Continue along the gently undulating trail for another 1.25 miles to a hard-to-spot junction (8127´; 11S 356303 4012024) with a poorly signed, faint trail right (east) toward Mowery Meadow and down Mountaineer Creek. About 150 yards down this trail—interrupted by a great deal of deadfall—is a pleasant, fire-safe campsite at beautiful Mowery Meadow. Find water well downstream here. This is a good choice for small parties to break their journey; larger parties should continue to Alpine Meadow, another half mile away (see the first part of Day 2).

DAY 2 (Mowery Meadow to Maggie Lakes, 4.9 miles): Shortly after the Mowery junction, the trail begins climbing generally northwest and steeply—the only sustained steep climb on this trip, with a relatively level section in the middle of the climb. The ascent leads to a forested ridgetop where the trail levels, following the ridge for a short distance before reaching the upper end of Alpine Meadow on the left (east) (8465´; 11S 356089 4012574).

CAMPING AT ALPINE MEADOW

This is a popular camping area for youth groups and equestrians. If you intend to camp here, look for a use trail eastward and follow it about 150 yards to the first and largest of three close-together campsites on dry "islands" in the meadow. These are heavily used, fire-safe sites with picnic tables that are somewhat to very dilapidated. The meadow's stream conveniently winds between the first two "islands."

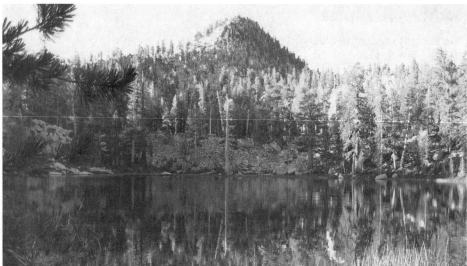

Kathy Morey

Lower Maggie Lake

From Alpine Meadow's edge, stay on Summit National Recreation Trail and climb past a large hillside meadow. Presently reach a junction on the left (west) with the vanished Griswold Trail; on the right (east) is lovely Griswold Meadow, with a fire-safe campsite. Get water here for the climb ahead; the next reliable water is more than 2 miles away.

Continue ahead (generally north) past bouldery outcrops to begin a shady, gradual-to-moderate climb of Maggie Mountain's northeast shoulder. (Peakbaggers may want to add the trailless, 10,042-foot summit to their lists.) From the trail's high point, make a moderate, rocky descent to ford a tributary of Pecks Canyon's creek. Just beyond the ford, there's a signed junction where Summit National Recreation Trail branches left (initially west, then northwest) to the Maggie Lakes.

Head for the Maggie Lakes on this winding, up-and-down, often rocky track that finally leads up a flower-dotted rockfall, across the top of a meadow, and then over the Maggie Lakes' outlet to Lower Maggie Lake's north shore (9060'; 11S 354494 4016101). Here, there are good but well-used campsites under scattered lodgepoles—sites with fine views across the lake to a handsome little peak to the south that blocks Maggie Mountain from view. Unlike the forest and meadow country the route has passed through to get here, these lakes certainly have the "feel" of the High Sierra. Fishing at the lakes for golden trout is reportedly excellent.

A use trail begins a few yards west of the lake, before the main trail has climbed entirely out of Lower Maggie Lake's basin. The use trail crosses the lake's marshy inlet area and winds to the upper lake; about halfway up, it passes a spur left (southeast) toward the second lake (the spur peters out near that lake). The upper lake also has campsites, but deadfall along the shoreline can be a nuisance.

Days 3–4 (Maggie Lakes to Summit National Recreation Trailhead, 9.9 miles): Retrace your steps.

HWY 190

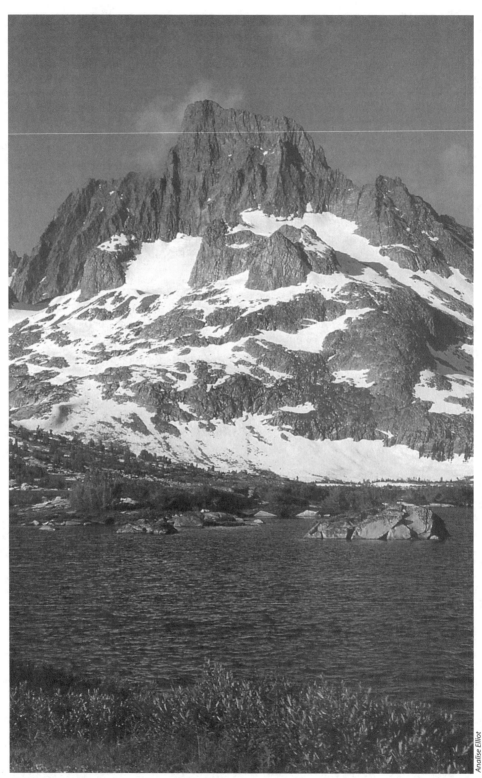

INTRODUCTION TO THE EAST SIDE

US Hwy. 395, which roughly parallels the Sierra's tall eastern escarpment, is the major road from which you take the lesser roads to starting trailheads. These drives start at 4000 to 7000 feet (or more!), they are typically short compared to west-side drives, and they are very scenic. A few shuttle trips end at roads not listed below. Small, charming towns along Hwy. 395 provide lodging, gas, and stores.

On the east side, you'll enter the Sierra on these roads and highways:

Horse Meadow Road (just east of Yosemite and south of State Hwy. 120)

State Hwy. 158 (the June Lakes Loop)

State Hwy. 203 (through Mammoth Lakes)

McGee Creek Road (between Mammoth Lakes and Bishop)

Rock Creek Road (also between Mammoth Lakes and Bishop)

State Hwy. 168 East Side (through Bishop)

Glacier Lodge Road (through Big Pine)

Sawmill Creek Road (between Big Pine and Independence)

Onion Valley Road (through Independence)

Whitney Portal Road (through Lone Pine)

Horseshoe Meadow Road (also through Lone Pine)

Kennedy Meadows Road (between Olancha and Pearsonville; unlike the other east-side roads, this is a long drive)

opposite: **The jagged skyline of Banner Peak rises above Thousand Island Lake (Trip 39).**

HORSE MDW

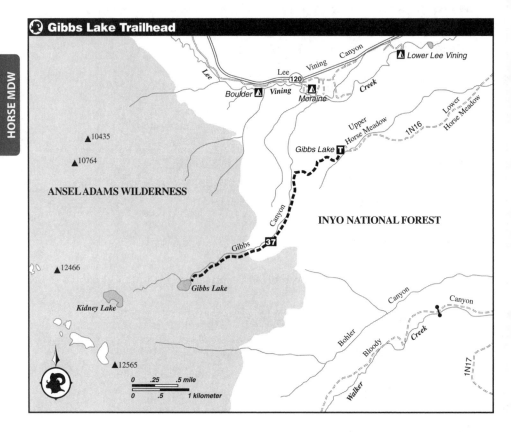

Gibbs Lake Trailhead

Lower Lee Vining

Lee Vining Canyon

Lee Vining

120

Boulder   Vining   Moraine

Creek

Upper Horse Meadow

Lower Horse Meadow

1N16

Gibbs Lake   T

▲10435

▲10764

ANSEL ADAMS WILDERNESS

Canyon

INYO NATIONAL FOREST

▲12466

Gibbs   37

Gibbs Lake

Kidney Lake

Canyon   Canyon

Bohler   Bloody   Creek

▲12565

1N17

0   .25   .5 mile

0   .5   1 kilometer

Walker

HORSE MEADOW ROAD TRIP

Gibbs Lake Trailhead

7953'; 11S 310792 4199130

DESTINATION/ UTM COORDINATES	TRIP TYPE	BEST SEASON	PACE (HIKING/ LAYOVER DAYS)	TOTAL MILEAGE
37 Gibbs Lake 11S 308113 4196978	Out & back	Mid to late	2/1 Leisurely	6.6

Information and Permits: This trailhead is in Inyo National Forest: 351 Pacu Lane, Suite 200, Bishop, CA 93514, 760-873-2400, www.fs.fed.us/r5/inyo/. Quotas apply, and permits are required for overnight stays and are available at Inyo National Forest ranger stations in Lone Pine, Bishop, Mammoth Lakes, and Mono Basin Scenic Area Visitors Center.

Driving Directions: You'll need a high-clearance 4WD vehicle to get all the way to the trailhead on this road. Nerves of steel help, too. Without such a vehicle, stop at the west end of Lower Horse Meadow, park off the road as best you can, and walk the rest of the way (1.2 miles).

From its northern junction with Hwy. 158 (June Lakes Loop), take Hwy. 395 for 3.1 miles north to the unsigned turnoff for Horse Meadow Road, the road to this trailhead. (The junction is also 1.2 miles south of Hwy. 395's junction with westbound Hwy. 120, also known as Tioga Road, from Yosemite.) Turn west onto this dirt road and follow it toward the mountains in spite of the huge number of intersecting roads. Horse Meadow Road immediately intersects another dirt road and then passes between tumbledown buildings on Native American tribal land. After climbing, the road skirts large Lower Horse Meadow on its north side. You may have to find parking at this meadow's far (west) end, about 2.1 miles from Hwy. 395.

If your car is up to the next stretch, which can be nerve-racking, continue up the narrow, steep, deeply rutted road and presently skirt Upper Horse Meadow on its south side before curving right (north) around its west end, dipping through a grove of trees, and meeting one and then another rough dirt road that climbs west to parking at the trailhead. Take either; the second one may be less chewed-up. The drive is a total of 3.3 miles; the trail begins at the lot's northwest edge, where a locked gate bars vehicles.

37 Gibbs Lake

Trip Data: 11S 308113 4196978; 6.6 miles; 2/1 days

Topos: *Mount Dana*

Highlights: The destination of this trip is a little-known lake in Ansel Adams Wilderness on the dramatic east slope of the Sierra, just east of Yosemite. It's a great place to find peace and quiet, and for serious anglers, there is a chance to catch some beautiful golden trout.

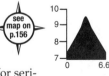

see map on p.156

HEADS UP! Don't forget that if your car can't make it to the trailhead and you must park at Lower Horse Meadows, the hike to Gibbs Lake will be 1.2 miles longer (4.5 miles).

DAY 1 (Gibbs Lake Trailhead to Gibbs Lake, 3.3 miles): Circumvent the gate and climb steeply up an old road on a north-trending ridge. Forest cover permitting, there may be over-the-shoulder views of Mono Lake here and there. Beyond a gentle dip, continue the steep climb, walking through mixed forest. The road levels out near a ruined flume; cross the flume and pick up a footpath on the left as the road ends on the right.

Climb to a ridge above Gibbs Canyon's unnamed creek and then leave the ridge to trudge up a dry wash lined with stunted aspens. At nearly 1.6 miles, the trail levels out on a dry shoulder offering views of Mt. Dana and Mt. Gibbs to the west-southwest. Back under forest cover, the path more or less parallels the creek and, at 2.5 miles, reaches the signed border of Ansel Adams Wilderness, where the creek is bright with currant, Labrador tea, and fragrant red heather.

The remaining climb is gradual to moderate until just before the lake there's a brief, steep climb to the outlet (9530´; 11S 308113 4196978). There are fair-to-good campsites south of the outlet and west of the inlet.

KIDNEY LAKE

Above and west of Gibbs Lake lies Kidney Lake (10,388´; 11S 306856 4196779). Adventurous hikers will find an easy if steep route to Kidney Lake up the forested south side of Gibbs Lake's inlet stream, and the expansive views of Mono Lake and the mountains around it are worth the climb. Most of the shore of Kidney Lake is barren, but some whitebark pines at the east end provide shelter for a Spartan camp.

DAY 2 (Gibbs Lake to Gibbs Lake Trailhead, 3.3 miles): Retrace your steps to the trailhead.

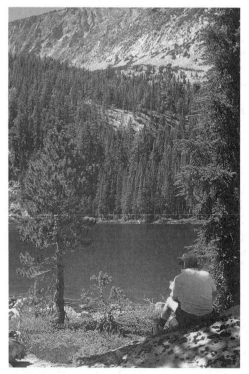

At Gibbs Lake

Rush Creek Trailhead

7220´; 11S 312464 4183408

DESTINATION/ UTM COORDINATES	TRIP TYPE	BEST SEASON	PACE (HIKING/ LAYOVER DAYS)	TOTAL MILEAGE
38 Thousand Island Lake-Rush Creek 11S 308650 4177836	Semiloop	Early to mid	3/1 Moderate	21

Information and Permits: This trailhead is in Inyo National Forest: 351 Pacu Lane, Suite 200, Bishop, CA 93514, 760-873-2400, www.fs.fed.us/r5/inyo/. Quotas apply, and permits are required for overnight stays and are available at Inyo National Forest ranger stations in Lone Pine, Bishop, Mammoth Lakes, and Mono Basin Scenic Area Visitors Center.

Driving Directions: Take Hwy. 395 to the June Lake Junction at the intersection of Hwy. 158 that is about 10 miles south of Hwy. 395's junction with Hwy. 120 (Tioga Road). This is the more southerly of the two junctions of Hwy. 158 with Hwy. 395. At the junction, take Hwy. 158 (the June Lakes Loop) toward the mountains and through June Lake Village to the northeast end of Silver Lake (7.3 miles from June Lake Junction). The trailhead is on the west side of the road between Frontier Pack Station and a mobile-home park. There are toilets, water, and a trailhead host/information kiosk. The trailhead host does not issue permits. Stop to show the host your permit; if you do not, the host is likely to find you and demand it.

HWY 158

38 Thousand Island Lake-Rush Creek

Trip Data: 11S 308650 4177836; 21 miles; 3/1 days

Topos: *Devils Postpile, Koip Peak, Mt. Ritter*

Highlights: Although this trip can be made in a weekend, the unforgettable scenery—from splendid Thousand Island Lake to the intimate

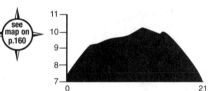

little Clark Lakes—warrants a slower pace. The biggest challenge may be deciding in which splendid spot to spend the layover day; perhaps the trip needs more layover days!

HEADS UP! Camping is prohibited within a quarter mile of Thousand Island Lake's outlet. Bears are very serious problems here.

DAY 1 (Rush Creek Trailhead to Waugh Lake, 7 miles): The rough, rocky, and heavily stock-traveled Rush Creek Trail begins at the Rush Creek Trailhead parking lot (7220´). Head west, cross a bridge over Alger Creek, bear left (south), and step across a tributary of Alger Creek. Leaving the aspen-lined creek, the route begins a long, steady, shadeless ascent south away from Silver Lake. At first, several use trails dart downslope toward Silver Lake Resort. Beyond, it's simply a long, moderate, uphill slog with good views.

At a juniper-shaded switchback turn and look for the long, white ribbon of Rush Creek dashing down to the Southern California Edison buildings below (upcoming Agnew, Gem, and Waugh lakes are dammed for power). Continuing, the trail has been blasted out of the rock; tall, poured-concrete "steps" hold the tread in place. Twice, the trail crosses the tracks of a cable railway (funicular) used to haul personnel and material to the dams on Rush Creek; watch for moving cars and stay off the tracks.

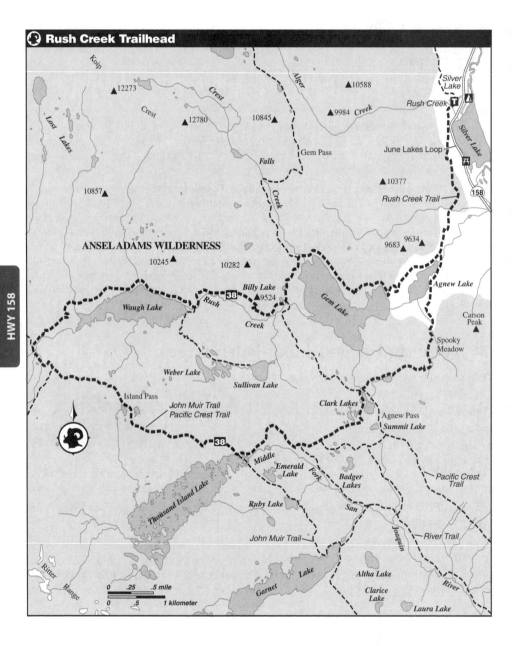

HWY 158

The trail bears right to begin another exposed series of switchbacks before briefly passing Agnew's dam and a signed junction (8466´) to Clark Lake, where hikers will close the loop part of this trip on Day 3. The return trail on the other side of the lake looks like a pencil line sketched across the rocky slope. Go right (southwest) at this junction and climb high above Agnew Lake (no campsites; there are some poor campsites back near the junction, below Agnew's dam).

The trail soon tops out at a knob above beautiful Gem Lake, and, from there, the track dips down to the shoreline. Next, hikers enjoy a long, undulating stroll along the lake's east and north shores (9058´). Eventually, the trail crosses Crest Creek (one of Gem's inlets), beyond which is the signed junction with the trail north to Alger Lakes. There are poor-to-fair campsites nearby on the lakeshore—about the only campsites at Gem.

Go ahead (south-southwest) to stay the Rush Creek Trail, which quickly climbs away from Gem Lake and then descends past a couple of tiny lakes. At the signed junction with another trail to the Clark Lakes, turn right (west) toward Waugh Lake. A circuitous, rocky climb brings hikers to Rush Creek. In a very marshy area where the creek broadens and slows, there are two huge packer campsites.

Beyond, the trail begins a final, stony climb to Waugh Lake, passing the lateral to Weber Lake; go ahead (west). Soon, the trail reaches the dam at the outlet of Waugh Lake (9442´; 307723 4180438). Campsites near the trail are poor and few until the trail is almost abreast of some granite islets near the west end of the lake, and there are more sites beyond here. Mt. Davis dominates the western skyline from here.

DAY 2 (Waugh Lake to Thousand Island Lake, 6.5 miles): The trail along the Waugh Lake's northwest shore passes through beautiful lodgepole pines to a wet ford of Lost Lakes' outlet. Now climb steeply away from Waugh Lake. As the grade eases, cross two forks of Rush Creek, the first on an impressive log bridge and the second by a wet ford. Just beyond the second ford, find the junction of the Rush Creek Trail and PCT/JMT. There are campsites in this vicinity (9607´).

Turn left (southeast) toward Island Pass; right goes northwest to Donohue Pass and into Yosemite. Begin a steady ascent under a continuing forest cover of lodgepole and mountain hemlock. Passing a junction (9677´) with a faint trail right (south-southwest) to Davis Lakes, climb ahead (southeast) to Island Pass (10,200´). Just south of this pass, the trail skirts two small lakes (locally called Ham and Eggs lakes; campsites) and then veers eastward. The views from this relatively low pass are magnificent.

Now descending, the trail emerges from dense stands of lodgepole and hemlock (the latter easily identified by their droopy tips) to a metamorphic slope above Thousand Island Lake.

VIEWS AND GEOLOGY NEAR THOUSAND ISLAND LAKE

Savor the panoramic views from the rocky slopes, and notice the striking differences between the predominantly darker rock of the Ritter Range and the lighter granite of the Sierra Crest's peaks. Geologically, the Ritter Range is made up of older rocks, originally volcanic in nature, and the spectacularly jagged skyline from Banner Peak southward has been captured in many a photo.

As the trail switchbacks down to the outlet of Thousand Island Lake, there are classic views across the island-studded waters to the imposing east faces of Banner Peak and Mt. Ritter. Shortly before the outlet, reach a junction where the PCT and JMT temporarily diverge (9865´). A few more steps on the JMT bring hikers to a junction (9836´; 11S 308650 4177836) with a use trail that branches right (southwest) through a no-camping zone to campsites on Thousand Island Lake's north shore. Read and follow all regulations posted here. Now take this trail along the lakeshore; the campsites get better the farther you go

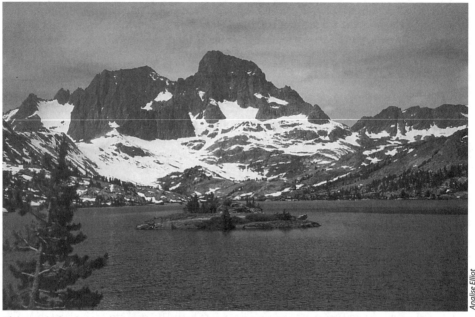

Analise Elliot

Thousand Island Lake sits in a broad basin nestled under massive Banner Peak.

toward the head of the lake, where the scenery is some of the most memorable in the central Sierra, and Indian paintbrush carpets summer's meadows. There are almost no acceptable campsites along the lake's southeast shore.

DAY 3 (Thousand Island Lake to Rush Creek Trailhead, 7.5 miles): Return to the junction where the PCT and JMT diverge and take the PCT northeast (9865'). Pass several attractive tarns before curving southeast and downhill. The trail swings east to a junction (9635') with the River Trail right (southeast) to Agnew Meadows. Continue ahead (left, northeast) on the PCT and climb to a little bench with another junction (9643'). Here, the left fork goes ahead (northeast) toward the Clark Lakes.

Take the left fork, ascending steeply through lodgepoles to cross the Sierra Crest at an unsigned, unnamed pass. Looking back, view the San Joaquin River's canyon, with the Minarets crowning the far ridge, and Ritter and Banner closer on the right. Directly below are the Badger Lakes.

After an extremely steep but short descent, pass three small Clark Lakes (9810'), one of which is guarded by a sheer and beautiful rock wall. The descent continues along the west side of the largest Clark Lake, where windswept grass and wild onion border the west end of this lake. There are a number of good campsites scattered around these lovely lakes. For a more leisurely trip, stop here.

At the outflow of the largest lake, there is a junction (9820'): The left (northwest) branch descends to Gem Lake; the right (southwest) one skirts Clark Lakes on their east side and leads up over Agnew Pass to the High Trail and thence to Agnew Meadows. This trip's route is the middle branch (northeast), which ascends to a tarn that hosts a poor campsite and a signed junction with a spur trail hard right (southwest) toward Agnew Pass—seemingly straight into the face of Banner Peak. Go left (ahead, east-northeast), skirting the tarn through a volcanic landscape and climbing a little to a second, much smaller tarn with a good campsite on the opposite side of the trail (9930').

Continue climbing, skirting a meadow with views of Gem Lake below on the left and briefly of Mono Lake ahead in the distance; dark Negit Island is prominent. The climb is almost over, and hikers top one last shoulder before descending moderately, then steeply, through the beautiful meadow and woodland at the foot of Spooky Meadow, nestled in a deep cirque on Carson Peak's west side.

The trail crosses Spooky Meadow's stream (9430′) once by a campsite and then again shortly after beginning a long, steep, loose, rocky descent to the next lower meadow, where the grade eases briefly at streamside amid stands of lodgepoles and mountain hemlocks. Soon the trail plunges down again, leaving Ansel Adams Wilderness and crossing the stream for the last time as it descends a narrow, rocky canyon. Early in this descent there are surprising views of Gem Lake, impossibly blue and barely constrained by its thin, shell-like dam. Below it, Agnew Lake is a long, green pool backed by reddish slopes, across which the Rush Creek Trail that you began on seems a mere scratch.

Next, the trail exits the canyon and continues downward gradually to moderately on switchbacks in and out of aspen and hemlock, occasionally dipping into cool nooks where moisture-loving wildflowers flourish. At the bottom of the switchbacks, descend moderately on the rocky "pencil line" trail noted on Day 1.

The descent ends in lodgepole and western white pine, and hikers climb steeply up a knob, around a gully, and past a fine picnic spot under a mature, forked lodgepole.

A brief, very stony descent takes you to a bridge over the dam's primary outlet and then to a much smaller bridge over another stream. In early season, there may be a third braid. The trail leads up to the flat on which some Southern California Edison buildings sit. This area is the last chance for campsites and water before the trailhead.

Now cross the funicular tracks and pick up a rocky lateral that climbs to meet the Rush Creek Trail. Here, close the loop part of this trip, turn right (northeast) toward Silver Lake and Reversed Peak, and retrace the first part of Day 1.

HWY 158

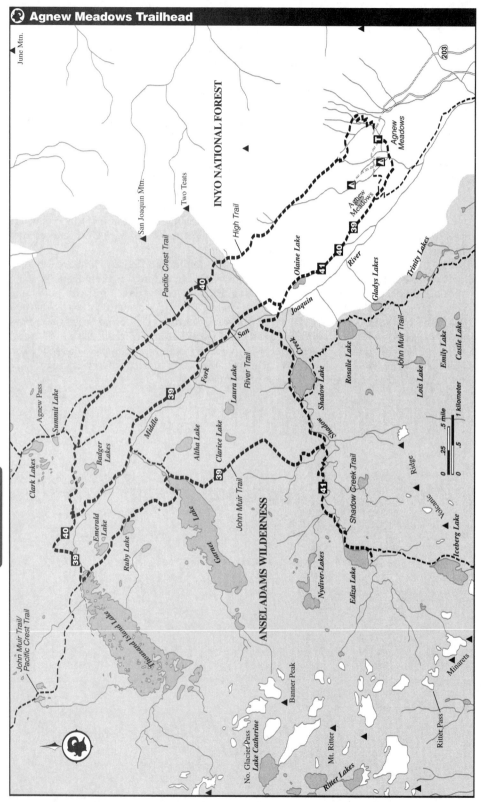

Agnew Meadows Trailhead

8325'; 11S 315496 4172684

DESTINATION/ UTM COORDINATES	TRIP TYPE	BEST SEASON	PACE (HIKING/ LAYOVER DAYS)	TOTAL MILEAGE
39 Thousand Island Lake-JMT 11S 308650 4177836	Semiloop	Mid to late	2/1 Moderate	17.6
40 Thousand Island Lake-PCT 11S 308650 4177836	Loop	Mid to late	2/1 Moderate	17.6
41 Ediza Lake 11S 309131 4173295	Out & back	Mid to late	2/1 Moderate	14

Information and Permits: This trailhead is in Inyo National Forest: 351 Pacu Lane, Suite 200, Bishop, CA 93514, 760-873-2400, www.fs.fed.us/r5/inyo/. Quotas apply, and permits are required for overnight stays and are available at Inyo National Forest ranger stations in Lone Pine, Bishop, Mammoth Lakes, and Mono Basin Scenic Area Visitors Center.

Driving Directions: From the intersection of Hwy. 395 and Hwy. 203 (the Mammoth junction), drive 3.8 miles west on Hwy. 203 through the town of Mammoth Lakes. At the second traffic light, with Minaret Road (also Hwy. 203), turn right onto Minaret Road and go 4.2 miles farther to the main lodge of Mammoth Mountain Ski Area. Here you will have to park your car and take a shuttle bus (fee), unless you arrive before or after operating hours or qualify for certain exceptions (contact the Mammoth Lakes ranger station for current regulations). Get off at the Agnew Meadows stop and walk about a quarter mile farther north on the dirt road, past a pack station and a trailhead for the northbound PCT on the right, and then about 100 yards farther to the roadend parking lot.

Or, if timing permits driving your own car, continue up Hwy. 203 to Minaret Summit for 1.4 miles. Go 2.7 miles past Minaret Summit down the narrow, mostly one-lane road into the Devils Postpile area and find the turnoff to Agnew Meadows on the right at the switchback turn. Turn right here and drive the quarter mile down this dirt road, past a pack station and a trailhead for the northbound PCT, to the roadend parking lot.

The starting trailhead for this trip, for the southbound PCT, the JMT, and the River Trail (your initial route), is on the south edge of this parking lot (toilets, water).

Note: In this area, between Thousand Island Lake on the north and Devils Postpile on the south, the JMT and PCT do not coincide. From Thousand Island Lake, the JMT stays west of Middle Fork San Joaquin. The PCT (also called the High Trail here) climbs and

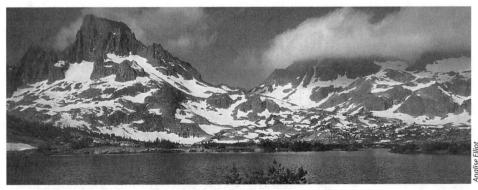

Jagged Banner Peak from the shore of Thousand Island Lake

Andlise Elliot

traverses the south side of San Joaquin Ridge, east of the river, before dropping to the river through Agnew Meadows and crossing it near Soda Springs Campground. The trails reunite just north of Devils Postpile.

39 Thousand Island Lake-JMT

Trip Data: 11S 308650 4177836; 17.6 miles; 2/1 days

Topos: *Mammoth Mountain, Mt. Ritter*

Highlights: Thousand Island Lake, with its numerous granite islands, is set in a broad, barren basin and backdropped by massive Banner Peak. This

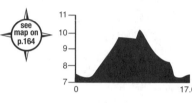

very popular area is a favorite of photographers and naturalists alike for its superlative scenery and dayhiking opportunities.

HEADS UP! *Camping is prohibited within a quarter mile of Thousand Island Lake's outlet. Bears are very serious problems here.*

DAY 1 (Agnew Meadows Trailhead to Thousand Island Lake, 7.1 miles): The route begins by heading south over a couple of little fords before curving west-northwest to pass a fenced meadow. The trail goes another half mile to a fork whose left branch is a connector to the PCT.

Continue straight ahead (northwest) to descend a dry, sun-exposed slope blanketed in chaparral. At the bottom of this descent, pass another connector trail to the PCT on the left as this trip continues straight ahead (northwest) and skirts the northeast shore of Olaine Lake (8070´). Just beyond the lake and 2 miles from the trailhead, the path meets a junction (8085´) with the trail ascending to Shadow and Ediza lakes (see Trip 41).

Go right (northwest) on the River Trail, make a switchback, and walk gradually to moderately uphill under dense lodgepole and fir, with Middle Fork San Joaquin River bubbling along on your left (southwest). Over the next few miles, there are occasional poor-to-fair campsites between the trail and the river. Numerous streams crease San Joaquin Ridge, above your trail on the right (north), and the trail fords several of them.

Presently, the path comes to a signed junction with a spur trail to the PCT, here also known as the High Trail (9020´): left (west) toward Thousand Island Lake; right (east) toward the Badger Lakes and the PCT. Go left, staying on the River Trail, and curve northwest and then west. Shortly beyond, there's a junction with a lateral going left (southwest) across the river to Garnet Lake and the JMT. Continue ahead (northwest) here.

At the next junction, with the PCT, turn left (west, soon curving northwest) toward Thousand Island Lake. Passing several snowmelt tarns, the trail reaches the meadow-lined outlet of Thousand Island Lake (9836´; 11S 308650 4177836) and a junction with the JMT (9865´): right (northwest) to Island Pass; left (southeast) to cross the lake's outlet on a footbridge; ahead (west) on a use trail along the lake's northwest shore. Read and observe all local regulations at this junction, including the no-camping area.

Go ahead, following the use trail along the lakeshore. The campsites get better the farther you go toward the head of the lake. There are almost no acceptable campsites along the lake's southeast shore.

GARNET LAKE

A layover day would permit an adventurous, part cross-country, looping dayhike to Garnet Lake via the obvious saddle that's the low point (10,100´) on the ridge to the southeast. Return on the JMT, past Ruby and Emerald lakes, reversing part of Day 2.

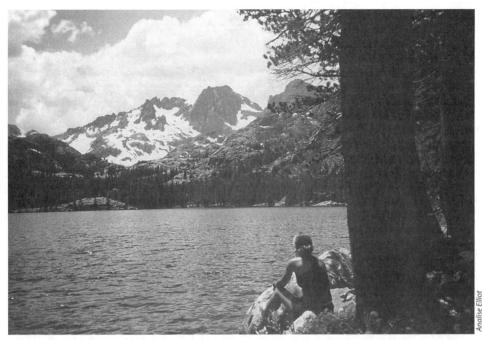

Shadow Lake is a no-camping zone, but it offers one of the Sierra's most spectacular scenic vistas.

DAY 2 (Thousand Island Lake to Agnew Meadows Trailhead, 10.5 miles): Return to the JMT and turn right (southeast) to cross the bridge over the outlet. Following the JMT, pass first Emerald Lake (9865′) and its neighboring tarn and then the more strikingly sapphire and picturesque Ruby Lake (9910′).

The trail descends to and then traces Garnet's east shore, crossing its outlet on a rickety bridge and passing the invisible junction with the lateral from the River Trail, before climbing some 500 feet to a saddle (10,105′) with a little tarn. From here, the trail drops 1100 rocky, dusty feet, mostly in forest, to Shadow Creek. Pass potential campsites on this descent; however, the area may be dry by late season. Just before Shadow Creek, a flat along the JMT offers a campsite or two.

Down in Shadow Creek's canyon, the trail reaches a junction (9055′): right (generally west) up Shadow Creek to Ediza Lake (Trip 41); left (northeast) on the JMT down Shadow Creek to Shadow Lake. Read and observe all posted regulations for this area; camping is prohibited due to severe overuse.

Follow the JMT as it descends along Shadow Creek toward Shadow Lake (also no camping). At a junction just before the lake, the JMT turns right to cross the lake's inlet. This trip's route continues ahead (east) along the lake's north shore and, beyond the lake, begins sunny, rocky, dusty, incredibly scenic switchbacks that drop nearly 700 feet along the thundering cascades of Shadow Creek as it plunges to join Middle Fork San Joaquin River below.

Cross the turbulent river on a stout footbridge and pass a packer campsite before reaching the signed junction with the River Trail (Day 1's route). Turn right (southeast) here and retrace your steps of Day 1 past Olaine Lake to the trailhead (8325′; 11S 315496 4172684).

40 Thousand Island Lake-PCT

Trip Data: 11S 308650 4177836; 17.6 miles;
2/1 days

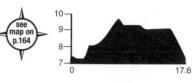

Topos: *Mammoth Mountain, Mt. Ritter*

Highlights: Very scenic and justly popular Thous-
and Island Lake is your destination. On the return,
enjoy the magnificent views from and flower gardens of the PCT (High Trail).

*HEADS UP! Camping is prohibited within a quarter mile of Thousand Island Lake's outlet. Bears are
very serious problems here.*

DAY 1 (Agnew Meadows Trailhead to Thousand Island Lake, 7.1 miles): *(Recap: Trip 39, Day
1.)* Go south and then west to a fork; continue straight ahead (northwest) to descend and,
at the bottom, pass another connector trail to the PCT. Go straight ahead (northwest) and
skirt Olaine Lake (8070´) to a junction (8085´) with the trail ascending to Shadow and Ediza
lakes (see Trip 41).

Turn right (northwest) on the River Trail, make a switchback, and ascend with Middle
Fork San Joaquin River on your left (southwest), fording several small streams from San
Joaquin Ridge above. At the next junction, go left (west-northwest) toward Thousand
Island Lake and soon find a junction with a lateral going left (southwest) across the river
to Garnet Lake and the JMT. Continue ahead (northwest) here.

At the next junction, with the PCT, turn left (west, soon curving northwest) toward
Thousand Island Lake to the lake's outlet (9836´; 11S 308650 4177836) and a junction with
the JMT (9865´). Read and observe all local regulations at this junction, including the no-
camping area. Ahead, take the use trail along the lake's north shore. The campsites get better the farther you go toward the head of the lake. There are almost no acceptable
campsites along the lake's southeast shore.

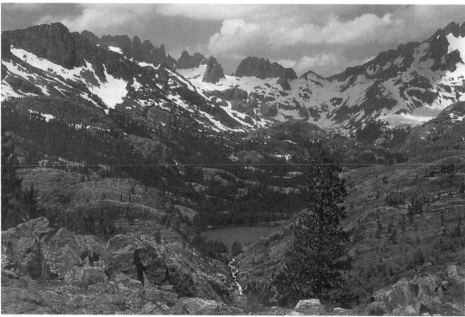

From the High Trail, Shadow Lake appears impossibly blue under the Ritter Range.

DAY 2 (Thousand Island Lake to Agnew Meadows Trailhead, 10.5 miles): Return to the JMT junction at the lake's outlet (9865´) and then go ahead (northeast and then southeast), retracing Day 1's steps to the PCT (High Trail)-River Trail junction.

Turn left (east) on the PCT, begin climbing moderately, and shortly reach the next junction (9690´): right (east, then southeast) on the High Trail to the Badger Lakes and Agnew Meadows; left (east-northeast) to the Clark Lakes and Rush Creek Trailhead. Go right on the High Trail, through lodgepole pine stands and past an unsigned lateral right (southwest) to mosquito-haven Badger Lakes (poor to fair camping). Stay on the High Trail here.

Emerging from dense forest, the trail winds up and down through a ground cover that, except for a few scattered stands of pine, is sagebrush, bitterbrush, willow, and some mountain alder. Go ahead (east and then southeast) on the High Trail at the three junctions in the mile beyond the Badger Lakes turnoff (the lateral right to the River Trail and a couple of spurs left and upslope to Summit Lake and Agnew Pass). Although the 7.5´ topo shows the PCT going to Summit Lake, in fact, it does not. You'll stay on it by following this trip's directions.

The High Trail then contours along the southwest side of San Joaquin Mountain, where slopes are fragrant with sage and slashed by streams that support a colorful tapestry of wildflowers: larkspur, lupine, shooting star, columbine, penstemon, monkeyflower, scarlet gilia, and tiger lily. Views are excellent of the Ritter Range to the west, particularly Garnet Lake and its long, cascading outlet and the notched view of Shadow Lake directly across the San Joaquin River canyon.

The trail then loses its cross-canyon views as it descends through a forest of pine and massive red fir. Five hundred feet of well-graded switchbacks bring hikers to the parking lot north of the pack station. Turn right (west) on the road that runs by the pack station and follow it a short distance farther to the parking lot (8325´; 11S 315496 4172684).

41 Ediza Lake

Trip Data: 11S 309131 4173295; 14 miles; 2/1 days

Topos: *Mammoth Mountain, Mt. Ritter*

Highlights: If we had to pick a favorite hike in the 2 million acres that encompass Inyo National Forest, the jaunt to Ediza Lake would be at the top of the list. Its

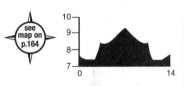

alpine scenery is so spectacular you will wish for one more layover day to explore surrounding peaks, fish, swim, and appreciate the awe that Ansel Adams experienced while photographing this inspiring wilderness now named in his honor.

DAY 1 (Agnew Meadows Trailhead to Ediza Lake, 7 miles): Go south and then west to a fork; continue straight ahead (northwest) to descend and, at the bottom, pass another connector trail to the PCT. Go straight ahead (northwest) and skirt Olaine Lake (8070´) to a junction (8085´) with the trail ascending to Shadow and Ediza lakes.

Turn left (west-southwest) through aspens, shortly arriving at a bridge over Middle Fork San Joaquin River. Cross the bridge, leave the river, hike briefly south, and then begin a 700-foot climb up juniper- and sagebrush-studded slopes beside cascading Shadow Creek.

Past the last beautiful cascade, arrive at Shadow Lake through a notch in the heavily glaciated, metavolcanic rocks. Shadow Lake (8755´), 3.5 miles from the trailhead, is closed to all overnight camping but makes a great dayhiking destination. Read and follow all regulations posted to protect this very overused area. The trail continues southwest along Shadow Lake's north shore to a junction with the JMT by a bridge over the inlet.

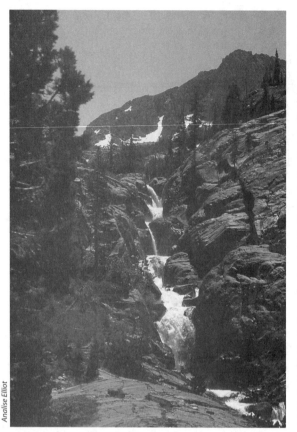

Go ahead (southwest) on the JMT for a mile, ascending near rushing Shadow Creek. Numerous deep holes in the smooth, sun-baked granite slabs are ideal for fishing, swimming, and lounging. No camping is allowed between Shadow Creek and the trail. At the next junction, the JMT branches north toward Thousand Island Lake, while this trip continues upstream (ahead, west) near Shadow Creek for 1.5 miles farther. Climb high into subalpine stands of lodgepole and mountain hemlock and to the outlet of Ediza Lake (9320′; 11S 309131 4173295), from whose west side jut dark, jagged peaks of the Ritter Range.

To get to the legal campsites on the lake's west end, go around the south side, which has the more established trail. (The north-side route is shorter, but much of the trail's tread was obliterated by rockslides and now requires extensive boulder-hopping.) Ediza Lake makes a fine base for exploring the basin above.

Andlise Elliot

Shadow Creek plunges 700 feet through a narrow gorge.

OPTIONAL CROSS-COUNTRY SHUTTLE

Experienced cross-country hikers can turn this trip into a scenic shuttle by returning via Minaret Lake and exiting at Devils Postpile instead of retracing their steps. This route is approximately 3 miles long but because it is very rough, it generally takes a day. Follow an unmaintained route from the southeast corner of Ediza Lake to Iceberg Lake. From Iceberg Lake's outlet (9790′), follow the faint tread along the eastern shore and ascend talus slopes to Cecile Lake's outlet (10,240′). This stretch may be impassable until late season due to steep, icy slopes. From the southeast end of the lake, adventurous hikers are rewarded with spectacular views of Clyde Minaret, Minaret Lake, and Minaret Creek's canyon. From Cecile Lake, the cross-country route (which occasionally looks like a faint trail to the east) descends 500 tough feet to Minaret Lake (9820′), at the east end of which is the maintained trail to Devils Postpile (as described in Trip 42). Take that trail south, then generally east along Minaret Creek to Middle Fork San Joaquin River, and finally south again, crossing the river on the bridge near Devils Postpile and reaching the trailhead shortly thereafter.

DAY 2 (Ediza Lake to Agnew Meadows Trailhead, 7 miles): Retrace your steps to the trailhead.

Devils Postpile Trailhead
7600´; 11S 316045 4166770

DESTINATION/ UTM COORDINATES	TRIP TYPE	BEST SEASON	PACE (HIKING/ LAYOVER DAYS)	TOTAL MILEAGE
42 Minaret Lake 11S 309536 4170320	Out & back	Mid to late	2/1 Moderate	16
43 King Creek Lakes 11S 311156 4167329 (Superior Lake)	Loop	Mid to late	3/1 Moderate	16.5

Information and Permits: This trailhead is in Inyo National Forest: 351 Pacu Lane, Suite 200, Bishop, CA 93514, 760-873-2400, www.fs.fed.us/r5/inyo/. Quotas apply, and permits are required for overnight stays and are available at Inyo National Forest ranger stations in Lone Pine, Bishop, Mammoth Lakes, and Mono Basin Scenic Area Visitors Center.

Driving Directions: From the intersection of Hwy. 395 and Hwy. 203 (the Mammoth junction), drive 3.8 miles west on Hwy. 203 through the town of Mammoth Lakes. At the second traffic light, with Minaret Road (also Hwy. 203), turn right onto Minaret Road and go 4.2 miles farther to the main lodge of Mammoth Mountain Ski Area. Here you will have to park your car and take a shuttle bus (fee), unless you arrive before or after operating hours or qualify for certain exceptions (contact the Mammoth Lakes ranger station for current regulations). Get off at the Devils Postpile stop, right in front of the ranger station.

Or, if timing permits driving your own car, continue up Hwy. 203 to Minaret Summit for 1.4 miles. Go past Minaret Summit down the narrow, mostly one-lane road into the Devils Postpile area, and continue to the signed turnoff for Devils Postpile, 6.7 miles beyond Minaret Summit. Turn right here, down a 0.3-mile spur road to the Postpile ranger station and parking lot. Overnight parking isn't permitted there; overnighters must park in a lot on the right side of the spur road just a few yards after the turnoff. You may wish to leave your party and all the packs at the end of the spur road, in front of the ranger station, and then drive back to the overnighters' lot and walk back from there to the ranger station, which is right at the trailhead.

42 Minaret Lake

Trip Data: 11S 309536 4170320; 16 miles; 2/1 days

Topos: *Mammoth Mtn., Mt. Ritter*

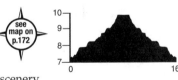

Highlights: Minaret Lake is a popular destination for climbers, but it's also a great choice for backpackers who want to get up close to some of the most dramatic scenery in the Sierra.

HEADS UP! Campfires are prohibited at Minaret Lake.

DAY 1 (Devils Postpile Trailhead to Minaret Lake, 8 miles): From the Devils Postpile ranger station, follow the well-worn path south a short distance to a junction. Detour to see Devils Postpile if you wish; see the "Devils Postpile Detour" sidebar on page 173.

If you don't take the detour, turn right (west) and shortly cross a sturdy footbridge across the Middle Fork San Joaquin. Follow the trail as it veers right (north) upstream and then west, quickly reaching the next junction, between the King Creek Trail (left, southwest) and a spur to the PCT/JMT (right, north).

Turn right toward the PCT/JMT and traverse a sandy slope to junction where the northbound JMT and PCT diverge. Head northwest on the JMT (not northeast on the PCT), ascending through dusty pumice. After a little more than a mile, find a junction with the Beck Lakes Trail on the left; stay right (northwest) on the JMT and ford Minaret Creek.

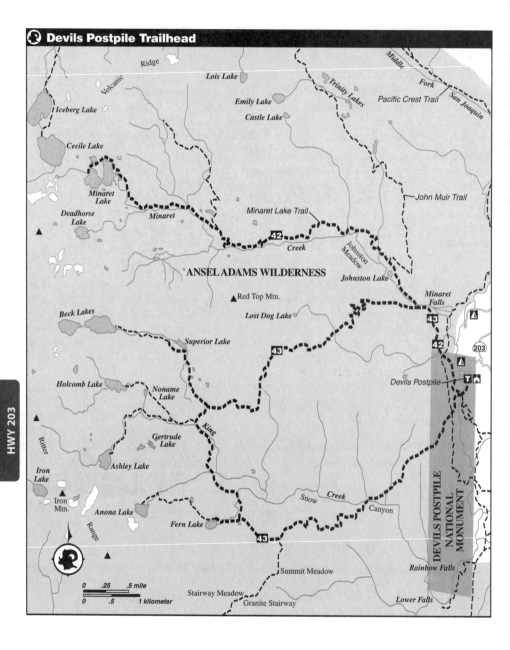

Devils Postpile Trailhead

Ridge

Lois Lake

Middle

Fork

Emily Lake

Trinity Lakes

Pacific Crest Trail

San Joaquin

Iceberg Lake

Castle Lake

Cecile Lake

John Muir Trail

Minaret Lake

Deadhorse Lake

Minaret

Minaret Lake Trail

42

Creek

Johnston Meadow

ANSEL ADAMS WILDERNESS

Johnston Lake

▲ Red Top Mtn.

Minaret Falls

43

Beck Lakes

Lost Dog Lake

▲

Superior Lake

43

42

203

Holcomb Lake

Noname Lake

▲

Devils Postpile

T

Ritter

King

Gertrude Lake

Iron Lake

▲

Iron Mtn.

Ashley Lake

Snow   Creek

Canyon

DEVILS POSTPILE NATIONAL MONUMENT

Anona Lake

Fern Lake

43

Range

▲

Summit Meadow

Rainbow Falls

0   .25   .5 mile

Stairway Meadow

0   .5   1 kilometer

Granite Stairway

Lower Falls

HWY 203

DEVILS POSTPILE DETOUR

From the junction after the ranger station, go ahead (south) a short distance, ascending to the base of the eponymous volcanic formation, where there are interpretive displays explaining the Postpile's origin better than we can do it here. The tall, slender, basalt "columns" soaring high into the blue mountain skies are a striking sight. A short use trail loops from here around the top of the Postpile, where a small, glacially polished slice through the formation reveals the columns' predominantly hexagonal (though irregular) cross section. To continue this trip, return to the first junction and turn left (west) to cross the footbridge.

The grasses of Johnston Meadow soon appear on the left. Just past marshy, reedy Johnston Lake (8100´; 11S 314747 4168729; possible campsites), leave the JMT, which continues right (northwest). This trip goes left (west), following Minaret Creek on pumice-covered trail. The going gets steeper and the cascading creek more dramatic, and the trail alternates between exposed switchbacks with nice views and dense fir forest for about 2 miles. There are campsites hidden under the trees near the creek on this stretch of trail.

The climb intensifies at a rocky outcrop; catch your breath and admire the beautiful cascade on the left. The trail widens above the cascade—you're on the old Minaret Mine Road, getting peekaboo views of the peaks ahead. Three miles and 1000 feet of elevation gain from the junction where this trip left the JMT, reach an intersection with a trail going up to the abandoned mine; ignore it. Continue ahead, generally west, along the creek, before curving north-northwest on a forested flat (damp, buggy campsites).

Leave the flat to make a final ascent on long switchbacks to Minaret Lake's outlet (9822´; 11S 310067 4170293), where you come face to face with the imposing Minarets, which rise behind Minaret Lake and are dominated by 12,281-foot Clyde Minaret. The trail skirts the north side of the lake to the most crowded and overused campsites, but there are fine campsites (no fires) all around, reached by use trails. The most secluded may be at the various tarns south of and overlooking the lake.

FUN AT MINARET LAKE

There's lots to do on a layover day here. For experienced cross-country navigators only, scramble cross-country from Minaret Lake to Cecile and Iceberg lakes and then follow a trail to Ediza Lake (Trip 41's destination). Climb the Class 2 route from Minaret Lake to Volcanic Ridge. Explore the lakeshore. Or simply enjoy the amazing views right from your camp.

DAY 2 (Minaret Lake to Devils Postpile Trailhead, 8 miles): Retrace your steps.

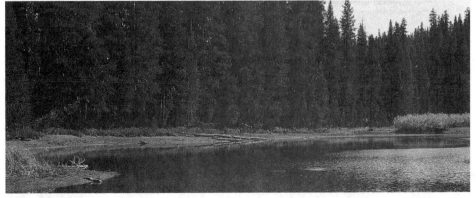

Peaceful Johnston Lake

43 King Creek Lakes

Trip Data: 11S 311156 4167329; 16.5; 3/1 days

Topos: *Mammoth Mtn., Mount Ritter, Cattle Mtn., Crystal Crag*

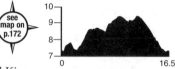

Highlights: Just east of more famous terrain— Minaret and Ediza lakes, the Minarets—the less-traveled King Creek Loop boasts a half-dozen lakes, polished granite, and great camping. This is a low-mileage trip with excellent subalpine scenery. We recommend starting this loop on the trail to Superior Lake for the shade on the uphill, but you can easily reverse the trip and spend the first night at Fern Lake.

HEADS UP! On the hike from Devils Postpile to Superior Lake, there's little to no water between Minaret Creek and Superior Lake. Plan accordingly.

DAY 1 (Devils Postpile Trailhead to Superior Lake, 7 miles): Head toward Devils Postpile, turning right (west) to cross Middle Fork San Joaquin River on the footbridge. At the junction with the King Creek Trail, take the spur to the PCT/JMT right (north). At the next junction, an X-junction where the northbound JMT and PCT diverge, ascend the JMT northwest through dusty pumice to a junction with the trail to Beck Lakes.

Go left (west) toward Beck Lakes and soon begin an ascending traverse on deep pumice in dense forest cover. Admire the filtered view down to Johnston Meadow and beyond to Volcanic Ridge as the trail switchbacks farther up. About 2 miles of fairly flat trail—viewless and dry forest that gives way to occasional meadows—end at the edge of Snow Canyon, bordered by Iron Mountain to the east and the Ritter Range to the north. Views open up, and there is a "preview" of the next day's hiking.

Descend to meet the trail to Superior and Beck lakes just beyond the remains of Beck Cabin (9113'; 11S 311526 4166352). Turn right (north) onto that trail, and walk about a mile, passing tarns and a sweet little meadow, before the few switchbacks up to Superior Lake (9372'; 11S 311156 4167329), today's destination, which is tucked beneath Red Top Mountain and the spiny ridges separating this drainage from Deadhorse and Minaret lakes. There is hemlock-shaded camping near the outlet or by the inlet (marshy in early season).

More austere camping in a high alpine environment with bigger views can be found a mile upstream at Lower Beck Lake (9890'; 11S 310007 4167724). Contrary to the topo, there's only a wandering, rocky, often invisible, use route between Superior Lake and Lower Beck Lake.

DAY 2 (Superior Lake to Fern Lake, 3.5 miles): Retrace yesterday's steps back to the junction with the main King Creek Trail, and go right (south-southwest) to immediately meet another junction to Holcomb and Ashley lakes.

HOLCOMB AND ASHLEY LAKES

These lakes are both quite scenic but fairly well used by horse packers, although packers have so abused Holcomb that they're now forbidden there. Follow a straightforward trail west and then northwest to Holcomb, a trail from which a use trail to Ashley Lake (9544'; 11S 309824 4165621) departs southwestward partway to Holcomb. Early on, there's a small campsite just above and right (north) of the Holcomb Trail, where the creek drops in a low but showy cascade. The trail to Ashley departs from the Holcomb Trail westward at first and then arcs southward through a large meadow (campsites in the rocks) and over rises to Ashley's outlet, which you follow to that lake. Ashley is perfectly framed by Iron Mountain and surrounding peaks. There's a good campsite south of the outlet (when the site is not full of horse manure).

If you're heading directly to Fern Lake, go left (south) at the junction to cross King Creek (difficult in early season; slippery at any season; just above a waterfall). Heading generally south, descend to ford Anona Lake's outlet in a scrubby, open area, and then climb away, presently returning to forest. On the climb, be sure to puase for an over-the-shoulder view of the foaming waterfall on King Creek. The open and pleasant, 2-mile trip to Fern stays high on the southwest edge of Snow Canyon, crossing some talus before meeting the signed side trail to Fern.

Turn right (west) to walk on the often muddy path to pretty Fern Lake (8720´; 11S 311650 4164369), where numerous wooded campsites can be found on both sides of the outlet. If you fancy a swim, jump in—lower-altitude Fern is one of the warmer lakes in the region.

Solitude seekers and granite hounds might want to set up camp higher up at beautiful Anona Lake (9107´; 11S 310359 4164724), accessible via an unsigned, faint use trail that skirts Fern's north shore before making a rocky ascent to Anona, that, like Ashley, sits in Iron Mountain's shadow.

DAY 3 (Fern Lake to Devils Postpile Trailhead, 6 miles): Walk back to the main King Creek Trail, turn right (south), and climb for less than a mile to meet the trail to Summit Meadow and Granite Stairway (a route that goes across the Sierra to Clover Meadow; see Trip 3 for details). Go left (northeast) to stay on the King Creek Trail, and start the descent on loose pumice that soon gives way to a stony path. Views are far-reaching from the many switchbacks down to lower King Creek, and seasonal flowers add splashes of color.

Lower King Creek is a welcome sight more than halfway back to Devils Postpile; rest and get water here for the dusty and surprisingly uphill journey back. Ford the creek (campsites on the east side) and start a moderate climb through a forest burned in the 1992 lightning-caused Rainbow Fire before curving north and dropping to the intersection with the trail from Devils Postpile to close the loop.

Go ahead (north-northeast) and retrace your steps to Middle Fork San Joaquin River and over the footbridge to the ranger station and shuttle stop. (If you drove down, your car is up the spur road.)

Fish Creek Trailhead

DESTINATION/ UTM COORDINATES	TRIP TYPE	BEST SEASON	PACE (HIKING/ LAYOVER DAYS)	TOTAL MILEAGE
44 Silver Divide Lakes 11S 325109 4148983 (at Peter Pande Lake)	Semiloop	Early to late	6/1 Moderate	45

Information and Permits: This trailhead (also called the Rainbow Falls Trailhead) is in Inyo National Forest: 351 Pacu Lane, Suite 200, Bishop, CA 93514, 760-873-2400, www.fs.fed.us/r5/inyo/. Quotas apply, and permits are required for overnight stays and are available at Inyo National Forest ranger stations in Lone Pine, Bishop, Mammoth Lakes, and Mono Basin Scenic Area Visitors Center.

Driving Directions: From the intersection of Hwy. 395 and Hwy. 203 (the Mammoth junction), drive 3.8 miles west on Hwy. 203 through the town of Mammoth Lakes. At the second traffic light, with Minaret Road (also Hwy. 203), turn right onto Minaret Road and go 4.2 miles farther to the main lodge of Mammoth Mountain Ski Area. Here you will have to park your car and take a shuttle bus (fee), unless you arrive before or after operating hours or qualify for certain exceptions (contact the Mammoth Lakes ranger station for current regulations). Get off at the Rainbow Falls stop and walk south 0.1 mile down a short, dirt spur road and through a parking lot to the trailhead (toilet, water).

Or, if timing permits driving your own car, continue up Hwy. 203 to Minaret Summit for 1.4 miles. Go past Minaret Summit down the narrow, mostly one-lane road into the Devils Postpile area, and continue 8.1 miles from Minaret Summit to a Y whose right fork is a signed turnoff south for Rainbow Falls. Go 0.1 mile on this dirt road to a parking lot and the signed trailhead.

Note: While popularly known as the Rainbow Falls Trailhead, this is also the Fish Creek Trailhead. Mercifully for you, the huge summertime throngs here are almost all headed for Rainbow Falls.

44 Silver Divide Lakes

Trip Data: 11S 325109 4148983 (at Peter Pande Lake); 45 miles; 6/1 days

see map on p.178

Topos: *Crystal Crag, Bloody Mountain, Graveyard Peak*

Highlights: This scenic trip travels through some lesser-known corners of John Muir Wilderness. From the wonders of the Middle Fork San Joaquin River's canyon and backcountry hot springs, walk to a string of lakes set beneath the sharp, granite "shark's teeth" (or perhaps "tombstones") of the Silver Divide. The all-trail route (with one short cross-country option) stays below 10,000 feet, making it an early-season possibility—all the better to avoid seasonal crowds at Iva Bell Hot Springs!

HEADS UP! *Early-season hikers may encounter very difficult fords on this route.*

DAY 1 (Fish Creek Trailhead to Island Crossing, 8 miles): Take the Fish Creek Trail as it heads south, and soon step across the PCT/JMT, continuing ahead (south). Be alert for your southbound Fish Creek Trail here; this heavily used area is full of junctions with use trails as well as maintained trails. Continue straight ahead (south) again at a junction with a spur trail arcing north toward Reds Meadow Resort, and yet again at a junction with a trail angling north to Devils Postpile. Ford Boundary Creek and then go ahead (south) at a junction with a horse trail north to Reds Meadow Resort.

Reach a junction with the trail to Rainbow Falls in just under 1 mile; if you've not seen 101-foot Rainbow Falls, the half-mile round-trip detour is worth the effort. Following the Fish Creek Trail ahead (south) from this intersection, leave almost everyone else behind and presently enter John Muir Wilderness. For the next 2 to 3 miles, the trail goes through an often exposed section of forest that burned in the 1992 lightning-caused Rainbow Fire. Descend on pumice-covered trail through manzanita, past granite walls popular with climbers, to a very soothing cascade on Crater Creek. The trail meanders along the west side of the creek and then crosses it. The footing changes from pumice to granite, and the path crosses two tributaries of Crater Creek at approximately 4 miles; there are several nice campsites in this area.

Views open up as the track begins a traverse on a sloping granite ledge high above Middle Fork San Joaquin River, and Crater Creek dives spectacularly off the canyon's lip; this dramatic section of trail alone is worth the trip. The trail curves away from the canyon to ford Cold Creek (6790′; 11S 315492 4158485), climb a rocky, flowery outcrop, and pass through spring-fed aspen groves and meadows. Another gentle ascent brings hikers under a changing forest canopy that now includes oak.

Finally, the trail levels off and curves east toward Fish Creek Valley. Switchback steeply down the valley's north wall (watch for rattlesnakes) to meet roaring Fish Creek and find a sturdy bridge at Island Crossing (6340′; 11S317530 4156232). There are campsites on the creek's south side, near the junction with the Silver Creek Trail.

DAY 2 (Island Crossing to Lost Keys Lakes, 6 miles): Today's hike involves the biggest elevation gain of the trip: about 3000 feet from Island Crossing to Lost Keys Lakes.

From the bridge at Island Crossing, note the signed intersection with the Silver Creek Trail: left (east) to Iva Bell Hot Springs and Minnow Creek; right (west) up to Silver Creek. Go left to make a gentle, bucolic, eastward ascent up Fish Valley, roughly paralleling Fish Creek on its south side and trying not to trip over tree roots or soak your feet in the several stream crossings as you stare up at the valley's impressive granite walls. Near 6693 feet, upper Fish Creek descends the valley walls from the north, while Sharktooth Creek flows into Fish Creek from the east (the confluence is at about 11S 319365 4156287). The eastbound trail now traces Sharktooth Creek's south bank

At the next intersection (7140′; 11S 320965 4155883), hikers face these choices: left (north) across the creek to Iva Bell Hot Springs and Cascade Valley, or right (south) to Lost Keys Lakes and Minnow Creek.

HWY 203

IVA BELL HOT SPRINGS

Although it's not on this trip's itinerary (but it is the goal of Trip 46), most people who have come this far will want to detour to Iva Bell, or Fish Creek, Hot Springs (7169′; 11S 321042 4155961). They'll have a second chance to visit the springs on Day 5.

It's a magical place in danger of being loved to death. Tread lightly here! To reach the hot springs from the Minnow Creek/Cascade Valley trail junction, cross Sharktooth Creek on a log bridge and look for an unsigned path at the next tributary stream that crosses the trail. That path leads uphill (east), passing good but heavily used campsites on the left about a quarter mile to a large, wet meadow, in which a hot spring flows directly out of a granite outcrop into a small pool.

According to Peter Browning's *Place Names of the Sierra Nevada* (Wilderness Press), these springs are named for "Iva Bell Clark [who] was born unexpectedly at the springs in July 1936, surprising both parents; Mrs. Clark had thought she had a tumor."

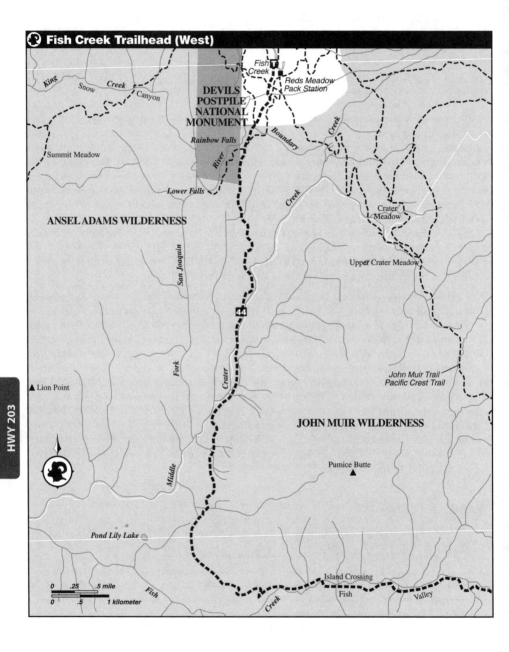

Fish Creek Trailhead (West)

King
Snow   Creek   Canyon
Fish Creek
Reds Meadow Pack Station
DEVILS POSTPILE NATIONAL MONUMENT
Boundary
Creek
Rainbow Falls
River
Summit Meadow
Lower Falls
Creek
Crater Meadow
ANSEL ADAMS WILDERNESS
San Joaquin
Upper Crater Meadow
44
Fork
Crater
John Muir Trail
Pacific Crest Trail
▲ Lion Point
JOHN MUIR WILDERNESS
Middle
Pumice Butte
▲
Pond Lily Lake
0   .25   .5 mile
0   .5   1 kilometer
Fish
Island Crossing
Creek   Fish   Valley

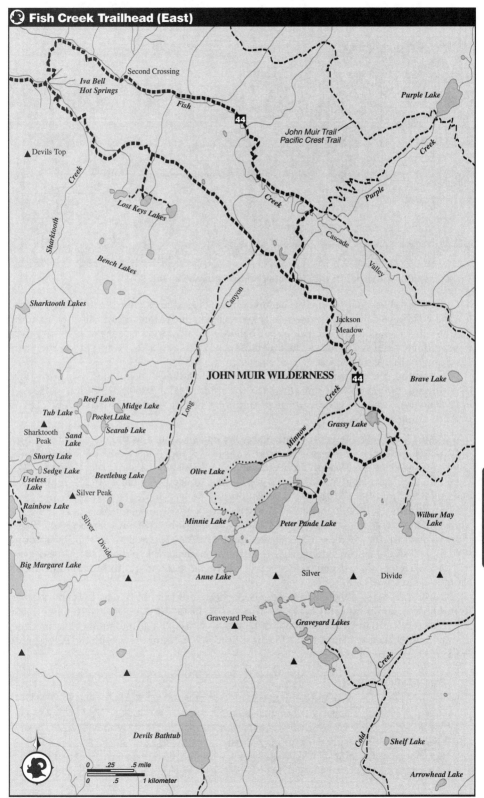

Iva Bell
Hot Springs

Second Crossing

Fish

Purple Lake

44

John Muir Trail
Pacific Crest Trail

Devils Top

Creek

Purple

Creek

Sharktooth

Lost Keys Lakes

Creek

Cascade

Bench Lakes

Valley

Sharktooth Lakes

Canyon

Jackson
Meadow

JOHN MUIR WILDERNESS

44

Brave Lake

Reef Lake
Midge Lake

Long

Creek

Tub Lake
Pocket Lake

Scarab Lake

Minnow

Grassy Lake

Sharktooth
Peak
Sand
Lake

Shorty Lake

Olive Lake

Sedge Lake
Useless
Lake

Beetlebug Lake

Silver Peak

Minnie Lake

Peter Pande Lake

Wilbur May
Lake

Rainbow Lake

Silver

Divide

Big Margaret Lake

▲

Silver

▲

Divide

▲

Anne Lake

▲

Graveyard Peak

Graveyard Lakes

▲

Creek

▲

Cold

Devils Bathtub

Shelf Lake

0   .25   .5 mile

0   .5   1 kilometer

Arrowhead Lake

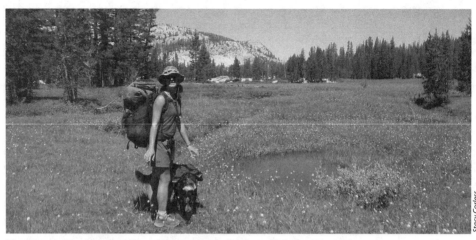

The Minnow Creek Trail passes wide, granite-rimmed meadows on Day 3.

Ignoring the temptation to visit the hot springs, begin the loop part of this trip: Go right toward Lost Keys Lakes and immediately switchback, under forest cover, steeply up along Sharktooth Creek. Cross the creek about halfway up the steep ascent out of Fish Valley. After another set of switchbacks, the trail crosses a Lost Keys Lakes outlet stream and veers east, coming to a saddle.

Continuing, the signed lateral trail to Lost Keys Lakes appears, and you turn right (south) and continue a half mile to reach the middle lake (9350´; 11S 322603 4153894). Follow anglers' trails to good campsites and good fishing at any of these lovely, heavily wooded, hanging-valley lakes.

DAY 3 (Lost Keys Lakes to Peter Pande Lake, 7.5 miles): Return to the main trail and turn right (east) to start a gentle ascent toward Minnow Creek Valley and the Silver Divide Lakes. You cross and recross an outlet stream from Beetlebug Lake in Long Canyon, passing a trail that leads right (southwest) some 3 miles to Beetlebug Lake. At 2.75 miles, meet a lateral (9030´; 11S 325170 4152502) descending left (north) to Cascade Valley.

Temporarily end the loop part of this trip and begin an out-and-back part along the Minnow Creek Trail to and from Peter Pande Lake: Go right (east) and climb some 200 feet more to meet Minnow Creek and enter its sublime valley. The trail skirts southwest along verdant Jackson Meadow, staying near the oxbow-shaped creek, passing abandoned-looking packer camps that, if you're lucky, will be the closest you get to human encounters along this stretch of trail.

Nearly 2 miles from the Cascade lateral junction, ford Minnow Creek as it pours down from Olive Lake and meet a lateral trail going right (southwest) to lovely Olive Lake. Continue left (southeast) on the main trail, passing Grassy Lake and another picturesque, granite-lined meadow. In just under 1 more mile, come to the junction with the Peter Pande Trail (9527´; 11S 32695 4149731).

OTHER CAMPING OPTIONS

If you don't want to make the climb to Peter Pande or the other high-country lakes with your pack on, look for established though less scenic campsites in Jackson Meadow, on the north and west shores of marshy Grassy Lake, or at Wilbur May Lake. Get to Wilbur May Lake by staying southeastbound on the Minnow Creek Trail at the turnoff to Peter Pande Lake; in a half mile, turn right (south) onto the spur that leads in a little under a half mile to Wilbur May Lake (9730´; 11S 327075 4148607). Going to Wilbur May Lake adds about 2 miles total to this trip.

Take the Peter Pande Lake lateral right (southwest), crossing the meadow to make the pleasant 2-mile, 500-foot climb to Peter Pande Lake. At the trail's crest above Peter Pande, veer right (west) to descend to its basin (9981'; 11S 325142 4148931). Find fine camping along the lake's north and northwest shores, with up-close views of Graveyard Peak and the Silver Divide.

AROUND PETER PANDE LAKE

On a layover day, hike cross-country to Minnie, Anne, and Olive lakes, taking a use trail around Peter Pande's northwest shore to the inlet stream from Anne and Minnie, then following that stream southwest to Anne Lake. From Anne Lake, go cross-country generally northwest to Minnie Lake and over the divide between Minnie and Olive lakes. Descend, still generally northwest, to one pond and then another, and finally veer northeast along the second pond's outlet, which becomes Olive Lake's inlet, down to Olive Lake's northwest shore. (This route is a good alternative for strong hikers for Day 4's return trip; you can take the trail from Olive Lake 1.5 miles northeast to the main Minnow Creek Trail. The junction is a little northwest of Grassy Lake.) If you're comfortable on talus and with Class 2-3 hiking, head cross-country south from Peter Pande Lake to "Silver Fox" or "Graveyard" Pass, just east of Graveyard Peak, to catch a glimpse of the Graveyard Lakes (Trip 19) on the other side of the Silver Divide.

DAY 4 (Peter Pande Lake to Cascade Valley, 6.5 miles): Leave Peter Pande Lake and head back to the Minnow Creek Trail. At that junction, turn left (northwest) and retrace your steps past Jackson Meadow to the junction with the Cascade Valley lateral trail.

Take that trail right (north) to reopen the loop part of this trip. Make a short, steep descent to meet Fish Creek in aptly named Cascade Valley. There is one nice campsite on the creek's south bank, with a tempting beach. Stop there for a very short day or cross the creek (difficult in early season) to meet the Cascade Valley Trail at a junction: left (northwest) toward Iva Bell Hot Springs and Reds Meadow, or right (southeast) toward the PCT/JMT.

Turn left and descend the narrow valley for almost 3.5 scenic miles, playing hide and seek with Fish Creek. Choose one of the campsites between here and Second Crossing; this day's mileage assumes a camp near Second Crossing (7871'; 11S 322316 4155968).

DAY 5 (Cascade Valley to Island Crossing, 9 miles): The trail fords Fish Creek at Second Crossing (very difficult in early season) and then continues down the polished granite canyon. Turning south, the route steeply ascends the canyon wall and then breaks out onto a granite saddle with vistas back toward Cascade Valley. The slopes of Sharktooth Ridge rise to the south, and directly below is the intense green foliage marking the outflow of Iva Bell Hot Springs.

From the saddle, follow the trail south as it steeply descends switchbacks on Fish Creek Valley's north wall into a dense, wet forest, heading toward the confluence of Fish and Sharktooth creeks. This stretch passes west of Iva Bell Hot Springs (turn left, east, on an unmarked lateral to soak or camp at Iva Bell; see the sidebar on page 177 for directions and information).

Otherwise, continue on the main trail to ford Sharktooth Creek and meet the Fish Creek Trail. At this junction, close the loop part of this trip and turn right (generally west) to retrace your steps on the Fish Valley Trail to campsites near Island Crossing.

DAY 6 (Island Crossing to Fish Creek Trailhead, 8 miles): Retrace the steps of Day 1. Get an early start up the hot, steep switchbacks out of Fish Valley. The trailhead is a short walk from the store and café at Reds Meadow Resort, as well as from hiker sites and free hot-spring-fed showers at nearby Reds Meadow Campground.

Duck Pass Trailhead

9120´; 11S 324402 4162265

DESTINATION/ UTM COORDINATES	TRIP TYPE	BEST SEASON	PACE (HIKING/ LAYOVER DAYS)	TOTAL MILEAGE
45 Lake Virginia 11S 329309 4153440	Semiloop	Mid to late	4/1 Moderate, part cross-country	25.5/26.5
46 Iva Bell Hot Springs 11S 321042 4155961	Shuttle	Early to late	4/1 Moderate	28
47 Upper Crater Meadow 11S 319195 4161678	Shuttle	Mid to late	3/1 Leisurely	17.4

Information and Permits: This trailhead is in Inyo National Forest: 351 Pacu Lane, Suite 200, Bishop, CA 93514, 760-873-2400, www.fs.fed.us/r5/inyo/. Quotas apply, and permits are required for overnight stays and are available at Inyo National Forest ranger stations in Lone Pine, Bishop, Mammoth Lakes, and Mono Basin Scenic Area Visitors Center. Bear canisters are required.

Driving Directions: From the junction of Hwy. 395 and Hwy. 203, take Hwy. 203 west, where it becomes Main Street and heads into the town of Mammoth Lakes. Continue southwest on Main Street through all traffic lights as it becomes the Lake Mary Road and curves south into the Mammoth Lakes Basin. Stay on the Lake Mary Road at the turnoff to Twin Lakes. At the signed Y past the pack station and just before Lake Mary, turn left and follow this unnamed road along Mary's eastern shore to the Coldwater Campground/Duck Pass Trailhead road. Turn left up this road and follow it southeast-ward as it climbs through the campground to its end at a large parking area. There are three trailheads here; the Duck Pass Trailhead is the middle one, near the east side of the lot (toilets, water).

45 Lake Virginia

Trip Data: 11S 329309 4153440; 25.5/26.5 miles; 4/1 days

Topos: *Bloody Mountain*

Highlights: Spectacular high alpine terrain is the reward for venturing off the beaten path. This semiloop takes you to Lake Virginia on the PCT/JMT via Ram Lake, a less frequently visited spot in a lofty granite basin dotted with sparkling lakes and serene meadows. If you're a strong backpacker looking to explore off trail, this trip is a good place to start.

HEADS UP! *After a heavy winter, the Duck Pass Trail may be under snow beyond Skelton Lake well into July; check at the Mammoth Lakes ranger station before setting out. The journey from Ram Lake to Lake Virginia is cross-country; route-finding and map-and-compass skills are a must.*

DAY 1 (Duck Pass Trailhead to Pika Lake, 5 miles): Head southeast past an information sign, crossing an unmapped streamlet to enter John Muir Wilderness at a junction: left (north) to Mammoth Consolidated Mine, right (southeast) to Duck Pass. Turn right and follow the dusty Duck Pass Trail as it climbs gradually to moderately before beginning a series of lazy switchbacks.

At 1 mile, reach a marked junction: left (southeast) to Arrowhead Lake (barely visible below), right (south, ahead) to Duck Pass. Stay on the trail to Duck Pass, climbing through granite outcrops to pass lovely Skelton Lake (9915´). Although there are campsites throughout this drainage, the area is overused; it's better to spend a night acclimating at a front-country campground and get over the pass today.

Climb moderately past alpine meadows and presently top a rise overlooking pretty Barney Lake (10,203´; campsites). Little Red Lake is visible on the left as the tread skirts Barney's east shore. The trail crosses Barney's outlet before attacking the steep, winding, rocky, view-rich ascent to Duck Pass. At unsigned Duck Pass (10,797´), enjoy the spectacular overlook of huge Duck Lake and its companion to the east, smaller Pika Lake. Take a spur trail left (east) along Duck's northeastern shore to Pika (10,530´; 11S 327273 4157864), where there are fair-to-good campsites. No camping is permitted within 300 feet of Duck's outlet.

DAY 2 (Pika Lake to Ram Lake, 6.5 miles): Return to the main trail below Duck Pass, turn left (south), skirt Duck Lake's western shore, cross the outlet, and descend to an intersection with the PCT/JMT that's above an extremely popular camping area along Duck Creek (poor-to-fair sites). Turn left (south) on the PCT/JMT and climb out of the basin to make a waterless, pumice-covered traverse high above Cascade Valley, with astonishing views west and south of the Silver Divide.

The trail eventually curves east into the valley holding Purple Lake and descends to a junction: left (north) to Ram Lake and campsites along Purple Lake's west shore, right (southeast) to stay on the PCT/JMT and cross Purple's outlet. Take the left fork along lovely Purple Lake (9928´), where fishing is fair to good for rainbow and some golden and brook. Purple Lake's partly timbered, rocky shoreline gives way to meadow at the northern end of the lake. Follow the trail as it gradually ascends along the left (northwest) bank of Purple Creek, the stream flowing from Ram to Purple Lake.

As the trail inches closer to the imposing ridge that separates Ram's basin from Duck and Pika lakes' basin, cross the stream and follow the ever fainter trail to a high alpine meadow just below a series of tarns. To reach rockbound Ram Lake (10,810´; 11S 329661 4156861), cross back over the stream and follow it east about a half mile up to the lake with its spectacular, sparsely visited campsites and great fishing just below the jagged Sierra Crest.

To reach Glen and Glenette lakes (both with nice camping and impressive scenery), stay south of the stream and go southeast over a small rise to the tarns. Glen (10,675´; 11S 329402 4156593) beckons about a half mile beyond. Walk uphill along the stream connecting the two lakes to find Glenette.

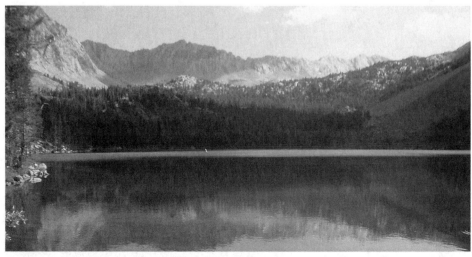

Stacy Corless

Purple Lake reflects the high peaks above Ram Lake's basin.

HWY 203

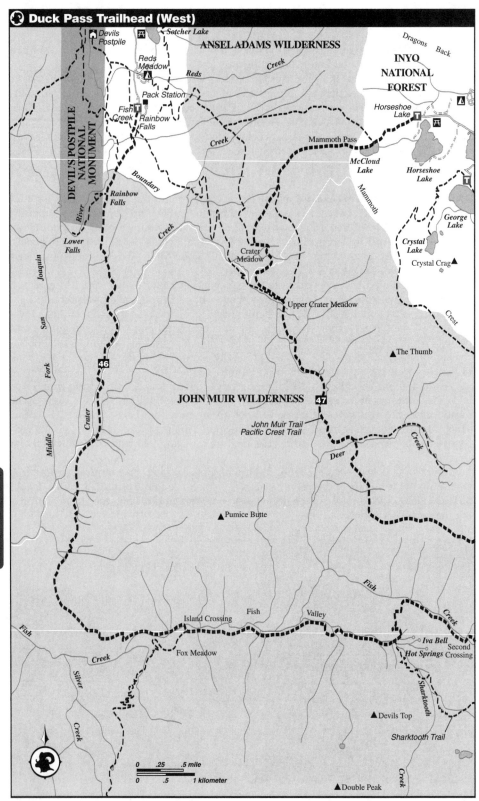

ANSEL ADAMS WILDERNESS

Dragons Back

INYO NATIONAL FOREST

Devils Postpile

Sotcher Lake

Reds Meadow

Reds

Creek

Pack Station

Fish Creek

Rainbow Falls

Horseshoe Lake

Mammoth Pass

McCloud Lake

Horseshoe Lake

Boundary

Rainbow Falls

River

Creek

Crater Meadow

Mammoth

George Lake

Crystal Lake

Crater

Lower Falls

San

Joaquin

Upper Crater Meadow

Crystal Crag

Crest

The Thumb

46

Fork

Middle

JOHN MUIR WILDERNESS

47

John Muir Trail
Pacific Crest Trail

Creek

Deer

Pumice Butte

Fish

Island Crossing

Fish

Valley

Creek

Fish

Fox Meadow

Creek

Iva Bell
Hot Springs

Second Crossing

Silver

Creek

Devils Top

Sharktooth

Sharktooth Trail

0   .25   .5 mile
0   .5   1 kilometer

Double Peak

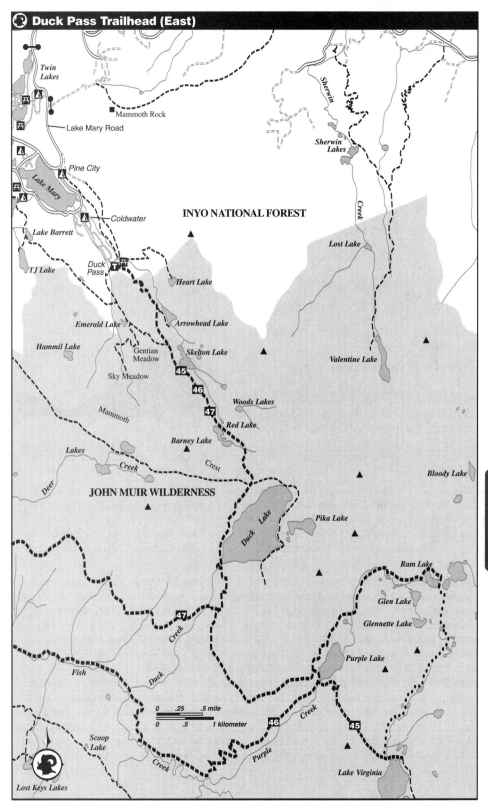

Twin Lakes

Mammoth Rock

Lake Mary Road

Pine City

Lake Mary

Coldwater

Lake Barrett

TJ Lake

Duck Pass

T

Heart Lake

Sherwin

Sherwin Lakes

INYO NATIONAL FOREST

Lost Lake

Creek

Emerald Lake

Arrowhead Lake

Hammil Lake

Gentian Meadow

Skelton Lake

Valentine Lake

Sky Meadow

45

46

Mammoth

47

Woods Lakes

Red Lake

Barney Lake

Lakes

Creek

Crest

Deer

JOHN MUIR WILDERNESS

Duck Lake

Pika Lake

Bloody Lake

Ram Lake

Glen Lake

47

Creek

Glennette Lake

Fish

Duck

Purple Lake

46

Purple

Creek

45

Scoop Lake

Creek

Lost Keys Lakes

Lake Virginia

0   .25   .5 mile
0   .5   1 kilometer

DAY 3 (Ram Lake to Lake Virginia, 3–4 miles, cross-country): From Ram's southeast shore, take a short hike to gain the ridge to the south for a view of what's ahead: nice and easy—albeit high elevation—cross-country travel. Descend south over firm but rocky footing, aiming for a series of tarns above Glenette Lake's basin.

Starting to climb, reach the first tarn (10,859′; 11S 329926 4156007) and follow the stream south-southwest to the low point in the ridge ahead. There are use trails to help with route finding, and soon you're at the top, enjoying a breathtaking view of the distant Silver Divide peaks, Lake Virginia, and the series of lakelets that will guide you down.

Meander approximately 1.5 miles generally south-southwestward through charming little meadows until the green gives way to forest duff near Lake Virginia's north shore (10,357′; 11S 328912 4153858) and the PCT/JMT. Turn left on the trail to go to the many campsites on this large lake's southeast shore (10,403′; 11S 329309 4153440).

DAY 4: (Lake Virginia to Duck Pass Trailhead, 11 miles): Head north on the PCT/JMT, leaving Lake Virginia to make a modest ascent before dropping into Purple Lake's basin to close the loop. Retrace your steps from here.

46 Iva Bell Hot Springs

Trip Data: 11S 321042 4155961;
28 miles; 4/1 days

Topos: *Devils Postpile, Bloody Mtn.,
Crystal Crag*

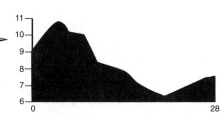

Highlights: This trip offers beautiful views along much of the route, good trails, and idyllic cold-water pools. But the real treat is one of the handful of wilderness hot springs in the entire High Sierra. Iva Bell, or Fish Creek, Hot Springs is a magical Shangri-la of a place that is in danger of being loved to death. Tread lightly here.

HEADS UP! *After a heavy winter, the Duck Pass Trail may be under snow beyond Skelton Lake well into July; check at the Mammoth Lakes ranger station before setting out. To have a more solitary experience, visit Iva Bell early or late in the season, skipping the Duck Pass Trailhead if snow prohibits passage over Duck Pass, and instead doing an out-an-back trip from the much lower Devils Postpile/Reds Meadow area on the Fish Creek Trail (7673′; 11S 316723 4165032; see the shuttle directions).*

Shuttle Directions: From the intersection of Hwy. 395 and Hwy. 203 (the Mammoth junction), drive 3.8 miles west on Hwy. 203 through the town of Mammoth Lakes. At the second traffic light, with Minaret Road (also Hwy. 203), turn right onto Minaret Road and go 4.2 miles farther to the main lodge of Mammoth Mountain Ski Area. Here you will have to park your car and take a shuttle bus (fee), unless you arrive before or after operating hours or qualify for certain exceptions (contact the Mammoth Lakes ranger station for current regulations). Get off at the Rainbow Falls stop and walk south 0.1 mile down a short, dirt spur road and through a parking lot to the trailhead (toilet, water). If timing permits driving your own car, continue up Hwy. 203 to Minaret Summit for 1.4 miles. Go past Minaret Summit down the narrow, mostly one-lane road into the Devils Postpile area, and continue 8.1 miles from Minaret Summit to a Y whose right fork is a signed turnoff south for Rainbow Falls. Go 0.1 mile on this dirt road to a parking lot and the signed trailhead. **Note:** While popularly known as the Rainbow Falls Trailhead, this is also the Fish Creek Trailhead.

DAY 1 (Duck Pass Trailhead to Duck Creek, 6 miles): Hike generally southeast up the deservedly popular Duck Pass Trail, bypassing a spur trail to Arrowhead Lake at 1 mile, then skirting Skelton and Barney lakes before tackling the switchbacks leading southward to Duck Pass (10,797´; 11S 326641 4158655). Descend from the pass and veer right (southwest) to stay on the Duck Pass Trail as it skirts around the northwest shore of large and lovely Duck Lake before crossing its outlet (no camping within 300 feet of the outlet) and descending to the junction where the trail meets the PCT/JMT (10,100´; 11S 326064 4156410).

Turn right (west) onto the northbound JMT to drop to the very popular camping area on the bench flanking Duck Creek, where there are poor-to-fair campsites and fine views across Cascade Valley to the Silver Divide.

DAY 2 (Duck Creek to Fish Creek, 5 miles): Retrace your steps to the junction of the PCT/JMT with the Duck Pass Trail. Turn right (south) to stay on the PCT/JMT, climbing over pumice to make the scenic southeast traverse above Cascade Valley toward Purple Lake. At the lake's southwest shore, meet the Ram Lake use trail heading north to campsites (no camping within 300 feet of Purple's outlet).

Go right (southeast) on the PCT/JMT. Shortly, the trail reaches another junction (9930´; 11S327723 4155152): left (ahead, east) to stay on the PCT/JMT, right (southwest) to Cascade Valley and Fish Creek.

Take the right fork to descend, gently at first, parallel to Purple Creek, enjoying fine views of the Silver Divide and some of the waterfalls that give the valley its name. The going gets steeper, and the long switchbacks terminate at last on the valley floor, where, in a few more steps, this route meets the Cascade Valley Trail (8361´; 11S 325797 4153622) and Fish Creek: left (southeast) to meet the PCT/JMT again upstream, right (northwest) to Iva Bell Hot Springs and Reds Meadow.

Turn right and pass a junction with a trail going left to Minnow Creek. Continue ahead (northwest), staying on the Cascade Valley Trail. Descend the dusty path through a beautiful, mixed forest, playing hide and seek with Fish Creek, which cascades in smooth sheets over boulders into glorious pools. Choose one of the many idyllic campsites between here and Second Crossing; this day's mileage assumes a camp near Second Crossing (7871´; 11S 322316 4155968).

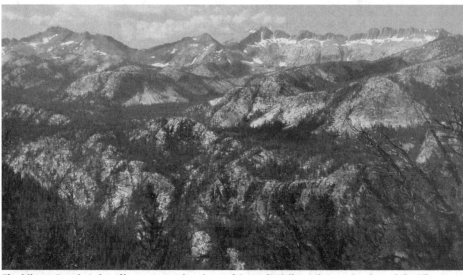

The hike to Purple Lake offers spectacular views of Cascade Valley, Minnow Creek, and the Silver Divide.

DAY 3 (Fish Creek to Island Crossing, 9 miles): On this day, you visit Iva Bell Hot Springs; however, we recommend that you do not camp there, even though there are campsites, because the area is very overused.

The trail fords Fish Creek at Second Crossing (very difficult in early season) and then continues down the polished granite canyon. Turning south, the route steeply ascends the canyon wall and then breaks out onto a granite saddle with vistas up Cascade Valley. To the south rise the slopes of Sharktooth Ridge, and directly below is the intense green foliage marking the outflow of the hot springs.

The trail drops steeply through manzanita and then levels out abruptly in dense, wet forest, with a ground cover of ferns and wildflowers. At a small tributary stream, an unsigned path leads uphill (east), passing good but heavily used campsites on the left, about a quarter mile to a large, wet meadow and Iva Bell (or Fish Creek) Hot Springs (7169´; 11S 321042 4155961; see the sidebar on page 177).The trail ends in a meadow where a hot spring flows directly out of a granite outcrop into a small pool, offering luxurious bathing at 100°F. Soak up improbable views in the tub and amazing Clark Range sunsets from atop the rock. A second pool is located a little higher in the meadow. If you camp at Iva Bell, opt for the sturdier campsites you passed on your way to the tub, avoiding the sites in the meadow and illegal sites down on the trail. Hardy souls can look for campsites and hidden springs in the granite ledges high above the meadow.

Regain the main trail and cross Sharktooth Creek at a log bridge. Beyond, the route comes to a signed junction: left (south) and up, up, up to Lost Keys Lakes and Minnow Creek (see the sidebar below), or right (west) on the Fish Valley Trail to Island Crossing and Reds Meadow. Go right on the Fish Valley Trail. The trail gently descends the granite-rimmed valley, following Sharktooth Creek and then Fish Creek through large Jeffrey pines and firs to Fox Meadow and the bridge at Island Crossing (6340´; 11S 317530 4156232). Many laterals lead to campsites here.

HWY 203

MINNOW CREEK TRAIL

Hikers familiar with the Duck Pass backcountry might want to add a few days onto the Iva Bell or Lake Virginia trips and explore the Minnow Creek area (described in Trip 44). Above and west of Cascade Valley, the main Minnow Creek Trail skirts wide, verdant meadows. Lateral trails lead up to lakes nestled up to the Silver Divide (Peter Pande Lake is one of the largest and most scenic). Minnow Creek isn't really the fastest way to get anywhere—a fact that makes your chances of solitude quite good.

Commandeer an old packer's camp in the valley, hide out in a gorgeous high country basin, or fish for legendary trout at Bench Lakes—Minnow Creek is a worthy detour. Reach Minnow Creek from the south by continuing on the PCT/JMT south from Lake Virginia 6 miles through Tully Hole to a junction above Squaw Lake; turn right and head west to good camping at Lake of the Lone Indian. The Minnow Creek Trail climbs the lake's west shore before beginning its descent into the valley. From there, the trail veers north for 5.5 miles. At a junction near Marsh Lake, you can turn right (north) to drop into Cascade Valley, or go ahead (west) to reach Fish Valley and Iva Bell Hot Springs.

DAY 4 (Island Crossing to Fish Creek Trailhead, 8 miles): *(Recap in Reverse: Trip 44, Day 1.)* The outdated 1994 7.5´ topo map shows Island Crossing east of Fox Meadow, but it's west. So, just west of Fox Meadow at a signed junction, turn right (west and then north) over a sturdy bridge at Island Crossing. Fill your hydration system here: There's no drinking water until Cold Creek, about 4 miles and a stiff climb away.

Now the trail switchbacks steeply up the hot, exposed north slope of the canyon— watch for rattlesnakes as you take in expanding views up and down Fish Creek, and eventually into Middle Fork San Joaquin River. The route levels off through a mixed forest, including oak. Aspens, springs, and a riot of flowers appear just before the outcropping and switchbacks southwest of Cold Creek.

After a welcome pause at Cold Creek (6790´; 11S 315492 4158485), the track breaks out onto exposed ledges of continuously sloping granite. The dramatic views from this section of trail alone are worth the trip: glimpses to the Middle Fork San Joaquin River below and its carved valley west, and a breathtaking waterfall where Crater Creek spills over the edge of the canyon. There are several campsites near the first creek crossing and beyond on the west side of the creek.

The trail follows Crater Creek, mostly in forest, crosses the creek on a large log, and then ascends on dusty pumice as it passes several granite walls and another spectacular waterfall. Here, hikers begin to see trees charred by the 1992 lightning-caused Rainbow Fire. The last section trudges through manzanita before reaching a junction with trails to Rainbow Falls (left, west) and to Devils Postpile, the Rainbow Falls Trailhead, and Red's Meadow Resort (right, north). Rainbow Falls is only a quarter mile away from this junction; if you can muster the energy, it's worth a detour to the 101-foot cascade.

Take the broad, right fork north toward the Fish Creek Trailhead and Red's Meadow. Crossing Boundary Creek, the trail enters Devils Postpile National Monument; for hikers with dogs, leashes are required here.

Just beyond the creek, reach a fork: left (north) to Devils Postpile, right (northeast) to the trailhead. Go right, shortly reaching another junction: left (north) to the trailhead, right (northeast) to Reds Meadow Resort. Go left to hop over an unnamed creeklet, step across the intersecting PCT/JMT, and reach the Fish Creek Trailhead and parking lot (7,644´; 11S 316712 4165029), where you can catch the shuttle back to your car at Mammoth Mountain. This lot is a short walk from the store and café at Reds Meadow Resort and also from hiker sites in the adjacent campground.

47 Upper Crater Meadow

Trip Data: 11S 319195 4161678; 17.4 miles; 3/1 days

Topos: *Devils Postpile, Bloody Mountain, Crystal Crag*

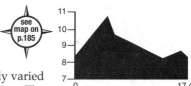

Highlights: Moderate trails lead through wonderfully varied scenery, including a pair of cinder cones, the Red Cones. The eastern Sierra has many fascinating volcanic features like the Red Cones, though it's been hundreds of years since there's been a volcanic event, other than an occasional tremor, in this area. The trailheads are only a few miles apart, so this is an easy shuttle to set up.

HEADS UP! After a heavy winter, the Duck Pass Trail may be under snow beyond Skelton Lake well into July; check at the Mammoth Lakes ranger station before setting out.

Shuttle Directions: From the junction of Hwy. 395 and Hwy. 203, take Hwy. 203 west, where it becomes Main Street and heads into the town of Mammoth Lakes. Continue southwest on Main Street through all traffic lights as it becomes Lake Mary Road and curves south into the Mammoth Lakes Basin. At the signed Y just before Lake Mary, take the right fork and follow the road, still Lake Mary Road, north past lakes Mary and Mamie (don't turn off to Lake George). Continue to roadend parking at Horseshoe Lake; the trailhead is near the cinderblock restrooms at the lake's north end (toilets, water).

DAY 1 (Duck Pass Trailhead to Duck Creek, 6 miles): *(Recap: Trip 46, Day 1.)* Hike generally southeast up the deservedly popular Duck Pass Trail, bypassing a spur trail to Arrowhead Lake at 1 mile, then skirting Skelton and Barney lakes before tackling the switchbacks leading southward to Duck Pass (10,797´; 11S 326641 4158655). Descend from the pass but don't go to Pika Lake.

Veer right (southwest) to stay on the Duck Pass Trail as it skirts around the northwest shore of large and lovely Duck Lake before crossing the outlet (no camping within 300 feet of the outlet) and descending to the junction where the trail meets the PCT/JMT (10,100´; 11S 326064 4156410).

Turn right (west) onto the northbound JMT to drop to the very popular camping area on the bench flanking Duck Creek, where there are poor-to-fair campsites and fine views across Cascade Valley to the Silver Divide.

DAY 2 (Duck Creek to Upper Crater Meadow, 7.7 miles): Late in the year, or in a dry year, there may be no water between Duck Creek and Deer Creek, almost 6 miles away, so fill up water bottles at Duck Creek.

The northbound PCT/JMT leaves the bench and begins a long, gradual, northwest-ward traverse on lightly wooded slopes high above Cascade Valley. Views south to the Silver Divide are awe inspiring. The footing changes from dirt to pumice—volcanic rock so light it floats on water, though here it simply slips and crunches underfoot.

Approaching Deer Creek, the trail veers away from the valley's rim, curves over low knolls, and descends a little to ford the well-forested creek (overused campsites), nearly 5.6 miles from Duck Creek. Just beyond is a junction with a spur trail right (east) up Deer Creek; stay on the PCT/JMT (left, west). The gradually graded trail curves north and soon begins to pass through one charming meadow and over one pretty stream after another. The gentle, forested slopes cupping these meadows offer the occasional campsite.

Arriving at flowery Upper Crater Meadow (8921´; 11S 319195 4161678), find a two-way junction. The right fork goes north to Mammoth Pass and Horseshoe Lake and the left fork is the northbound PCT/JMT to Reds Meadow.

> **MAP ERROR**
>
> The *Crystal Crag* topo shows this as a three-way junction, with the rightmost fork going to Mammoth Pass, the middle fork heading along the PCT/JMT, and the leftmost fork going to the Red Cones and Crater Meadow. However, the PCT/JMT has been rerouted onto the left-most fork, and the old middle fork is growing very faint from erosion and disuse. You may not even notice it.

Look for good campsites on the forested slopes around the meadow, especially on a rise reached by briefly following the faint old middle fork described in the sidebar.

DAY 3 (Upper Crater Meadow to Horseshoe Lake, 3.7 miles): Although you could head directly to Mammoth Pass and Horseshoe Lake by taking the rightmost fork at the junction in Upper Crater Meadow, don't miss the Red Cones. Return to the PCT/JMT and descend a sandy ravine northwest along Crater Creek, fording the creek and passing the less striking, forested, southern Red Cone. The Red Cones get their name from the pre-dominantly brick red color of the volcanic cinders forming them.

Ford Crater Creek again at the base of the northern Red Cone and reach a junction with another trail right (northeast) to Mammoth Pass. Near this junction, an obvious use trail takes off up the open, red cinder slopes of the striking, northern Red Cone, from whose cratered summit hikers enjoy wide-ranging views back to the Silver Divide; of the bare hulk of Mammoth Mountain, an 11,053-foot remnant of a 400,000-year-old volcano that's a major ski area in winter and a busy mountain bike park in summer; of the Middle Fork San Joaquin River; and of the dark, jagged Ritter Range. This is a classic cinder cone, fit to occu-py a spot in Maui's famed Haleakala Crater, except for its sprinkling of conifers. The ascent is optional but highly recommended.

Back on the PCT/JMT at the junction, turn right (east-northeast) onto the trail to Mammoth Pass to continue this trip. Passing more use trails up the cone, the main trail climbs gently along blooming Crater Meadow, fed by a fork of Crater Creek, to a faint junction with the old PCT/JMT segment from Upper Crater Meadow. Turn left (west), away from the meadow and creek, and shortly reach another junction: left (northwest) to Reds Meadow, right (north) to Mammoth Pass.

Turn right to climb gradually to moderately to a junction by a noisy spring with the trail that was the rightmost fork at the junction in Upper Crater Meadow: right (south) to Upper Crater Meadow, left (ahead, north) to Mammoth Pass and Horseshoe Lake.

Go ahead to cross broad, forested, viewless Mammoth Pass, leaving designated wilderness behind. The gradient is so gradual that hikers may not notice the pass. Presently, skirt beautiful McCloud Lake (no camping), tucked picturesquely under the light-colored cliffs of the Mammoth Crest, and reach a junction: left on a different route over Mammoth Pass, right (ahead, east-northeast) to Horseshoe Lake. Take the right fork ahead to descend to the parking lot at Horseshoe Lake.

HORSESHOE LAKE'S DEAD TREES

Studies have shown that the trees around the parking lot at Horseshoe Lake died because their roots were smothered by carbon dioxide seeping up in measurable amounts from some underground source related to the magma body beneath this volcanic area. There are other, similarly caused tree-kill sites here and on Mammoth Mountain. The seepage is small enough that (so far) it poses no threat to people when they're in the open air. Read and heed all warnings here.

HWY 203

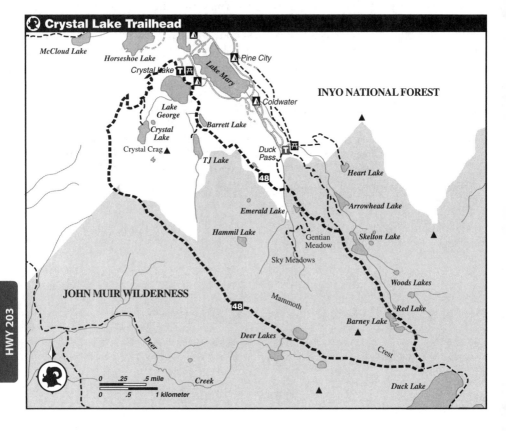

Crystal Lake Trailhead

McCloud Lake

Horseshoe Lake

Crystal Lake

Pine City

Lake Mary

INYO NATIONAL FOREST

Coldwater

Lake George

Barrett Lake

Crystal Lake

Crystal Crag

Duck Pass

Heart Lake

TJ Lake

Arrowhead Lake

Emerald Lake

Skelton Lake

Hammil Lake

Gentian Meadow

Sky Meadows

JOHN MUIR WILDERNESS

Woods Lakes

Mammoth

Red Lake

Barney Lake

Deer Lakes

Crest

Deer

Creek

Duck Lake

0   .25   .5 mile
0   .5   1 kilometer

Crystal Lake Trailhead   9038´; 11S 322473 4163681

DESTINATION/ UTM COORDINATES	TRIP TYPE	BEST SEASON	PACE (HIKING/ LAYOVER DAYS)	TOTAL MILEAGE
48 Deer Lakes 11S 324420 4159117	Loop	Mid	2/0 Moderate	15

Information and Permits: This trailhead is in Inyo National Forest: 351 Pacu Lane, Suite 200, Bishop, CA 93514, 760-873-2400, www.fs.fed.us/r5/inyo/. Quotas apply, and permits are required for overnight stays and are available at Inyo National Forest ranger stations in Lone Pine, Bishop, Mammoth Lakes, and Mono Basin Scenic Area Visitors Center.

Driving Directions: From the intersection of Hwy. 395 and Hwy. 203, take Hwy. 203 (Main Street) west into the town of Mammoth Lakes. Continue ahead at all traffic lights and follow Main Street as it turns into Lake Mary Road and curves south into the Mammoth Lakes Basin. Cross the outlet of Twin Lakes (on the right) on a bridge and continue ahead at the turnoff right to Twin Lakes. At the signed Y past the pack station and just before Lake Mary, take the right fork and follow the road, still Lake Mary Road, along Lake Mary's northeast corner to a junction at the Pokenobe Store/Marina with a spur road left to Lake George. Turn left here and head past the Lake Mary Campground and over the stream between lakes Mary and Mamie, to a T-junction. Here, turn right and drive up to Lake George and a paved parking area. The signed Crystal Lake/Mammoth Crest Trailhead is on the right (north) side of this lot (toilet on other side of lot, water in adjacent Lake George Campground).

48 Deer Lakes

Trip Data: 11S 324420 4159117; 15 miles; 2/0 days

Topos: *Devils Postpile, Crystal Crag, Bloody Mtn.*

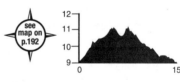

Highlights: The Deer Lakes Loop makes an ideal weekend trip or an ambitious, strenuous dayhike. In the journey from Lake George down Duck Pass, hikers encounter both stark alpine and dense forest terrains. The lightly traveled route to Deer Lakes follows the spine of the Mammoth Crest, with expansive views in every direction. The trip is described as a loop; for a shuttle trip, leave a car at the nearby Duck Pass Trailhead (see page 182 for directions) and shave 2 miles off the hike.

HEADS UP! *There is no water (and no acceptable camping) on the trail before you reach the Deer Lakes basin. Part of this trip on Day 2, from Deer Lakes to Duck Pass, follows an unmaintained use trail. Hikers should be comfortable on Class 2 terrain and with route finding.*

DAY 1 (Crystal Lake Trailhead to Deer Lakes, 7 miles): The trail leaves the Lake George parking lot at its north end and heads north at first but then gradually arcs southwest. Climbing above the resort cabins there, it switchbacks fairly steeply up through tall mountain hemlocks and lodgepole pines, affording views down to Lake George and eastward to Red and Gold Mountain. At a signed junction with the trail left to Crystal Lake, this trip's route continues ahead (southwest) and up toward Mammoth Crest. Views get better and better as the route climbs.

Just past the John Muir Wilderness boundary, the trail descends briefly and passes a pair of unsigned use trails to the right (one of these ascends a red cinder cone for fabulous, 360-degree views). Continue south, dip through the remnant of a crater, bypass another unsigned use trail to the right, and reach the crest. From this point, excellent views take in the Ritter Range to the west, and, to the southwest, the Silver Divide and the Middle Fork

San Joaquin River's canyon converging with Fish Creek's canyon. The rocky-sandy route continues south, and the crest broadens into a moonscape of red and white pumice.

The trail climbs moderately, then steeply, just west of the crestline, offering views down to lush Crater Meadow before briefly touching the crest on an eastward-facing knife edge with a dizzying view east down a sheer, often snowy chute. The crest then curves left (eastward) and so does the trail before it descends into the Deer Lakes basin. The trail terminates near the middle (northernmost) Deer Lake (10,700'). Find a campsite near this lake or along the stream connecting it with the lowest Deer Lake.

DAY 2 (Deer Lakes to Crystal Lake Trailhead via Duck Pass, 8 miles): Over gentle, high-alpine terrain, several indistinct trails head toward the pass to Duck Lake, directly east of the highest (easternmost) Deer Lake. Take the trail that leaves just east of the outlet of Middle Deer Lake. If you lose that trail, continue in a straight line generally east toward the very obvious low point just east of the highest Deer Lake. At the edge of the talus, walk along its base, almost reaching a small tarn not shown on the topo map.

From this point, a very steep use trail snakes 200 feet up on loose scree and dirt footing to a lovely, wide meadow. The trail crosses this meadow eastward past a lone, very large boulder in a low saddle. Continue directly ahead (generally east-southeast) toward Duck Lake. If you lose the sometimes faint trail, head straight downhill (avoid contouring leftward); this route soon intersects the well-maintained Duck Pass Trail (11S 326702 4158587 at the northwest end of Duck Lake).

Turn left (north) onto the trail, which shortly leads to Duck Pass, 350 yards ahead. The solitude of the previous day's hike is long gone on the beautiful but busy Duck Pass Trail. Take it approximately 2.5 miles downhill and north-northwest, passing Barney and Skelton lakes (overused campsites at both). Under forest cover, the trail levels off after leaving Skelton's basin.

Almost abreast of a broad track that angles right to popular campsites on Skelton Lake, find a trail left (west) at an unsigned junction (11S 325284 4160889) with sometimes faint lateral that leads over rocky outcrops to the Emerald Lake/Sky Meadows Trail. Its start is usually picked out by parallel rows of rocks. Follow the lateral west-northwest above a few unmapped tarns (in early season, these may be a single, huge tarn). Where this track appears to lead ahead onto an outcrop where the beaten path vanishes, the real trail veers right (north) and down tight switchbacks into a small gully. The trail curves westward after exiting the gully, leads along the base of an outcrop, drops to a seasonal tributary of Emerald Lake, and roughly parallels that tributary to Emerald Lake's basin.

Upon reaching that basin at a signed junction, turn right (north) on the Emerald Lake/Sky Meadows Trail to quickly reach pretty little Emerald Lake (no campsites). Below Emerald, continue for about a half mile to an abrupt descent leftward (west), down to an angler's trail along Coldwater Creek and a signed junction. Turn right (north-northwest and then west) on the angler's trail and downstream along the creek, and soon come to a small footbridge. Cross the creek and bear left (southwest, briefly upstream), following a well-maintained, obvious trail that doesn't appear on older topos.

Head toward a meadow (possibly the last legal camping) before veering right (northwest) into forest and leaving John Muir Wilderness. There's no camping allowed between here and the trailhead. The trail passes an unnamed pond and then continues northwest almost a mile to Barrett Lake ("Lake Barrett" on the topo). Avoid a turnoff left to TJ Lake as the main trail contours around Barrett Lake's west shore before dropping down the final half mile to Lake George, soon visible ahead. The final drop to the lakeshore is steep and rocky.

At a signed junction with a use trail around Lake George, go right (east) below a cabin, cross an outlet stream, and walk through a picnic area on the lake's east shore to the Barrett/TJ Lakes Trailhead on the parking lot's south side; your starting trailhead is a few steps away, on the lot's north side.

McGee Creek Roadend Trailhead

10,250′; 11S 340796 4157548

DESTINATION/ UTM COORDINATES	TRIP TYPE	BEST SEASON	PACE (HIKING/ LAYOVER DAYS)	TOTAL MILEAGE
49 Steelhead Lake 11S 341299 4151119	Out & back	Mid to late	2/1 Leisurely	12
50 Pioneer Basin 11S 341245 4148576	Semiloop	Late	5/1 Strenuous, part cross-country	26
51 Big McGee Lake 11S 337039 4150662	Out & back	Mid to late	2/1 Leisurely	14
52 Rock Creek 11S 345426 4144580	Shuttle	Mid to late	5/2 Strenuous, part cross-country	30.6

Information and Permits: This trailhead is in Inyo National Forest: 351 Pacu Lane, Suite 200, Bishop, CA 93514, 760-873-2400, www.fs.fed.us/r5/inyo/. Quotas apply, and permits are required for overnight stays and are available at Inyo National Forest ranger stations in Lone Pine, Bishop, Mammoth Lakes, and Mono Basin Scenic Area Visitors Center.

Driving Directions: From Hwy. 395, 32 miles north of Bishop or 8 miles south of the Mammoth Lakes junction, turn southwest onto McGee Creek Road. Follow paved road across Crowley Lake Drive, past McGee Creek Campground, and continue on dirt surface past McGee Creek Pack Station to a paved parking loop at the road's end. The trailhead is equipped with vault toilet and horse-loading facilities.

49 Steelhead Lake

Trip Data: 11S 341299 4151119; 12 miles; 2/1 days

Topos: *Convict Lake, Mt. Abbot*

Highlights: Travelers new to entering the Sierra from its eastern escarpment will discover the ascent of McGee Creek fascinating because of the swirling patterns in the

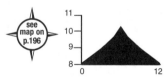

highly fractured, red, metamorphic rocks of the canyon wall. An early start is good, as the first few miles travel up a narrow, essentially shadeless canyon and can be stiflingly hot in the middle of the day. The scenic lakeshore offers splendid campsites and excellent fishing.

HEADS UP! The Convict Lake *topo doesn't show the trailhead correctly. The trailhead is now significantly farther east. "Upper McGee Creek Campground" doesn't exist anymore, but the road that went to it is now one of the two trails leaving the parking lot—in this case, the wide track that stays near the creek. Don't take it. The trail you need is the dusty, narrower one to the right of the wider track; it heads up the chaparral-clad slopes and is soon well above the creek.*

DAY 1 (McGee Creek Roadend Trailhead to Steelhead Lake, 6 miles): Leave the parking area near the restrooms and the trailhead signboard; take the narrower, dusty footpath that heads up chaparral-clad slopes and west into McGee Creek's canyon. Ahead to the west, the multicolored, contorted rock layers composing the canyon walls contrast pleasantly with the open, shrub-covered moraine the trail traverses.

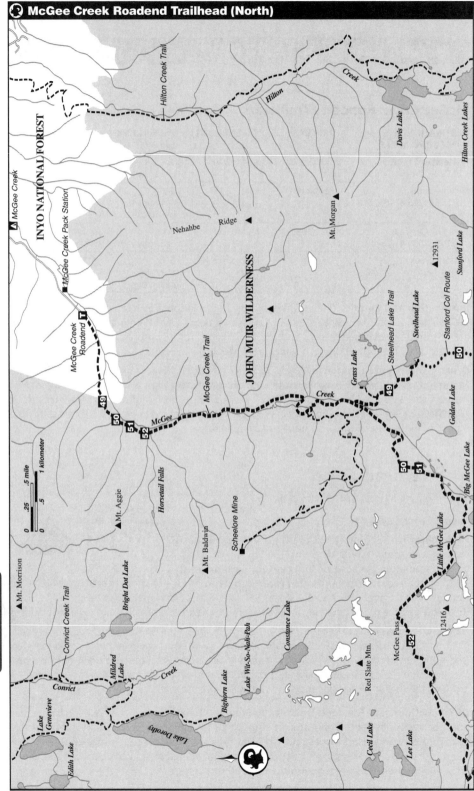

McGee Creek

INYO NATIONAL FOREST

△ McGee Creek

■ McGee Creek Pack Station

Hilton Creek Trail

Hilton

Creek

Davis Lake

Hilton Creek Lakes

Nehahbe Ridge ◄

Mt. Morgan ▲

▲12931

Stanford Lake

▶ McGee Creek Roadend

McGee Creek Roadend

McGee Creek Trail

JOHN MUIR WILDERNESS

◄

Steelhead Lake Trail

Steelhead Lake

Stanford Col Route

50

49

50

51

52

McGee

Creek

Grass Lake

49

Golden Lake

50

51

.5 mile

.25

.5

1 kilometer

0

0

.5

1

▲ Mt. Aggie

McGee Creek Trail

Horsetail Falls

Scheelore Mine

■

▲ Mt. Baldwin

Big McGee Lake

Little McGee Lake

▲ Mt. Morrison

Convict Creek Trail

Bright Dot Lake

Mildred Lake

Convict

Creek

Bighorn Lake

Lake Wit-So-Nah-Pah

Constance Lake

Red Slate Mtn. ▲

McGee Pass

12416▲

52

Lake Genevieve

Lake Dorothy

Edith Lake

◄

Cecil Lake

Lee Lake

◄

◄

McGEE CR

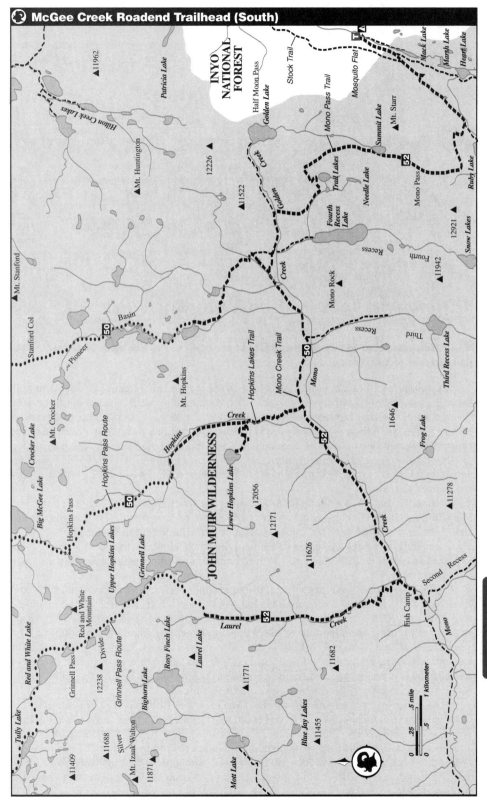

McGee Creek Roadend Trailhead (South)

INYO
NATIONAL
FOREST

Half Moon Pass
Stock Trail
Golden Lake
Mono Pass Trail
Mosquito Flat

Patricia Lake
▲11962

Hilton Creek Lakes
▲Mt. Huntington

12226 ▲

▲11522

Golden Creek

Trail Lakes
Needle Lake
Summit Lake
▲Mt. Starr
52
Mono Pass
Ruby Lake

Mack Lake
Manly Lake
Heart Lake

Fourth Recess Lake

Fourth Recess

12921 ▲
Snow Lakes

▲11942

Mono Rock ▲

▲Mt. Stanford

Stanford Col

Basin
50
Pioneer

Mono Creek Trail

Hopkins Lakes Trail

Mono Creek

50

Recess

Third

Third Recess Lake

▲Mt. Crocker

Mt. Hopkins ▲

Hopkins Pass Route

Crocker Lake

Hopkins Creek

52

1646 ▲
Frog Lake

Big McGee Lake

Hopkins Pass

50

Upper Hopkins Lakes

JOHN MUIR WILDERNESS

Lower Hopkins Lake
▲12056
▲12171

Creek

52

▲11278

Grinnell Lake

▲11626

Second Recess

Red and White Mountain ▲

Divide

Grinnell Pass Route

Rosy Finch Lake

Laurel Lake

52
Laurel

Creek

Fish Camp

Mono

McGEE CR

Red and White Lake

Grinnell Pass

12238 ▲

Silver
▲Mt. Izaak Walton

Bighorn Lake

▲11771

▲11682

Tully Lake

▲11688

11871 ▲

Blue Jay Lakes
▲11455

Mott Lake

0   .25   .5 mile
0   .5   1 kilometer

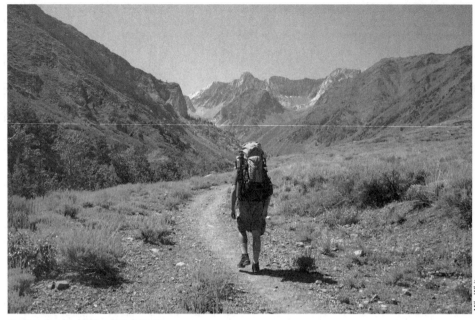

Mike White

Backpacker on McGee Creek Trail

A gradual-to-moderate ascent leads to a crossing of a thin stream trickling downhill from Buzztail Spring and then shortly to the signed John Muir Wilderness boundary. Beyond here, the trail curves slowly southward and proceeds deeper into the gorge of McGee Creek, with improving views of Horsetail Falls spilling down the west wall of the canyon. Seasonal flowers can be spectacular along this stretch. Presently, the trail curves south, and the views are temporarily obscured by a lengthy grove of aspen. Amid the aspen, cross a pair of close streams that overflow the trail, the second of which carries water from the falls.

Eventually, the aspen are left behind, allowing for fine views up the canyon on the way to a stout, flat-topped, twin-log bridge across McGee Creek (one wonders how logs of this size were transported this far into the wilderness without mechanized support). The shadeless trail continues along the east side of the creek, climbing to a shelf above a beautiful meadow, where, thanks to some industrious beavers, the stream meanders in sensuous curves.

Come to a second, smaller pair of flat-topped logs bridging McGee Creek again, and then head away from the west bank into lodgepole pine forest. The trail curves around a large outcrop past a pair of lodgepole-shaded campsites and passes by an obscure junction with an old mining road leading to the Scheelore Mine, the initial stretch doubling as a stock route to the McGee Creek Trail for the numerous pack trains that frequent the canyon. Following a sign for McGee Pass, you turn left (southeast) at the junction, cross a tributary on a wood-plank bridge, and proceed through shady forest up the main fork of McGee Creek to a Y-junction, 4.75 miles from the trailhead.

At the junction, turn left (south) and ford McGee Creek (difficult in early season) before starting a steep, switchbacking, 460-foot climb up the east wall of the canyon to a junction with the half-mile trail to Grass Lake (9826´; campsites). Bear right (east-southeast) here on a brief climb, follow and then cross a small brook, wind uphill to where the terrain eases near a couple of tarns, and then descend past good campsites to the northwest shore of 25-acre Steelhead Lake (10,380´). Look for good campsites atop the small peninsula above the southwest side of the lake.

> **AT STEELHEAD LAKE**
>
> Views from the lakeshore take in the granite grandeur of Mt. Stanford and Mt. Crocker to the south and west, and rust-and-buff-colored Mt. Baldwin in the north. Anglers will find the fishing for rainbow and brook trout excellent (best in early and late season). The name "Steelhead" is certainly a misnomer for this lake, as the term refers to ocean-going trout. The mistake may be somewhat understandable, as, over the years, rainbow trout from the lake have exhibited pale and faded markings similar in appearance to their silver cousins of coastal waters.

DAY 2 (Steelhead Lake to McGee Creek Roadend Trailhead, 6 miles): Retrace your steps to the trailhead.

50 Pioneer Basin

Trip Data: 11S 341245 4148576; 26 miles; 5/1 days

Topos: *Convict Lake, Mt. Abbot*

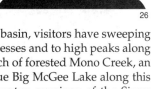

see map on p.196

Highlights: Pioneer Basin, holding a string of lakes surrounded by flower-dotted alpine meadows and ringed by gray granite peaks, is one of the most scenic spots in the central Sierra. From the basin, visitors have sweeping views across the deep cleft of Mono Creek into the Mono Recesses and to high peaks along the Mono Divide. Backpackers will also get to sample a stretch of forested Mono Creek, an ascent up the lush canyon of Hopkins Creek, and picturesque Big McGee Lake along this semiloop. This rugged route utilizes two difficult, cross-country crossings of the Sierra Crest: Stanford Col, above Steelhead Lake on the way into the basin, and Hopkins Pass, above Big McGee Lake, on the return to the McGee Creek Trail.

HEADS UP! *The Convict Lake topo doesn't show the trailhead correctly. The trailhead is now significantly farther east. "Upper McGee Creek Campground" doesn't exist anymore, but the road that went to it is now one of the two trails leaving the parking lot—in this case, the wide track that stays near the creek. Don't take it. The trail you need is the dusty, narrower one to the right of the wider track; it heads up the chaparral-clad slopes and is soon well above the creek.*

The difficult cross-country sections along this route, especially the climb over talus, loose rock, and scree from Steelhead Lake to Stanford Col, make this a trip for experienced mountaineers only. To avoid going to Pioneer Basin this way, take Trip 55 instead.

DAY 1 (McGee Creek Roadend Trailhead to Steelhead Lake, 6 miles): *(Recap: Trip 49, Day 1.)* Follow the narrower, dusty trail through sagebrush scrub up McGee Creek's canyon, as the trail heads west and then gradually curves south, crossing streams along the way. Beyond an extensive aspen grove, make a pair of log-bridge crossings of McGee Creek and proceed upstream past an obscure junction with an old mining road to a Y-junction of the Steelhead Lake and McGee Creek trails, 4.75 miles from the trailhead.

Veer left (south) at the junction, ford McGee Creek (difficult in early season), and climb steeply up the Steelhead Lake Trail to a junction with the lateral to Grass Lake. Bear right (east-southeast) and proceed past tarns and campsites to the north shore of Steelhead Lake (10,380′).

DAY 2 (Steelhead Lake to Pioneer Basin, 2 miles, cross-country): From the southwest shore of serene Steelhead Lake, head south to ascend the steep and rocky slope just above the lake to gain the more moderately sloping talus field below Stanford Col, the obvious low

McGEE CR

point at the head of the canyon that becomes visible after the initial climb. Carefully negotiate your way up the talus slope over large, blocky boulders—a climb made perhaps less
difficult if solid snowfields allow travel above the jumbled rocks.

Upon reaching the base of the final slope, a steep, loose collection of scree and rock,
begin a very steep climb generally south toward the col, making sure everyone in your
party is out of each other's fall line in order to avoid getting knocked in the head by a stray
projectile. After the 400-foot climb, more secure footing is gained at the col (11,611´; 11S
340023 4150425), where an impressive view sweeps across Pioneer Basin toward the
rugged peaks of the Mono Divide, a superlative vista that makes the steep and tedious
climb seem worthwhile. The view to the north of McGee Creek's multicolored canyon is
stunning as well.

With the most difficult part of the entire trip completed, leave the col and easily drop
southward down scree slopes toward the upper part of Pioneer Basin. Following the short
descent, head generally south cross-country over sandy soil sprinkled with boulders and
tiny alpine plants toward Lake 10862, the largest of the Pioneer Basin lakes. Along the way,
come alongside and then follow the main branch of the flower-and-meadow-lined creek
that drains the basin to the northeast shore of the long, irregularly shaped lake (10,862´). A
few windy campsites bordered by dwarf whitebark pines pepper the knoll above the east
shore.

Better campsites can be found near the south end of the lake and around Lake 11026,
but you're more likely to see other backpackers there who have accessed the basin via trail
over Mono Pass. Pioneer Basin is a fine place to spend additional days exploring the nooks
and crannies of the area on easy cross-country romps, or to simply relax and enjoy the
panoramic scenery. Although the lakes seem to hold a healthy population of brook and
rainbow trout, for some reason, fishing reports seem to be disappointing.

DAY 3 (Pioneer Basin to Lower Hopkins Lake, 6.5 miles): From Lake 10862, follow a use trail
generally south along the the lakes on the basin's west side. If you notice it, ignore a well-
trod use trail from Lake 10862's southeastern peninsula to the basin's east side; it's fine for
exploring the basin but not for today's journey.

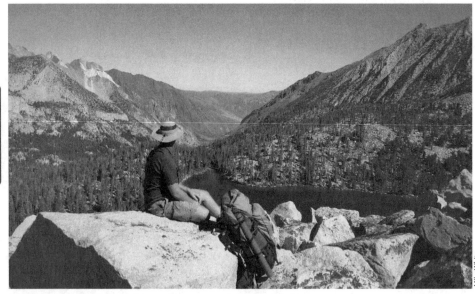

Gazing down McGee Creek Canyon from route to Stanford Col

From the southeast shore of the southwesternmost large lake in Pioneer Basin (the almost bathtub-shaped one a little southeast of Mt. Hopkins' peak at 10,820′; 11S 340547 4147480; also known as Lake 2), the trail leaves the idyllic upper basin and drops moderately to steeply away from the lakes into a scattered-to-light forest of lodgepole pines. The rate of descent eases where the trail traverses an open flat harboring the lowest lake, a shallow lake called Mud Lake, and then fords Mud Lake's outlet. Across this flat are good views of the massive hulk of towering Mono Rock and the deep cleft of Fourth Recess.

Heading back into the trees, the descent toward Mono Creek resumes across hillsides carpeted with lush foliage. Approaching the floor of the canyon, step across a brook and head downstream to an unsigned junction with twin laterals to the Mono Creek Trail, one on the left for eastbound hikers and one on the right for westbound hikers. Go right (southwest) and follow the lateral a short distance to an unsigned junction with the Mono Creek Trail (10,062′; 11S 341401 4146193).

Turn right (west) at the junction, following the dusty and sometimes rocky Mono Creek Trail through lodgepole pine forest adorned with a lush understory of plants and wildflowers. Make three close crossings of the same tributary stream and continue downstream along Mono Creek on gradually graded trail, hopping across the two streams draining Pioneer Basin and passing Mono Rock on the opposite side of the canyon. Several campsites are spread across the canyon floor, some of which can't be clearly seen from the trail (the ones that can be seen are often within 100 feet of the trail or Mono Creek and are therefore illegal).

Pass by a use trail to a packer's camp and break out of the forest into an open meadow where an unsigned trail heads south across the creek and into Third Recess. Continue downstream on the main trail, generally west, through alternating stands of trees and clearings to a signed Y-junction with the Hopkins Creek Trail.

Turn right (north) to leave the Mono Pass Trail and begin a moderately steep, zigzagging climb up the north wall of the canyon across boulder-studded slopes beneath lodgepole pines to the right of Hopkins Creek. At the top of the switchbacks, climb more moderately through luxuriant vegetation to a ford of the creek and then immediately reach a junction with the trail to Lower Hopkins Lake, a mile from the Mono Creek Trail junction.

Go left (west) at the junction and climb steeply on the winding trail to Lower Hopkins Lake. Eventually, the grade eases, and a short stroll leads past decent campsites to the roughly oval lake (10,354′; 11S 338418 4146835). A strip of meadow and a smattering of lodgepole pines surround the quiet lake, which has a rugged backdrop of steep granite cliffs. Rainbow and brook trout will tempt anglers.

DAY 4 (Lower Hopkins Lake to Big McGee Lake, 4.5 miles, part cross-country): Retrace your steps to the junction with the Hopkins Creek Trail, turn left (north) onto it, and then resume the moderate ascent up the canyon through thickly vegetated meadowlands and scattered lodgepole pines. The grade eases as the trail enters a long, flower-filled meadow with views up the canyon toward aptly named Red and White Mountain.

The tread progressively deteriorates across this meadow, revealing badly constructed sections of trail through soggy areas, which has resulted in parallel ruts in the soil.

MEADOW RUTS

As these roughly parallel ruts get deeper with repeated use, they fill with water, and then hikers create an adjacent path on higher soil that, over time, will suffer the same fate. Continuing across the meadow, notice several areas where three or more paths have been created by this unfortunate dilemma. This trail desperately needs to be rerouted to higher ground, but a path like the little used Hopkins Creek Trail is generally a low priority on the Forest Service's project list.

Farther up the meadow, the tread periodically disappears, but ducks should help lead the way generally north-northwest toward trailless Hopkins Pass; this route doesn't go to the Upper Hopkins Lakes.

UPPER HOPKINS LAKES

If Upper Hopkins Lakes are the goal, eventually you will have to leave the ducked trail and head west on a faint use trail, or simply strike off cross-country to access these scenic gems. Campsites at the lower lake appear to be more hospitable than ones at the windswept upper lake.

Today's ducked route bypasses the upper lakes and heads straight for Hopkins Pass, going higher into the alpine zone on its way toward the head of the canyon. As the slope becomes rocky and dotted with small, ground-hugging plants, the tread and the ducks completely vanish, but the way to the low point of the broad pass is obvious.

First-timers may reach the edge of Hopkins Pass (11,495′; 11S 336881 4149720) and determine there is absolutely no safe way down the far side, where the terrain drops precipitously 800 vertical feet to the upper part of McGee Creek's canyon. Fortunately, a large cairn on top of a boulder marks the beginning of a use trail down this steep slope. Before starting the descent, be sure to take in the colorful view down McGee Creek's canyon out to the White Mountains, and behind Hopkins Creek's canyon.

Exercising extreme caution, follow the use trail generally northwest away from Hopkins Pass on a dicey descent across steep, rocky slopes. Initially, there is no single, defined trail, so you'll have to choose the most suitable path for a secure descent—the set of wider switchbacks appears to be a better choice, as opposed to the short set of switchbacks that zigzag tightly straight down the slope. Eventually, the route becomes less traumatic on its way to a crossing of the outlet that drains the tarn at the head of the canyon. After crossing this outlet, the route continues the descent above the west side of the cascading stream, with picturesque views of the multicolored peaks and ridges that make up the upper part of McGee Creek's canyon, as well as the striking waterfall exiting Little McGee Lake. With the drop in elevation, grasses, sedges, clumps of willow, and colorful wildflowers begin to appear, a cheerful sight after the bleak and rocky surroundings above.

Dwarf whitebark pines herald the approach to a bench above Big McGee Lake (10,472′; 11S 337039, 4150662), which sits in a bowl composed of steep cliffs and high-angle slopes. There are good campsites on top of a cliff on the peninsula on the lake's west side. Although widely scattered whitebark pines and mountain hemlocks offer little protection from the wind, these campsites do offer outstanding views of the lake and the upper part of the canyon. Despite limited access to the shoreline, anglers enjoy good fishing for both rainbow and brook trout. Also, there are fair-to-poor campsites on the peninsula that juts southward from the lake's north side; these sites are very popular with those who've come to Big McGee Lake directly from the trailhead on the main McGee Creek Trail.

DAY 5 (Big McGee Lake to McGee Creek Roadend Trailhead, 7 miles): Pick up a use trail in the vicinity of the peninsula and proceed north through meadowlands up toward the well-defined tread of the McGee Creek Trail. Turn right (east) and follow the trail across a talus slope well above Big McGee Lake before dropping past use trails to the poor-to-fair campsites on the north-side peninsula, and then to an area of meadows and slabs just below the lake, where decent campsites are spread along the banks of the outlet.

Hop across a pretty rivulet and descend away from the lake and down the canyon, passing through alternating sections of lodgepole pine forest and verdant, meadow-covered benches. Drop more steeply to a forested junction with an unmaintained trail to Golden Lake and continue a short distance to a small pond just off the trail, known locally as Round Lake, where needy campers could find fair, overused campsites south of the pond.

Proceed on a stiff, switchbacking descent through granite cliffs shaded by hemlocks on a well-engineered section of trail that incorporates several granite stairs. The roar of McGee Creek becomes louder on the way to a creekside junction with the Steelhead Lake Trail at the close of the loop. Partway down, a use trail on the left leads west to a packer campsite.

At the junction with the Steelhead Lake Trail, turn left (north, downstream), and retrace Day 1's steps 4.75 miles to the trailhead.

51 Big McGee Lake

Trip Data: 11S 337039 4150662; 14 miles; 2/1 days

Topos: *Convict Lake, Mt. Abbot*

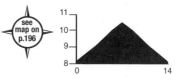

Highlights: In an alpine setting close under the Sierra Crest, Big McGee Lake shares a large granite basin with three other fishable lakes. This beautiful spot nestles below the sheer, colorful walls of 12,816-foot Red and White Mountain, and close to impressive 12,458-foot Mt. Crocker.

HEADS UP! *The Convict Lake topo doesn't show the trailhead correctly. The trailhead is now significantly farther east. "Upper McGee Creek Campground" doesn't exist anymore, but the road that went to it is now one of the two trails leaving the parking lot—in this case, the wide track that stays near the creek. Don't take it. The trail you need is the dusty, narrower one to the right of the wider track; it heads up the chaparral-clad slopes and is soon well above the creek.*

DAY 1 (McGee Creek Roadend Trailhead to Big McGee Lake, 7 miles): *(Recap in Reverse: Trip 50, Day 5.)* Follow the narrow, dusty trail through sagebrush scrub up McGee Creek's canyon, as the trail heads west and then gradually curves south, crossing streams along the

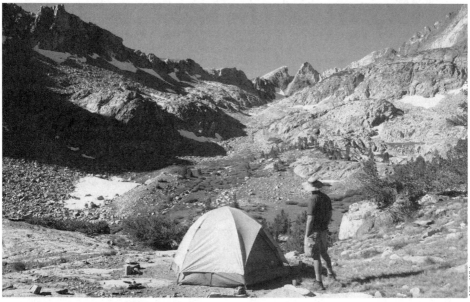

View from Big McGee Lake toward Hopkins Pass

way. Beyond an extensive aspen grove, make a pair of log-bridge crossings of McGee Creek and continue upstream past an obscure junction with an old mining road to a Y-junction of the Steelhead Lake and McGee Creek trails, 4.75 miles from the trailhead.

Go right (southwest) from the junction on the McGee Creek Trail, continuing south where the stock trail that split off earlier rejoins the main trail. Begin a moderate ascent that climbs about 450 vertical feet on numerous, short, rocky, hemlock-shaded switchbacks along granite cliffs. As you climb, 12,838-foot Mt. Stanford springs into view. Upon reaching the top of the switchbacks, the trail dips into a damp, forested hollow and arrives near a pond, known locally as Round Lake. Fair, overused campsites lie just south of this pond.

Beyond Round Lake, veer north past a verdant meadow and start a switchbacking climb to a series of meadow-covered benches that may become dry by late season and that offer surprisingly few campsites—practically none. The grade eases on these benches, where the trail carefully skirts the flowery meadows.

Reach an area of meadows and slabs below the north end of Big McGee Lake, where several campsites are spread along the banks of the creek. Just beyond and above the lake, use trails dart off to poor-to-fair, but very popular, campsites on the peninsula on Big McGee's north shore.

Above this area, the trail climbs across a lightly forested talus slope to more meadowlands, where a use trail splits away to the left (south) and accesses good campsites above a cliff on the peninsula that juts into the southwest side of the Big McGee Lake (10,472´; 11S 337039 4150662). Although the sparse whitebark pines and mountain hemlocks provide these campsites with little protection from the wind, the view of the aquamarine lake and the upper part of the canyon should more than make up for the potentially breezy conditions.

> **AT BIG McGEE LAKE**
> Although access to the shoreline is somewhat limited by the steep topography around much of the lake, anglers should enjoy good fishing for rainbow and brook trout. If time and inclination allow, anglers can explore the equally attractive fishing at Little McGee Lake (rockbound and campsite-less), Crocker Lake, or picture-book Golden Lake.

DAY 2 (Big McGee Lake to McGee Creek Roadend Trailhead, 7 miles): Retrace your steps to the trailhead.

52 Rock Creek

Trip Data: 11S 345426 4144580; 30.6 miles; 6/2 days

Topos: *Convict Lake, Mt. Abbot, Graveyard Peak, Mt. Morgan*

Highlights: This rugged route offers excitement and challenge sufficient to satisfy the most jaded appetite. High-country lakes surrounded by rampart-like peaks characterize this colorful route, and the fishing should be good to excellent.

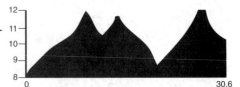

HEADS UP! The Convict Lake topo doesn't show the trailhead correctly. The trailhead is now significantly farther east. "Upper McGee Creek Campground" doesn't exist anymore, but the road that went to it is now one of the two trails leaving the parking lot—in this case, the wide track that stays near the creek. Don't take it. The trail you need is the dusty, narrower one to the right of the wider track; it heads up the chaparral-clad slopes and is soon well above the creek.

This trip is for experienced mountaineers only. If you're not, trips out of Rock Creek proper are more suitable (54, 55).

McGEE CR

Shuttle Directions: From Hwy. 395, 25 miles north of Bishop or 15 miles south of the Mammoth Lakes junction with Hwy. 203, turn west on Rock Creek Road at the small community of Tom's Place. Cross Crowley Lake Drive and follow the road past Rock Creek Lake 10.7 miles from Hwy. 395. Continue to the Mosquito Flat Trailhead at the end of the road (vault toilets). The road becomes very winding and narrow beyond the Hilton Lakes Trailhead; be prepared to yield to oncoming traffic. There is a small backpackers' campground across bridged Rock Creek from the parking lot, available only for one night before the start of your trip. You must show a valid wilderness permit from the Mosquito Flat Trailhead to demonstrate your eligibility for a campsite.

DAY 1 (McGee Creek Roadend Trailhead to Big McGee Lake, 7 miles): *(Recap in Reverse: Trip 50, Day 5.)* Follow the narrower, dusty trail through sagebrush scrub up McGee Creek's canyon as it heads west and then gradually curves south, crossing streams along the way. Beyond an extensive aspen grove, make a pair of log-bridge crossings of McGee Creek and proceed upstream past an obscure junction with an old mining road to a Y-junction of the Steelhead Lake and McGee Creek trails, 4.75 miles from the trailhead.

Go right (southwest) at the junction and follow a switchbacking, 450-foot climb through forest to a pond that locals refer to as Round Lake (campsites). Beyond the pond, the trail continues climbing to a series of meadow-covered benches before reaching meadows and slabs to the south of Big McGee Lake. Overnighters can find campsites in this area along the outlet. The main trail passes the lake's north shore; use trails go to fair-to-poor, overused campsites on the peninsula on this shore. Beyond, the tread climbs across a lightly forested talus slope above the west side of the lake to a use trail heading south to good campsites above some cliffs on a peninsula that juts into the lake's west side (10,472´; 11S 337039 4150662).

DAY 2 (Big McGee Lake to Tully Lake, 5.5 miles): Regain the main trail and turn west on it. From Big McGee Lake, follow the trail across steep meadows, pass above timberline on an exposed climb, and hop across a stream that drains the slopes below Corridor Pass. Pass above Little McGee Lake (rockbound and virtually campsite-less), and then climb steeply up the narrow canyon of the lake's inlet. Continue the ascent with the aid of an occasional switchback up the canyon through broken reddish rock toward 11,909-foot McGee Pass; snow may linger here until late season. Views from the pass across the headwaters of Fish Creek to the Silver Divide are breathtaking.

From the pass, a long, rocky, switchbacking descent ensues, leading nearly 1000 vertical feet down austere slopes to a large, lovely, meadow-floored basin at the headwaters of Fish Creek. The trail makes a gentle descent on a traverse of this basin, hopping across several seasonal rivulets along the way. Drop past a charming cascade and continue to a crossing of Fish Creek and a junction with a use trail to Tully Lake.

Turn left (south) away from the McGee Pass Trail and follow the use trail along the lake's outlet to the northwest shore of 10-acre Tully Lake (10,400´; 11S 333268 4150690). Good campsites may be found in the trees above the lake.

FISH CREEK ANGLING

Anglers should expect fair-to-good fishing for golden and brook trout. The headwaters of Fish Creek offer many other lakes, meadows, and creeks suitable for layover-day visits. Visitors may wish to try the waters of Red and White Lake, about a mile away over a ridge to the east, with fair-to-good fishing for rainbow trout. Those seeking stream fishing may find smaller rainbow, brook, and some golden along meandering Fish Creek.

DAY 3 (Tully Lake to Grinnell Lake, 3.5 miles, cross-country): From the east shore of Tully Lake, the route ascends the grassy swale that lies due east of the lake. At the outlet from Red and White Lake, the route turns right (southeast) and follows this stream to that lake (large rainbow). Although good campsites are virtually nonexistent, Red and White Lake offers an excellent vantage point from which to enjoy the spectacular and aptly named heights of Red and White Mountain. The saddle, called "Grinnell Pass," is high point of today's journey and is clearly visible as the low point on the peak's right (west) shoulder. The easiest route to the saddle follows the rocky east shore around the lake. The steepest part of the ascent is over treacherous shale (or snowfields in early to mid-season); travelers should proceed slowly and carefully. Carry a rope and use it when necessary, especially when ascending the west side of the pass.

GRINNELL PASS VIEWS

From Grinnell Pass (11,600'; 11S 335056 4149735), enjoy a well-deserved and stimulating view of the surrounding terrain. To the north, the immediate, dazzling blue waters of Red and White Lake set off the buff browns and ochre reds of the surrounding rock. Beyond this basin, the meadow-filled cirque forming the headwaters of Fish Creek is a large greensward that contrasts sharply with the austere, red-stained eminence of Red Slate Mountain, and the distant skyline offers sawtooth profiles of the renowned Ritter Range, with the readily identifiable Minarets, and the Mammoth Crest. To the south, the barren, rocky shores of the Grinnell chain of lakes occupy the foreground, and just beyond, the green-sheathed slopes of the Mono Creek watershed drop away, rising in the distance to the Mono Divide.

As with the ascent to the saddle, descend with care. The sudden, shale-filled drop terminates in a large "rock garden," a jumble of large boulders just above Little Grinnell Lake. The rock-hopping route leads along the east shore of this tiny lake to a long, grassy descent toward the west side of large Grinnell Lake (10,800'; 11S 6136 4148449). Midway along this side, where the most prominent peninsula infringes on the long lake, today's cross-country route strikes the distinct fisherman's trail veering southwest down a long swale to tiny Laurel Lake. Several fair campsites near this junction offer excellent views due to their location on a plateau above the lake. Anglers may find Grinnell Lake to have fair-to-good fishing for brook and rainbow. Other campsites can be found along the meadowed fringe of Laurel Lake (10,300'), about a mile to the southwest, where fishing for brook trout should be excellent.

DAY 4 (Grinnell Lake to Fish Camp, 4.5 miles): The fisherman's trail from Grinnell Lake to Laurel Lake descends southwest via a long scoop-like swale to the grassy meadows near the headwaters of Laurel Creek. The path, though initially very faint, becomes more distinct along the descent of slender Laurel Creek, which has abundant brook trout.

The gradual descent along the creek becomes somewhat steeper just above the larger meadows. This pleasant, timber-fringed grassland is divided by the serpentine curves of Laurel Creek. The trail across the meadow is hard to follow, but it can be found again across the creek in the vicinity of campsites at the south end of the meadow. The dense lodgepole cover at the end of the meadow soon gives way to manzanita thickets and occasional clumps of quaking aspen, as the trail reaches the top of switchbacks that lead steeply down toward Mono Creek. This unmaintained section of trail is prone to heavy erosion. However, the difficult tread is more than compensated for by the excellent views across the Mono Creek watershed into Second Recess. Particularly impressive are the heights of Mt. Gabb and Mt. Hilgard, which guard the upper end of that side canyon.

When the route strikes the Mono Creek Trail, turn right (west) for a gently descending half mile to the campsites at Fish Camp (8550'; 11S 335711 4143616), near the junction with the lateral to Second Recess. Fishing is generally good in Mono Creek for brook and rainbow trout.

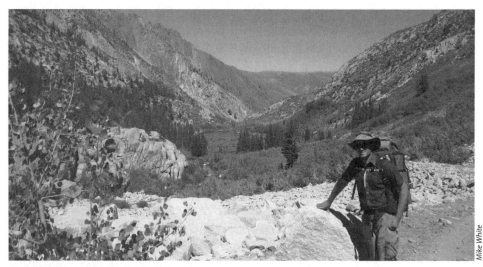

Mike White

Heading down McGee Creek Trail (Day 1)

DAY 5 (Fish Camp to Mosquito Flat, 10.1 miles): This is a long and strenuous day; get an early start.

From Fish Camp, head upstream and uphill east-northeast on the Mono Creek Trail a half mile back to the junction with the lateral to Grinnell Lakes. Continue ahead (northeast) on the Mono Creek Trail, now a dusty trail through a mixed forest of conifers and quaking aspens. In late season, the groves of aspen lining the creek create an incomparably colorful backdrop to an otherwise monotonous conifer green. Holes on Mono Creek offer good fishing for brook, rainbow, and some golden trout.

Reach the signed junction with the Hopkins Lake Trail and continue upstream (ahead, northeast on the Mono Creek Trail) through alternating stands of forest and open clearings to an unsigned junction on the right with the trail into Third Recess. Go ahead (east-northeast) and shortly bypass a use trail on the left that leads uphill to a large packer's camp.

Continuing up the canyon of Mono Creek, the trail passes several shady campsites on the way past the towering ramparts of Mono Rock, which can be seen through periodic breaks in the forest. Proceed through lodgepole pine forest with a thick understory of plants and wildflowers, and after several crossings of side streams, come to an unsigned junction on the left with the the a lateral to the trail into Pioneer Basin. Shortly, reach a second lateral to the Pioneer Basin Trail. At both junctions, go ahead (generally east), continuing up Mono Creek.

A short climb along the Mono Creek Trail from the lateral to Pioneer Basin leads to a junction with the trail right (southwest and then south) into Fourth Recess (a few campsites). For those who can afford the extra time, beautiful Fourth Recess Lake is well worth a visit. Thousand-foot walls frame the long lake on three sides, and its inlet is an 800-foot waterfall that plunges down the south wall.

Otherwise, continue east up Mono Creek as it eventually starts climbing more moderately on dusty and sometimes rocky tread to a junction with an unmapped trail east to Golden Lake (campsites) at a nearby ford of Golden Creek. Here the Mono Creek Trail turns south and begins a stiff climb toward the Trail Lakes, veering southeast after a while. The trail passes just below the lakes, a popular overnight destination for hikers crossing Mono Pass from the east. Along with campsites nestled in clumps of stunted whitebark pines, the Trail Lakes are home to the tiny stone hut of a California snow-survey shelter (no trespassing).

A steep, switchbacking climb from the Trail Lakes leads to the crest of a ridge.

VIEWS FROM THE RIDGE ABOVE THE TRAIL LAKES

Backpackers who take the time to pause here will be treated to a sweeping vista to the northwest of Pioneer Basin over the deep cleft of Mono Creek and bordered by the peaks of Mt. Stanford and Mt. Crocker. Immediately below are Trail Lakes and Needle Lake (the latter misspelled "Neelle" on the topo).

Leave the ridge and traverse a flat before a short climb that leads up to austere Summit Lake. Multiple paths lead past the lake, as snow often lingers in this basin and up to Mono Pass well into the season.

Reach Mono Pass (12,060´) on the Sierra Crest at the boundary between Sierra and Inyo national forests. Not only is the pass devoid of views, the stark landscape of shattered and decomposed granite appears lifeless.

WHAT'S TO SEE AT MONO PASS

Upon close inspection, the ground around Mono Pass soon dispels the impression of life-lessness by revealing an abundance of small, ground-hugging alpine plants. Some of these plants may seem familiar from lower elevations, but the extreme conditions at this elevation tend to dwarf their stature. Vista-starved peakbaggers can ascend a Class 2 route of Mt. Starr (12,835´) to the east for panoramic views. Note that there are two Mono Passes on the Sierra Crest; the other one is farther north, between Yosemite National Park and Inyo National Forest.

Leaving Mono Pass, the trail heads south, descending a rock-filled draw before arcing around to the east on a steep, switchbacking drop above Ruby Lake. Views along this descent of Little Lakes Valley and the impressive string of peaks to the west are quite dramatic. About 1.5 miles from the pass, the stiff descent momentarily abates at a junction with the Ruby Lake Trail alongside a verdant meadowland bisected by the lake's outlet.

From the Ruby Lake junction, zigzag down the west wall of the canyon, with fine views of Little Lakes Valley as nearly constant companions. Cross a number of flower-lined, seasonal streams and pass by a picturesque tarn. Nearing the floor of the valley, find a junction with a spur trail to the Rock Creek Pack Station; go right (east and then south) on a switchback. Shortly, reach a junction with the Morgan Pass Trail. Turn left (north) where the trail parallels Rock Creek downstream, descend and exit John Muir Wilderness, and soon arrive at the Mosquito Flat Trailhead parking lot (10,255´; 11S 345426 4144580).

McGEE CR

Hilton Lakes Trailhead

9845´; 11S 346030 4146799

DESTINATION/ UTM COORDINATES	TRIP TYPE	BEST SEASON	PACE (HIKING/ LAYOVER DAYS)	TOTAL MILEAGE
53 Hilton Lakes 11S 344811 4150098	Shuttle	Mid to late	2/1 Leisurely	12/13

Information and Permits: This trailhead is in Inyo National Forest: 351 Pacu Lane, Suite 200, Bishop, CA 93514, 760-873-2400, www.fs.fed.us/r5/inyo/. Quotas apply, and permits are required for overnight stays and are available at Inyo National Forest ranger stations in Lone Pine, Bishop, Mammoth Lakes, and Mono Basin Scenic Area Visitors Center. Bear canisters are required.

Driving Directions: From Hwy. 395 at Tom's Place, go south up Rock Creek Road approximately 9.5 miles, passing Rock Creek Lake on the left and Rock Creek Lakes Resort on the right. Just past the pack station, look for the Hilton Lakes Trailhead on the right and, just beyond that, the small parking area. Bears are very active in Rock Creek—don't leave food or toiletries in your car.

53 Hilton Lakes

Trip Data: 11S 344811 4150098; 12/13 miles; 2/1

Topos: *Mt. Abbot, Mt. Morgan, Convict Lake*

Highlights: Lovely Hilton Creek flows from rugged Sierra Crest peaks through a small basin, through the charming Hilton Lakes (or Hilton Creek Lakes), and finally out to Crowley Lake. Backpackers will find appealing campsites and good fishing at lakes 3 and 4 and fine dayhiking. The nearby pack station tends to send its clients to the closest lakes (Hilton Lakes 2 and 1; 1 is better known as Davis Lake), but it's still possible to find solitude up and down the basin. This shuttle trip follows Hilton Creek out of the basin through aspen groves to a seldom-used trailhead. (Or take the trip as a fine out-and-back from the Hilton Lakes Trailhead.)

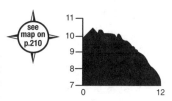

see map on p.210

Shuttle Directions: From the McGee Creek exit on Hwy. 395 (about 10 miles north of Tom's Place), turn south onto McGee Creek Road and, in a hundred feet, intersect Crowley Lake Drive. Turn left (east) on Crowley Lake Drive and go 2 miles. Just as you crest a very small rise, turn right onto a dirt road, signed for the Hilton Creek Trail. Trailhead parking is on the right at the end of the road (7175´; 11S 344979 4158928).

DAY 1 (Hilton Lakes Trailhead to Hilton Lake 3 or 4, 4 or 5 miles): The trail immediately begins a gradual-to-moderate climb on the ridge separating Rock and Hilton creeks, first through forest and then on exposed slopes that boast an amazing array of flowers in season. A switchback turn affords excellent views over Rock Creek Lake and the peaks south around Little Lakes Valley before the path begins a long, northward traverse and enters the John Muir Wilderness at a switchback turn.

The tread curves northwest and swings up to a junction at a little over 2 miles, where the left fork has been intentionally blocked off. Go right (northwest) through an open, sandy forest of lodgepoles, skirt a large meadow, and then curve generally west. After

ROCK CR

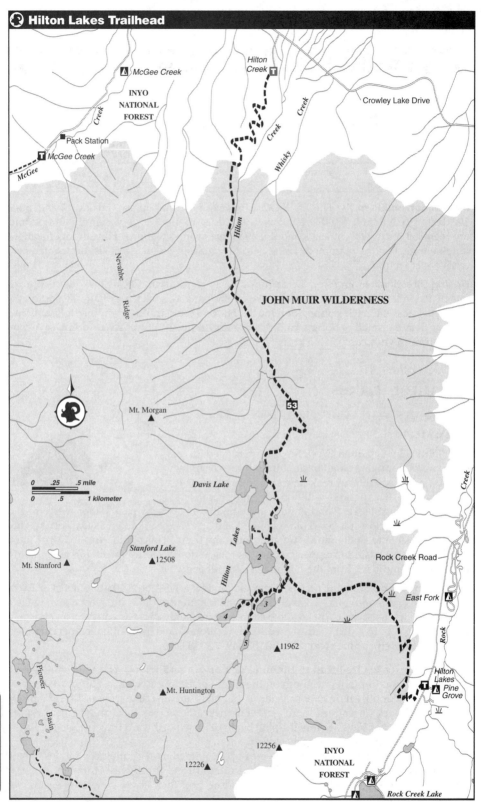

McGee Creek

**INYO
NATIONAL
FOREST**

Creek

Hilton
Creek

Crowley Lake Drive

Creek

Whisky

Pack Station

McGee Creek

McGee

Hilton

Creek

JOHN MUIR WILDERNESS

Mt. Morgan

53

Nevahbe
Ridge

0   .25   .5 mile
0   .5   1 kilometer

Davis Lake

Rock Creek Road

Hilton

Stanford Lake

Lakes

Mt. Stanford

12508

2

East Fork

3

4

Rock

5

11962

Hilton
Lakes

Pine
Grove

Pioneer

Mt. Huntington

Basin

12256

INYO
NATIONAL
FOREST

12226

Rock Creek Lake

another mile, the grade increases, and the trail soon tops out on a saddle at 10,380 feet above the Hilton Basin, looking at the impressive "railroad-baron peaks" of Mt. Stanford and Mt. Huntington.

From here, the route descends on gradual-to-moderate switchbacks to a trail junction at 4 miles: left (southwest) to Hilton Lakes 3 and 4; right (north) to Hilton Lake 2 and Davis Lake (a.k.a. Hilton Lake 1). Go left to cross a seasonal stream, pass a small meadow, and begin a short but steep series of switchbacks up, leveling out at fabulous views northward over Hilton Lake 2 and Davis Lake, and across Long Valley to Glass Mountain. At the stream connecting lakes 3 and 2, Hilton Lake 3 (10,300´; 11S 344811 4150098) is immediately upstream at 4.5 miles, with a dramatic backdrop of Mt. Huntington and Mt. Stanford. Take use trails from here to find campsites.

To continue to Hilton Lake 4, stay on the main trail to cross the stream and curve southwest along Hilton Lake 3's northwest shore. The trail veers west across a low ridge offering a fine view of the dashing cascades of Hilton Lake 5's outlet. Descend to cross the outlet in a meadow, bob over another ridgelet, and reach Hilton Lake 4 (10,353´; 11S 344155 4149852) at almost 5 miles. A layover day gives time for a cross-country scramble to the wild, scenic upper lakes, or for a move to a lower camp, perhaps near the northwest shore of Davis Lake.

DAY 2 (Upper Hilton Lakes to Hilton Creek Trailhead, 8 miles): Return to the main Hilton Lakes Trail junction below Lake 3. Go ahead (left, north) and descend toward Lake 2, passing above its east side. Where a use trail hooks left (west) around a little hill toward Lake 2's outlet, continue ahead (north) toward Davis Lake.

Pass a lovely meadow before curving around Davis Lake's outlet to leave the basin. Use trails here might be confusing, so continue to head northeast, staying on the east side of Hilton Creek. The terrain becomes sagebrush scrub, and the trail grows sandier as the trail descends the narrowing canyon, flanked on the west by imposing Mt. Morgan and Nevahbe Ridge.

After some 4 miles, ford Hilton Creek (difficult in early season). Beyond the crossing, turn right (north) to continue the easy descent, following an old mining road through the aspens. Especially striking along this stretch is the multicolored layering of Nevahbe Ridge's towering, fluted cliffs on the left (west). At the signed wilderness boundary, leave the creekside and come to an intersection (8621´; 11S 344167 4156955) with an old 4WD drive road to the left; the trail goes right (northeast) on a dusty, switchbacking descent.

Over the final 2-plus miles, the route takes in sweeping views of Crowley Lake, Glass Mountain, the Mono Craters, and surrounding peaks, before arriving at the Hilton Creek Trailhead (7175´; 11S 344979 4158928).

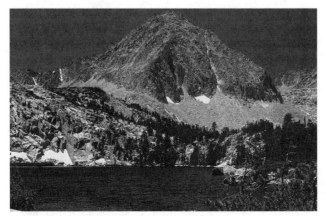

Mt. Huntington over Hilton Lake 3

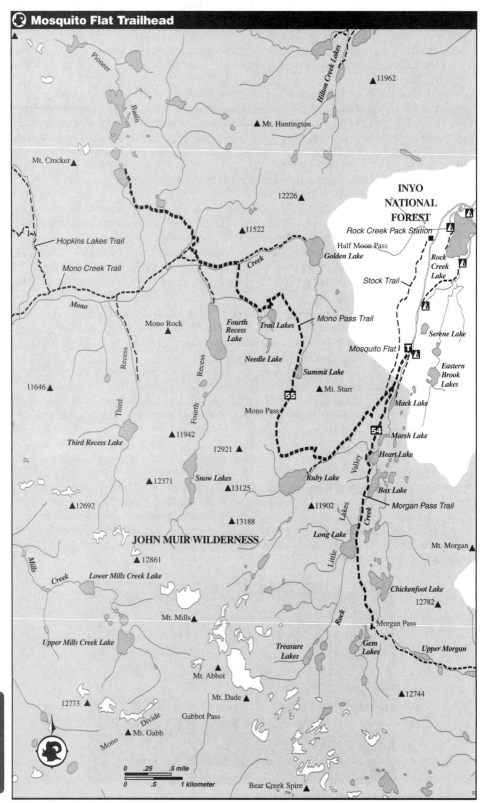

INYO
NATIONAL
FOREST

Rock Creek Pack Station

Half Moon Pass

Golden Lake

Stock Trail

Rock
Creek
Lake

Hilton Creek Lakes

▲11962

▲ Mt. Huntington

Mt. Crocker ▲

Pioneer

Basin

12226 ▲

▲11522

Creek

Hopkins Lakes Trail

Mono Creek Trail

Mono

Mono Rock
▲

Fourth
Recess
Lake

Trail Lakes

Mono Pass Trail

Mosquito Flat ⊤

Serene Lake

Eastern
Brook
Lakes

Needle Lake

Summit Lake

Mack Lake

11646▲

Third

Recess

Fourth Recess

▲11942

12921 ▲

▲ Mt. Starr

Mono Pass

55

54 Marsh Lake

Heart Lake

Box Lake

Morgan Pass Trail

Ruby Lake

Valley

Lakes

Little

Creek

Rock

Third Recess Lake

▲12371

Snow Lakes
▲13125

▲12692

▲13188

▲11902

Long Lake

JOHN MUIR WILDERNESS

▲12861

Mt. Morgan ▲

Mills

Creek

Lower Mills Creek Lake

Chickenfoot Lake

12782▲

Upper Mills Creek Lake

Mt. Mills▲

Treasure
Lakes

Gem
Lakes

Morgan Pass

Upper Morgan

12773 ▲

Divide

Mono ▲ Mt. Gabb

Mt. Abbot
▲

Mt. Dade ▲

Gabbot Pass

▲12744

0   .25   .5 mile

0   .5   1 kilometer

Bear Creek Spire ▲

ROCK CR

Mosquito Flat Trailhead

10,256′; 11S 345424 4144575

DESTINATION/ UTM COORDINATES	TRIP TYPE	BEST SEASON	PACE (HIKING/ LAYOVER DAYS)	TOTAL MILEAGE
54 Little Lakes Valley 11S 344473 4139674 (at Gem Lakes)	Out & back	Mid to late	2/1 Leisurely	6.6
55 Pioneer Basin 11S 341201 4147079 (Lake 1)	Out & back	Mid to late	4/2 Moderate	19

Information and Permits: This trailhead is in Inyo National Forest: 351 Pacu Lane, Suite 200, Bishop, CA 93514, 760-873-2400, www.fs.fed.us/r5/inyo/. Quotas apply, and permits are required for overnight stays and are available at Inyo National Forest ranger stations in Lone Pine, Bishop, Mammoth Lakes, and Mono Basin Scenic Area Visitors Center.

Driving Directions: From Hwy. 395 at Tom's Place, go south up Rock Creek Road and drive to its end, about 13 miles up-canyon, at Mosquito Flat.

54 Little Lakes Valley

Trip Data: 11S 344473 4139674; 6.6 miles; 2/1 days

Topos: *Mt. Abbot, Mt. Morgan*

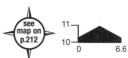

Highlights: Because of its majestic scenery, moderate terrain, good fishing, and high alpine feel, the route through Little Lakes Valley is a favorite with hikers.

HEADS UP! Campfires are prohibited. Dogs and goats are prohibited at the valley's south end, including the Treasure Lakes. Bear canisters are required. This area is very heavily used and is perhaps best seen on a dayhike. Carefully observe all closures and restoration sites.

DAY 1 (Mosquito Flat Trailhead to Gem Lakes, 3.3 miles): The wide, rocky-sandy trail starts southwest toward the imposing skyline dominated by soaring Bear Creek Spire. Shortly, the tread enters John Muir Wilderness, climbs a flowered slope, and reaches a junction. Take the left fork, the Morgan Pass Trail, south-southwest. Soon, the route tops a low, rocky ridge just west of Mack Lake, and from this ridge there are fine views of green-clad Little Lakes Valley and of the breathtaking peaks surrounding it. Flanked by Mt. Starr on the right and Mt. Morgan on the left, the valley terminates in the soaring heights of Mt. Mills, Mt. Abbot, Mt. Dade, Mt. Julius Caesar, and Bear Creek Spire, all over 13,000 feet. Still

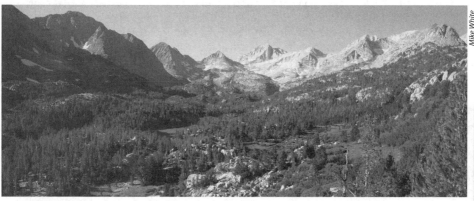

Little Lakes Valley

ROCK CR

active glaciers on the slopes of these great peaks are reminders of the enormous forces that shaped this valley eons ago.

Now the trail descends past Marsh Lake and presently fords the stream connecting much higher Ruby Lake with lovely little Heart Lake. Skirt Heart Lake on its west side and then ascend gently past the west side of Box Lake to the east side of aptly named Long Lake. Trace Long Lake's east shore and, beyond it, climb through a moderately dense forest cover of whitebark pines past a spur trail branching left (east) to Chickenfoot Lake. Dip across a seasonal stream, climb slightly, and dip again to the outlet stream of the Gem Lakes.

CAMPSITE OPTIONS

You'll inevitably see less considerate campers setting up tents directly in view of fellow visitors at illegal or barely legal sites in this area. If you are determined to camp in Little Lakes Valley, head to the more remote campsites away from the trail and the main lakes. (You still may feel like a zoo animal come morning when dayhikers and anglers walk through your camp.) Call the ranger station to get updates on any closures.

Here are some suggestions for campsites that are at least the legal distance from water and the main trail. There are doubtless others farther afield, including dry camps. Accessing the more remote campsites east of the trail and the main lakes requires you to cross the connecting streams, which form nascent Rock Creek. These fords may be difficult in early season. As noted earlier, Lower Morgan Lake has campsites. (Multiple flat spots within a few yards of each other constitute one campsite with multiple tent sites).

Box Lake: There are a few, fine, sandy campsites off trail at the north end of Box Lake. The obvious access is via a use trail that makes an abrupt exit hard left (north) off the main trail just where you first glimpse the lake. You'll have to scramble down the shoreline to campsites a little farther down the shore and back into the trees.

Chickenfoot Lake: This lake probably has the most sites, scattered on and between the rocky knolls around the shore. Where the signed spur trail approaches the lakeshore, you'll find a couple of campsites on the right and at least one on the knoll to the left. A use trail branches right from the spur trail well before you reach the lakeshore; this use trail leads past more knolls with additional campsites. Finally, a few remote campsites occupy the lake's northwest peninsula, reached by a rough angler's trail around the west shore of the lake.

Gem Lakes: A couple of campsites are found on the low ridge that rises southeast of the largest Gem Lake, between the inlet and outlet; both sites are above the trail, but the higher one is the better of the two.

Heart Lake: There are three campsites just north of the lake, between the trail and the outlet. Two are in the rocks above the lake and the third is below, at a just-barely-legal distance from the lakeshore and the inlet from Ruby Lake. Find more campsites nearby on a forested, sandy flat to the west of the inlet from Ruby Lake. The easiest access to those is to continue on the trail across the inlet, take the first use trail on the right, and then hook northward to sheltered and pleasant sites. Finally, a few hard-to-reach, trailless campsites occupy knolls east of Heart Lake.

Long Lake: Highly overused campsites reside on a sandy rise at the lake's north end and across the outlet; these may be the most popular sites in the basin. There are also a couple of trailless campsites high on the rise above the middle of the lake and on the west side. At the south end of the lake, there are three campsites high above the lake; two are on either side of the inlet from Treasure Lakes, and one is near the inlet from the tiny pond high above and well southwest of Long Lake. A faint use trail leads up a dry gully south of Long Lake and west of the main trail, south to a low rise with a campsite, flanked by a wet meadow.

Ahead on the left is the last switchback on the trail up Morgan Pass, through which the abandoned mining road that has been this trip's trail once reached the tungsten mines in the Pine Creek drainage. There's fair camping at pretty Lower Morgan Lake for those inclined to stay overnight and explore beyond the pass.

Just after a rockhop ford of Gem Lakes' outlet, reach a junction: left (ahead, east) to Morgan Pass and Morgan Lakes, right (south) to the Gem Lakes. Turn right and take this sometimes faint trail to those lakes, where there are a couple of campsites. See the sidebar on page 214 for campsite options.

DAY 2 (Gem Lakes to Mosquito Flat Trailhead, 3.3 miles): Retrace your steps.

55 Pioneer Basin

Trip Data: 11S 341201 4147079; 19 miles; 4/2

Topo maps: *Mt. Abbot, Mt. Morgan, Mt. Abbot*

Highlights: It's a tough hike into Pioneer Basin, but the spectacular views along the way and the

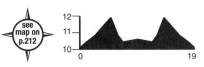

opportunities for superb dayhiking from a scenic base camp in the basin are ample rewards. Amateur botanists will delight in the variety of wildflowers. However, angling is generally poor.

HEADS UP! Bear canisters are required. Campfires are prohibited. Grazing is prohibited. Dogs may be prohibited in parts of this area to protect bighorn sheep; check with Inyo National Forest.

DAY 1 (Mosquito Flat Trailhead to Trail Lakes, 5.5 miles): Head south and ascend the scenic trail from Mosquito Flat. At the junction with the trail left (south) into Little Lakes Valley (Trip 54), turn right (ahead, south-southwest) for Mono Pass to begin a long climb of Mt. Starr's east slope on a sandy trail with increasingly excellent views. Shortly, pass a spur trail coming in on the right from the pack station—an almost invisible junction.

Continuing ahead, the trail intersects seasonal runoff nourishing surprising, seasonal flower gardens. Pass a pretty tarn, and, at almost 2 miles, turn into a swale and reach a junction with a signed lateral to Ruby Lake (campsites), a quarter mile away by turning left (southwest) on this lateral. Near this junction, Ruby Lake's outlet provides the last reliable opportunity for water until Summit Lake, a little beyond Mono Pass.

Bypassing Ruby Lake, take the right fork west and continue relentlessly up, with a view of Ruby Lake below and of the peaks around Little Lakes Valley. Finally, leaving the views behind, the trail turns into a sandy draw that may hold snow until very late in the season. For this reason, there may be multiple tracks between here and the far end of Summit Lake, made by hikers trying to avoid the retreating snow—though there may be no alternative to hiking through it.

At 4.5 miles, arrive at viewless Mono Pass (12,060′, though an old sign here says 11,970′) and step across the Sierra Crest, from Inyo National Forest into Sierra National Forest, in a stark landscape of shattered granite and decomposed-granite sand. Panoramic views are available by ascending Mt. Starr (12,835′; Class 2) to the east.

The trail descends a little toward the shore of Summit Lake, a turquoise oval set in cream-colored rock and gray-brown sand. The trail roughly parallels Summit Lake's outlet before its multiple tracks converge on a flat below the lake to veer northwest. (Don't drop into the meadow around the outlet stream unless you are desperate to find a campsite now.)

Climb a little ridge, possibly through more snow, and begin a switchbacking descent of a dry slope, from which there are breathtaking views over the great glacial canyon of Mono Creek. Especially prominent in these views are Needle Lake—misspelled "Neelle Lake" on the topo—to the west, with the Trail Lakes coming into view below it, and the lowest lake in Pioneer Basin to the northwest, set in a wide, inviting meadow.

Near the Trail Lakes, notice a tiny stone hut that's a California snow survey shelter; no trespassing! The main trail actually swings away from the Trail Lakes (11,200´) just before touching their shores, but the smaller lake is on the left as the path comes abreast of them. A rocky plateau a few feet above the larger lake provides several overused campsites (11,230´; 11S 342932 4145294) among stunted whitebark pines, and there is also a small flat about a tenth of a mile below the lakes, across the trail from the meadow bracketing the lakes' outlet.

DAY 2 (Trail Lakes to Pioneer Basin Lake 2, 4 miles): Return to the main trail to begin a dusty, stony descent of nearly 800 feet to a welcome ford of Golden Creek (10,420´), where a use trail on the north bank turns upstream (east) toward Golden Lake. This trip's route, also on the north bank, turns west and downstream, paralleling Golden Creek and generally staying well above it. The descent eases, though the trail remains deep in dust and full of loose rocks, and the path is soon in moderate forest cover.

The trail presently reaches the signed lateral left (south) to Fourth Recess, a beautiful cirque with a large lake fed by an 800-foot waterfall; it's an enjoyable dayhike from Pioneer Basin. Go right (ahead, west) on the Mono Creek Trail and shortly find the signed lateral that goes right (ahead, west) to Pioneer Basin. Take this lateral. At first, the lateral avoids climbing straight into Pioneer Basin, instead bobbing over a couple of little ridges. But soon the trail descends to a year-round stream at a junction where a use trail leads left (southwest, downstream) to a few campsites and back toward Mono Creek.

Staying on the lateral, curve right (northeast and upstream) through a moderate forest of lodgepole pines to begin a sometimes steep climb into Pioneer Basin. Ford the stream to ascend rocky switchbacks through patchy forest. The grade eases as the trail approaches

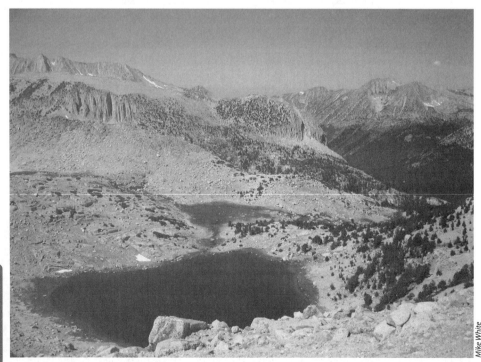

Mike White

Trail Lakes and Mono Creek Canyon from Mono Pass Trail

ROCK CR

the ridgetop east of Lake 1, and the trail soon dips into the meadow around the lake, ford-ing its outlet. This lake (10,400´; 11S 341201 4147079; called "Mud Lake" by packers) offers the most popular campsites in the basin because they're the easiest to reach and have mod-erate forest cover. Being the lowest lake, it has the most comfortable temperature for swim-ming.

However, many more scenic campsites lie above in the upper basin. Continue west on the trail to ford Lake 1's outlet and then begin a moderately steep, stony climb into forest, curving north. Nearing the lower lip of the higher basin, the trees begin to thin, allowing flowers and shrubs to flourish. The grade eases as the path nears the southeast shore of the lowest of the lakes in the upper basin (Lake 2; 10,820´; 11S 340547 4147480).

Or, also from Lake 1, a well-beaten trail a little before Lake 1 leads north toward lakes on the basin's east side; this trail isn't on the topo but is on the large USDA/USFS wilder-ness map.

View-rich campsites may be found on benches around the upper basin's lower lakes. Campsites are fewer the higher you go, but their potential for solitude is much higher. Use trails provide straightforward travel to the lower lakes, but reaching the highest lakes takes easy cross-country rambling through gorgeous terrain.

Pioneer Basin is spectacularly ringed by Mt. Hopkins, Mt. Crocker, Mt. Stanford, and Mt. Huntington, peaks named for the "Big Four" among California pioneers—hence the basin's name—who were builders of the Central Pacific Railroad.

DAYS 3–4 (Pioneer Basin Lake 1 to Mosquito Flat Trailhead, 9.5 miles): Retrace your steps to the trailhead.

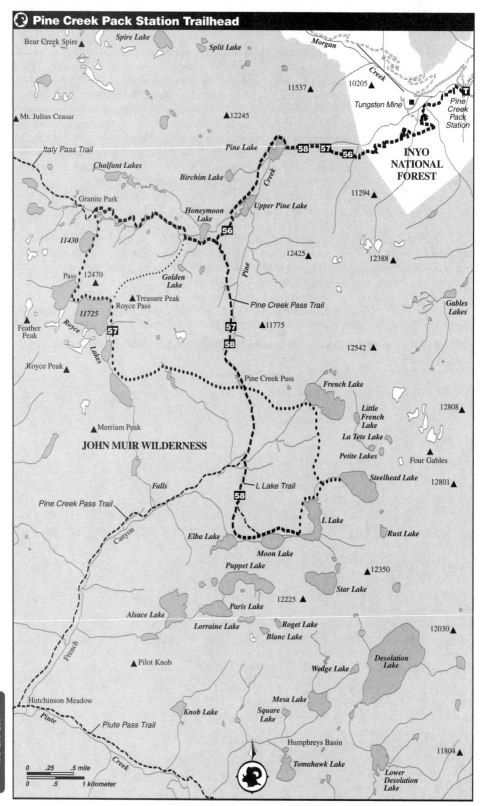

Bear Creek Spire ▲

Spire Lake

Split Lake

Morgan

Creek

11537 ▲

10205 ▲

Tungsten Mine

Pine Creek Pack Station

▲ Mt. Julius Ceasar

▲12245

Pine Lake

58 **57** **56**

INYO NATIONAL FOREST

Italy Pass Trail

Chalfant Lakes

Birchim Lake

Creek

11294 ▲

Granite Park

Honeymoon Lake

Upper Pine Lake

11430

56

12425 ▲

12388 ▲

Pass 12470 ▲

Golden Lake

Pine

Gables Lakes

▲ Treasure Peak
Royce Pass

11725

57

Pine Creek Pass Trail

▲11775

12542 ▲

Feather Peak

Royce

Lakes

Royce Peak ▲

Pine Creek Pass

French Lake

12808 ▲

JOHN MUIR WILDERNESS

▲ Merriam Peak

Little French Lake

La Tete Lake

Petite Lakes

Four Gables ▲

Falls

L Lake Trail

Steelhead Lake

12801 ▲

Pine Creek Pass Trail

58

Canyon

L Lake

Rust Lake

Elba Lake

Moon Lake

▲12350

Puppet Lake

12225 ▲

Star Lake

Paris Lake

Alsace Lake

Lorraine Lake

Roget Lake

12030 ▲

French

Blanc Lake

▲ Pilot Knob

Desolation Lake

Wedge Lake

Mesa Lake

Hutchinson Meadow

Piute

Square Lake

Piute Pass Trail

Knob Lake

Humphreys Basin

11804 ▲

Creek

Tomahawk Lake

Lower Desolation Lake

0   .25   .5 mile
0   .5   1 kilometer

Pine Creek Pack Station Trailhead
7435´; 11S 350167 4136301

DESTINATION/ UTM COORDINATES	TRIP TYPE	BEST SEASON	PACE (HIKING/ LAYOVER DAYS)	TOTAL MILEAGE
56 Upper Pine Lake 11S 346332 4134570	Out & back	Mid to late	2/2 Leisurely	9.5
57 Royce Lakes 11S 343883 4132196	Semiloop	Mid to late	4/1 Moderate, part cross-country	17.75
58 L Lake 11S 347151 4128737	Semiloop	Mid to late	3/1 Moderate, part cross-country	19.5

Information and Permits: This trailhead is in Inyo National Forest: 351 Pacu Lane, Suite 200, Bishop, CA 93514, 760-873-2400, www.fs.fed.us/r5/inyo/. Quotas apply, and permits are required for overnight stays and are available at Inyo National Forest ranger stations in Lone Pine, Bishop, Mammoth Lakes, and Mono Basin Scenic Area Visitors Center.

Driving directions: From Bishop, take Hwy. 395 northwest for 10 miles and turn west onto Pine Creek Road. Drive another 10 miles to a signed parking lot next to the Pine Creek Pack Station.

56 Upper Pine Lake

Trip Data: 11S 346332 4134570; 9.5 miles; 2/2 days

Topos: *Mount Tom*

Highlights: The tough, hairpin ascent to Upper Pine Lake offers breathtaking, over-the-shoulder views across Owens Valley to the White Mountains, and the campsite views from the shore of the Sierra Crest make this an outstanding choice for a base-camp location on the east side of the Sierra. Anglers should enjoy the chance to ply the waters for the resident trout without much competition from fellow anglers.

HEADS UP! The trail climbs nearly 3000 feet in 4.5 miles; don't attempt this strenuous elevation gain unless you're well acclimated and in very good shape. The start of the trip is diabolically steep: You go up 2000 feet in the first 2.5 miles, mostly on a dusty, shadeless old mining road that has deteriorated into a rocky jumble.

DAY 1 (Pine Creek Pack Station Trailhead to Upper Pine Lake, 4.75 miles): The trailhead is located at the pack station just south of Pine Creek. The dusty, duff trail heads generally southwest and ascends steeply from the pack station through a dense, mixed forest of Jeffrey pine, juniper, red fir, quaking aspen, and birch. Along the way, ford several branches of an unnamed tributary of Pine Creek, decorated with plentiful blossoms of wild rose, columbine, tiger lily, and Queen Anne's lace.

About 0.3 mile from the trailhead, the trail emerges from the forest cover and joins the rocky remnants of a 4WD road leading sharply uphill to the now closed Brownstone Mine. Now out in the open, a view of the defunct Union Carbide tungsten mill will be a constant companion for the next couple of miles.

The slope into Pine Creek canyon is steep and the footing is at times unpleasant, which makes this segment basically a slog-and-pant. Three welcome streams break the monotony of the climb, and the view (despite the ugly road cut that scars Morgan Creek) is spectacular. Gazing northeast down the Pine Creek drainage, you look across the Owens River drainage to the Volcanic Tableland and White Mountain (14,242´) on the skyline. Where the

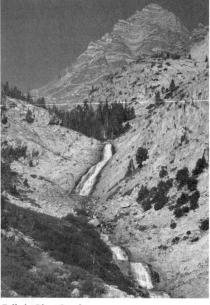

Falls in Pine Creek

road bends sharply left to the now quiet mine, single-track trail goes ahead (west) toward the dramatic cascades of Pine Creek, ascending over talus and scree via short, steep switchbacks. Scattered lodgepole pines dot the slope along with a sprinkling of junipers, some of which have left beautiful weathered snags of a dramatic golden hue.

Finally, with the steepest part of the ascent behind, the trail fords another unnamed tributary, switchbacks past a sign at the boundary of John Muir Wilderness, and then loses some of the hard-won elevation on a descent to the south bank of Pine Creek. Here, the creek alternates in cascades, falls, and chutes in a riot of whitewater.

Shortly, arriving at a signed junction with a stock ford, you veer right and cross the creek on a flattened-log bridge, 3.5 miles from the trailhead. Proceed upstream through moderate forest cover of lodgepole pines to the northeast end of Pine Lake (9942´). The medium-sized lake (16 acres) is a popular overnight camping destination for tired backpackers exhausted after the steep climb up the canyon (campsites on the northeast shore). Anglers may wish to tarry along the shore in order to sample the fair fishing for brook trout, but fishing is generally better at Upper Pine Lake.

The trail passes through a drift fence, skirts the rocky northeast side of Pine Lake and ascends through forest to ford the outlet from Birchim Lake. After climbing over a small ridge, the trail parallels the outlet from Upper Pine Lake to arrive at the northwest shore (10,214´; 11S 346160 4134352) and the first of many conifer-shaded campsites spread around the lake. Anglers will discover good fishing for brook, rainbow, and golden trout.

DAY 2 (Upper Pine Lake to Pine Creek Pack Station Trailhead, 4.75 miles): Retrace your steps to the trailhead.

57 Royce Lakes

Trip Data: 11S 343883 4132196; 17.75 miles; 4/1 days

Topos: *Mount Tom, Mt. Hilgard*

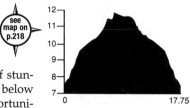

Highlights: A short, straightforward cross-country route leads from the Italy Pass Trail to a chain of stunningly scenic alpine lakes tucked into a rugged basin below a trio of 13,000-foot peaks. Anglers will find the opportunity to fish for a healthy population of golden trout to be quite alluring.

HEADS UP! *The steep climb from the Pine Creek Trailhead, along with the cross-country route to Royce Lakes, makes this a trip for experienced backpackers in good condition. Pack along a freestanding tent for campsites at Royce Lakes, as the few sandy spots suitable for campsites are on shallow soil (may not hold stakes).*

ROCK CR

DAY 1 (Pine Creek Pack Station Trailhead to Upper Pine Lake, 4.75 miles): *(Recap: Trip 56, Day 1.)* Follow the trail generally southwest through mixed forest until breaking out into the open, where the trail merges with an old 4WD road. Climb up the dusty and rocky road via steep switchbacks, fording an unnamed stream three times before leaving the road to continue climbing on single-track trail into scattered forest. After a brief descent to Pine Creek, the trail heads upstream a short distance to a bridged crossing of the creek, and then it proceeds to Pine Lake. Skirt around Pine Lake, cross the outlet of Birchim Lake, and then climb over a small ridge to Upper Pine Lake (10,214´; 11S 346160 4134352; good campsites).

DAY 2 (Upper Pine Lake to Granite Park, 2.5 miles): (For an alternate route to the Royce Lakes that bypasses Granite Park, see the sidebar on page 222.) After skirting the meadows around the north shore of Upper Pine Lake, cross the multibranched inlet stream via a long string of well-placed boulders (may be a wet ford in early season). A moderate ascent leads to the Pine Creek Pass/Honeymoon Lake junction.

Turn right (west), away from the Pine Creek Pass Trail, and follow the Italy Pass Trail a short distance to the top of a rise and then down to the outlet of very popular Honeymoon Lake (10,400´;11S 345553 4133784). At the top of the rise, a use trail provides access to fine though overused campsites on a knoll above the east side of the lake and beneath a grove of pines along the north shore. This lovely lake makes an excellent base camp for side excursions to 40 surrounding lakes in four drainages, or for climbing five nearby peaks that exceed 13,000 feet in elevation. Fishing for a healthy population of brook and rainbow trout is good.

Cross the willow-lined inlet of Honeymoon Lake on a steep but short climb over boulders to the resumption of dirt tread. Then continue climbing to a bench just west of the lake, where overnighters will find seldom-used but excellent campsites. Cross the creek on a log bridge and follow deteriorating tread up the canyon along the north bank of the stream that drains Granite Park through a diminishing forest of lodgepole and then whitebark pines.

Wind up the jumbled valley, passing many lovely diminutive swales and crossing sparkling rivulets. The trail arrives in aptly named Granite Park in a lovely timberline meadow, where the brook trout-filled stream momentarily adopts a lazy course through the verdant grassland. Continue climbing up the drainage on faint tread that continually disappears when crossing bedrock or talus and then reappears in areas of soil.

Reach a large, irregularly shaped tarn (11,340´; 11S 343830 4134219) and search for Spartan campsites tucked into small pockets of soil scattered around the basin. The extraordinary scenery and high probability of solitude will more than make up for the lack of highly developed campsites. The short day of backpacking allows plenty of time to explore the nooks and crannies of remarkable Granite Park. Italy Pass is visible on the ridgeline to the west; the tread to it becomes increasingly faint.

DAY 3 (Granite Park to Royce Lakes, 2 miles, cross-country): From the tarn, head south cross-country toward Lake 11430, 0.35 mile north-northwest of Peak 12470. Pass the lake on the east and leave the sublime surroundings of Granite Park on an increasingly steep climb over talus toward the obvious notch just west of Peak 12470. At the notch (11,851´; 11S 343395 4133226), the uppermost Royce Lake pops into view, nestled in an austere, rockbound, above-timberline basin towered over by Feather Peak. At these lofty heights, fingers of snow cling to the peak's shady crevices throughout the summer. Immediately striking is the crystal clarity of the lake's water and the aquamarine hue. Although the Royce Lakes are quite deep, thanks to the water's clarity, golden trout may be seen patrolling the shallower waters near the shore. Anglers will surely be tempted by the presence of this notable species.

Drop shortly to the lakeshore over blocky talus and proceed around the lower slopes of Peak 12470 toward Lake 11725, the largest of the Royce Lakes. Pass along the north shore

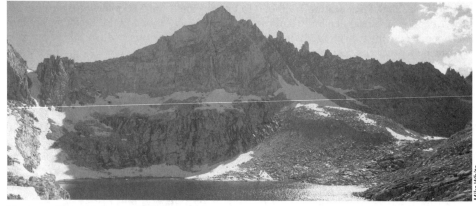

Mike White

Uppermost Royce Lake and Feather Peak

to the northeast tip of Lake 11725. Although much of the shoreline is a jumble of talus, there are a couple of Spartan campsites on small patches of sand above the northeast shore.

From Lake 11725, you must negotiate a steep slope of talus in order to head south toward the lower lakes. Beyond this minor obstacle, the way becomes much easier and traces of a use trail can be found toward the south end of the lake. All the while, the looming summits of Feather, Royce, and Merriam peaks dwarf the mere mortals who pass below them. In between Lake 11725 and the next lower lake, a few sandy campsites bordered by small patches of ground-hugging vegetation offer overnight sanctuary amid the dramatic scenery (11,705´; 11S 343883 4132196).

ALTERNATE ROUTE TO ROYCE LAKES

You can get to the Royce Lakes from Honeymoon Lake (without going to Granite Park): On the bench above Honeymoon Lake, leave the Italy Pass Trail immediately before fording the creek draining Granite Park and start climbing on a ducked route over granite slabs toward "Royce Pass," the obvious low point directly right (west) of Treasure Peak (12,563´). Through scattered pines, proceed along a ridge just to the left of a stream and then drop off the ridge around 10,385 feet onto a grassy ramp. Continue climbing toward the pass through open terrain covered with granite boulders and slabs and small pockets of meadow watered by trickling rivulets. Curve slightly around the base of Treasure Peak and then proceed directly to Royce Pass (11,580´; 11S 344023, 4132916). At the pass, Lake 11725, largest of the Royce Lakes, bursts into view immediately below the towering northeast faces of 13,240-foot Feather and 13,280-foot Royce peaks. Descend to the lake and pick up the route described above.

DAY 4 (Royce Lakes to Pine Creek Pack Station Trailhead, 8.5 miles, part cross-country): Continuing the cross-country leg, head south around the shoreline of the smallest of the lakes and continue toward Lake 11656, where the previously narrow basin widens eastward. In the shadow of Merriam Peak, leave Lake 11656 near its midpoint and head east over open, rock-and-sand slopes to the top of a rise. Here, a sweeping vista unfolds of a horseshoe of peaks, including the dark, imposing hulk of 13,986-foot Mt. Humphreys in the southeast and the row of peaks forming the Glacier Divide to the south. A bevy of lakes on benches above French Canyon also springs into view.

From the rise, descend an easy slope toward the ponds in the next drainage and cross spongy meadows just below the uppermost pond. Climb the sandy and rocky slope above the ponds to an even more impressive view of the surrounding peaks and lakes. Drop

ROCK CR

down to a large, flat area on a bench overlooking French Canyon and then descend more steeply toward the small tarns near Pine Creek Pass. Pick your way down slabs and past rock humps and boulders through a smattering of whitebark pines to the south side of a tarn and then swing around the tarn to intersect the trail just below Pine Creek Pass (11,160´; 11S 346215 4131347), the end of the cross-country section.

Now on the Pine Creek Pass Trail, head north across the pass's gentle terrain past the smaller of the two tarns, and then follow a steeper, winding descent on difficult tread down Pine Creek's boulder-studded canyon. Pass through a drift fence, descend to ford the creek, and then wind down across a talus slope. Beyond the talus, a growing number of whitebark pines, along with clumps of shoulder-high willows, a bevy of wildflowers, and meadows lining the stream soften the previously stark surroundings.

Continue downstream along the west bank to a good-size pond and cross its outlet. Gently graded trail moves away from the creek, passing through a scattered forest of lodgepole and whitebark pines, before a steep, dusty descent leads to the Pine Creek Pass/Italy Pass junction.

From the junction, turn right (northeast) and retrace your steps 5.25 miles to the trailhead. The many camping opportunities along the way make it easy to break this one long day into two shorter ones.

58 L Lake

Trip Data: 11S 347151 4128737; 19.5 miles; 3/1 days

Topos: *Mt. Abbot, Mount Tom*

Highlights: This trip samples picturesque alpine scenery near the lightly used lakes above French Canyon on a semiloop requiring minimal cross-country skills.

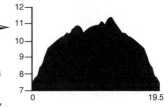

HEADS UP! Although the navigation along the cross-country section of this trip is straightforward, backpackers will have to negotiate a difficult stretch of talus between Steelhead and French lakes.

DAY 1 (Pine Creek Pack Station Trailhead to Upper Pine Lake, 4.75 miles): *(Recap: Trip 56, Day 1.)* Follow the trail generally southwest through mixed forest until breaking out into the open, where the trail merges with an old 4WD road. Climb up the dusty and rocky road via steep switchbacks, fording an unnamed stream three times before leaving the road to continue climbing on single-track trail into scattered forest. After a brief descent to Pine Creek, the trail heads upstream a short distance to a bridged crossing of the creek, and then proceeds to Pine Lake.

Skirt Pine Lake, cross the outlet of Birchim Lake, and then climb over a small ridge to Upper Pine Lake (10,214´; 11S 346160 4134352; good campsites).

DAY 2 (Upper Pine Lake to L Lake, 5.25 miles): Pass meadows at the north end of Upper Pine Lake, make a long boulder hop of the multibranched inlet, and climb moderately to the junction of the Pine Creek Pass and Italy Pass trails.

Turn left (south) and begin a steady, gradual climb toward Pine Creek Pass. Originally a Mono Indian trading route, this route over the pass has been in use by humans for nearly 500 years. The moderate forest cover of lodgepole and then whitebark pines thins as the trail climbs past a good-size pond to the right. Tiny, emerald green, subalpine meadows break the long granite slabs, and wildflower fanciers will find clumps of color from wallflower, shooting star, penstemon, lupine, primrose, and columbine.

The trail draws alongside a tumbling creek, the headwaters of Pine Creek, and ascends a long swale between steep granite walls. A final, rocky climb leads through a drift fence and up to a level area harboring two tarns before reaching Pine Creek Pass (11,160´; 11S 346215 4131347) on the Sierra Crest.

Descending from the pass through a rocky meadow, views open up of Elba Lake to the south, of Pilot Knob and the Glacier Divide to the southwest, and of Merriam and Royce peaks to the west. The trail skirts above a boggy meadow, crosses its outlet stream, and proceeds downhill across slopes covered predominantly by lush grasses, sedges, small plants, and wildflowers. Continue through the meadowlands of French Canyon to a Y-junction with the trail to L Lake (10,710´; 11S 346233 4130125), 1.25 miles from the pass.

Turn right (south) and follow a moderate climb across flower-filled slopes over a trio of rivulets for 0.6 mile to the Moon Lake-Elba Lake junction. Turn right (south) and follow the trail to Elba Lake, enjoying improving views of the dramatic waterfall spilling out of the Royce Lakes and down the north wall of French Canyon, along with the impressive ridge of spires known as the Pinnacles. Soon, you arrive at the northeast shore of island-dotted Elba Lake.

LIFE IN THE "MOONSCAPE"

Typical of these high, montane lakes, at first glance, Elba seems virtually devoid of life, and first-time visitors often describe the terrain as "moon country," but those who come to know and love it soon discover the beauty that hides close beneath the near-sterile veneer. Spots of green between the tumbled talus blocks indicate grassy tundra patches or clumps of willow, and occasionally the weathered landscape is broken by a dwarfed lodgepole or whitebark pine. Steady, silent scrutiny will usually discover movement indicating animal life. A bird is usually the first to be detected, oftentimes a rosy finch or a hummingbird. Four-footed movement among the rocks is most likely from a cony (pika) or marmot, or it could be a bushy-tailed wood rat. Anglers will soon find life, as Elba Lake has a good population of golden and golden hybrids.

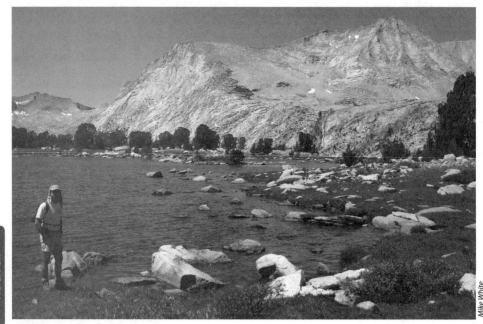

Hiker along the shore of Elba Lake

From Elba, ascend alongside the inlet stream steadily to a small pond and pick up the use trail that leads to larger Moon Lake (10,998′). Fair campsites can be found on the southeast side. Fishing for golden is excellent.

Continue on trail along the north side of Moon Lake and then over a hill toward the southwest end of L Lake. The path dead-ends near good campsites on a knoll above the outlet (11,090′; 11S 347151, 4128737).

DAY 3 (L Lake to Pine Creek Pack Station Trailhead, 9.5 miles, part cross-country): From the southwest end of L Lake, follow an easy cross-county course across open, sandy-and-rocky slopes west of the lake toward the north shore. Then, make a steady climb, generally northeast, away from the lake and toward the crest of a ridge directly east of Peak 11281. Before gaining the top of the ridge, veer east and follow the north side of Steelhead Lake's outlet on a short climb to the northwest shore of the 11,361-foot lake. One of the larger lakes in the area, Steelhead sits majestically in a basin below the rugged, rock-strewn slopes of Four Gables.

From the shore of Steelhead Lake, retrace your steps briefly back down the outlet and climb up to the crest of the ridge east of Peak 11281. Before continuing, take some time to plot the route to French Lake, selecting a course that attempts to minimize the amount of talus crossed en route. Drop off the ridge and descend generally northwest toward a small pond in the bottom of the canyon. Pass around the pond and begin an angling ascent up the far hillside to the southwest shore of French Lake (11,255′). Spartan campsites can be found on a rise just above the outlet (11,272′; 11S 347321 4131119).

Leaving French Lake, the object of the next cross-country part of the journey is to reach hidden Pine Creek Pass without losing a great deal of elevation along the way. The elevation difference between the lake and the pass is a mere 100 feet, but the pass is out of sight around a hill and across uneven terrain, which makes achieving this goal something of a challenge. Traverse as best you can, contouring generally west across the hillside toward the pass. Rounding the hill, the pass eventually comes into view, allowing you to set your bearings.

Once at Pine Creek Pass (11,160′; 11S 346215 4131347), take the Pine Creek Pass Trail generally north and retrace your steps to the trailhead. The many camping opportunities along the way make it easy to break this one long day into two shorter ones.

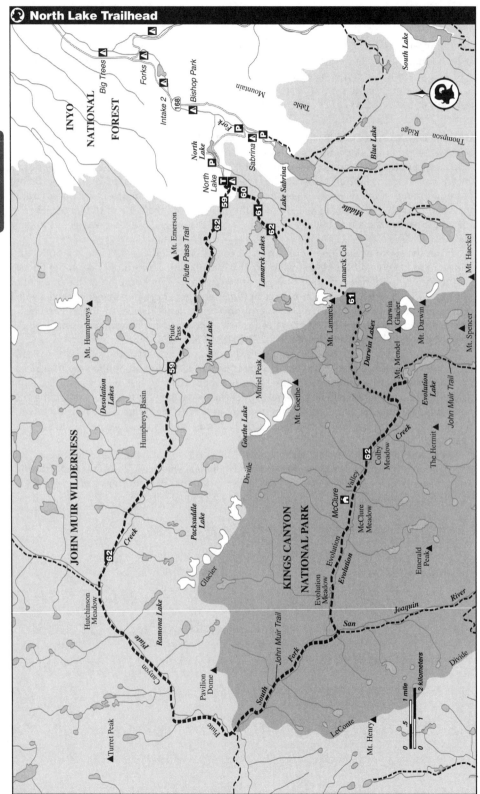

North Lake Trailhead

9344´; 11S 355642 4121338

DESTINATION/ UTM COORDINATES	TRIP TYPE	BEST SEASON	PACE (HIKING/ LAYOVER DAYS)	TOTAL MILEAGE
59 Humphreys Basin 11S 347832 4123135	Out & back	Mid to late	2/2 Moderate	14.4
60 Lamarck Lakes 11S 353936 4119707	Out & back	Mid to late	2/0 Leisurely	5.4
61 Darwin Lakes 11S 350640 4116953	Out & back	Mid to late	3/1 Moderate, part cross-country	14
62 Evolution Basin 11S 349107 4115269	Loop	Mid to late	6/1 Moderate, part cross-country	39

Information and Permits: This trailhead is in Inyo National Forest: 351 Pacu Lane, Suite 200, Bishop, CA 93514, 760-873-2400, www.fs.fed.us/r5/inyo/. Quotas apply, and permits are required for overnight stays and are available at Inyo National Forest ranger stations in Lone Pine, Bishop, Mammoth Lakes, and Mono Basin Scenic Area Visitors Center.

Driving Directions: In the town of Bishop, turn west from Hwy. 395 onto West Line Street (State Hwy. 168 East Side). Drive 18 miles southwest past the signed junction with South Lake Road and almost to Lake Sabrina. At the signed junction with dirt North Lake Road, turn right, cross the creek on a bridge, and continue 2 airy miles past little North Lake to a junction with the signed spur road to the pack station. Turn right here, pass the pack station's entrance, and shortly find the overnighters' parking lot. Alas, this lot is 0.7 mile from the true trailhead, which is farther up the road at the roadend and at the west end of North Lake Campground. So drop all the packs and most of the party at the true trailhead, and then designate someone to drive the car back to overnighters' parking and walk back up the road.

59 Humphreys Basin

Trip Data: 11S 347832 4123135; 14.4 miles; 2/2 days

Topos: *Mt. Darwin, Mount Tom*

Highlights: Humphreys Basin offers fine cross-country hiking to, and fishing in, dozens of lakes. Peakbaggers have a bevy of summits from which to choose, ranging

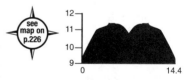

from difficult Mt. Humphreys—Class 4 by the easiest route—to gentle, unnamed knobs. A base camp in Humphreys Basin provides the gateway to countless high-country delights. Going only as far as Loch Leven or Piute Lake makes a great weekender.

HEADS UP! Away from maintained trail, be prepared for cross-country travel, ranging from easy off-trail to enjoyable but demanding bouldering.

DAY 1 (North Lake Trailhead to Humphreys Basin, 7.2 miles): From the true trailhead, go west and almost immediately reach a junction; go ahead (west) on the Piute Pass Trail. Soon entering John Muir Wilderness, the trail ascends gently along slopes dotted with patches of meadow, aspen groves, and stands of lodgepole pines. A wealth of wildflowers

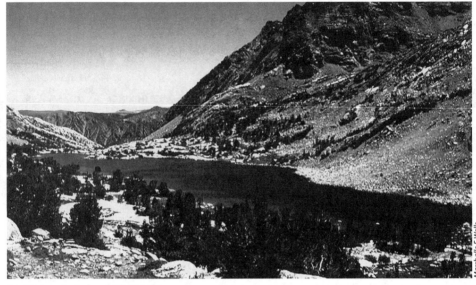

Looking eastward over Piute Lake

covers these meadows in season, including paintbrush, columbine, tiger lily, spirea, and penstemon.

After a pair of fords of North Fork Bishop Creek, the climb becomes moderate. As you climb, the aspen are left behind, the lodgepole become sparse, and some limber pine join the thinning forest. Flat-topped Peak 12691 on the south and 13,118-foot Mt. Emerson on the north flank the glaciated canyon. The trail switchbacks up a headwall with views of Loch Leven's cascading outlet and then follows gradual trail to that lake (10,700´), where picnic spots are scattered around the shoreline. There's a campsite off trail near its west end. Fishing is fair for brook, brown, and rainbow trout.

Beyond Loch Leven, the trail ascends moderately again through a sparse cover of lodgepole and whitebark pines, winding among large, rounded boulders, and skirting a pair of small lakes. Eventually, the climb abates, and the trail crosses a bench to Piute Lake's shore (10,958´; 11S 351971 4122378; brook and rainbow). Campsites can be windy here. Overused campsites are on the north side of the lake near the trail. (Solitude seekers might scramble cross-country southeast up a fairly steep, rocky slope to less-used sites at granite-bound Emerson Lake.)

From Piute Lake, follow the trail northwest toward timberline, ascending granite slabs, passing through meadowlands sliced by refreshing brooks, and skirting tiny ponds. Sooner than you might expect, a final traverse leads to Piute Pass (11,423´).

VIEWS FROM PIUTE PASS

Views from this aerie abound. Immediately below and to the west is the wide expanse of scenic, lake-dotted Humphreys Basin. In the southwest, the rugged Glacier Divide towers over the basin and is the northern boundary of Kings Canyon National Park. To the north is the dramatic summit of Mt. Humphreys—at 13,986 feet, the highest peak this far north in the Sierra. To the west lie Pilot Knob and the deep cleft of South Fork San Joaquin River.

From the pass, the rocky-dusty trail passes well above Summit Lake along the treeless edge of the great cirque that is Humphreys Basin. Below to the south, the headwaters of Piute Creek spill ribbonlike down the basin, forming a lake here and a pond there. Hidden from sight above and to the north lie Marmot Lake and the Humphreys Lakes, whose outlets the trail crosses where they nourish trailside patches of willows, shooting stars, and sneezeweed. Small, high campsites with panoramic views cling to the open slopes between the trail and these remote lakes. When searching for a campsite, seek a location well away from the main trail, as those close to the trail have become grotesquely overused.

Near a point where the Piute Pass Trail is above and north of a small lake with a green island, the route meets the unsigned but highly visible use trail that heads north to the Desolation Lakes. Those intrigued by the Desolation Lakes' reputation for fishing and who are fond of treeless, open camps will find some decent campsites above Lower Desolation Lake (11,200′) and on the wind-raked flats among the great white boulders surrounding aptly named Desolation Lake (11,375′; golden).

The Piute Pass Trail continues descending to the cascading outlet of the Desolation Lakes—the last reliable water source before Hutchinson Meadow during dry years. (If you missed the use trail to the Desolation Lakes, follow their outlet from here northward.) Below, the Golden Trout Lakes gleam down in the cirque bottom. If headed for the good campsites on the knolls around Upper Golden Trout Lake (10,835′; 11S 347832 4123135), descend about a half mile south to it. There, small whitebark pines shelter little flats overlooking the water, which gracefully mirrors the Glacier Divide. These sites offer fine views northeast to Mt. Humphreys and west to Pilot Knob as well. Lower Golden Trout Lake is closed to camping within 500 feet of the shoreline. Campsites in Humphreys Basin make fine base camps for exploring the area's wonders.

DAY 2 (Humphreys Basin to North Lake Trailhead, 7.2 miles): Retrace your steps to the trailhead.

60 Lamarck Lakes

Trip Data: 11S 353936 4119707; 5.4 miles; 2/0 days

Topos: *Mt. Darwin*

Highlights: This short trail leads to two attractive lakes and an optional cross-country tour of the seldom visited but highly scenic Lamarck Lakes.

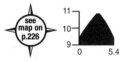

HEADS UP! While the 2.7-mile distance to the lakes is short, the elevation gain of 1700 feet makes this hike no easy chore.

DAY 1 (North Lake Trailhead to Upper Lamarck Lake, 2.7 miles): From the true trailhead, almost immediately find the junction with the Piute Pass Trail; for this trip, turn left (south) on the Lamarck Lakes Trail. Cross three bridges over branches of North Fork Bishop Creek and make a moderately steep, switchbacking climb through aspens, lodgepole pines, and limber pines to a junction with a 0.2-mile lateral to aptly named Grass Lake, 1 mile from the start of the trail. As the season progresses, Grass Lake, down in a deep hole, usually becomes less of a lake and more of a meadow.

Go right (west) at the junction and continue climbing toward the Lamarck Lakes. Switchbacks resume as the trail becomes steep and rocky near some exposed cliffs, where the open terrain allows good views of Grass and North lakes until obscured by the return of light forest. Beyond another set of switchbacks, pass a small pond and soon spy Lower Lamarck Lake (10,662′; 11S 354483 4120281). Make a short drop to ford the outlet and find the east shore of the 10,662-foot lake, 2.2 miles from the campground.

Lower Lamarck Lake is quite scenic, cradled below granite cliffs and backdropped by the pyramidal summit of Peak 12153. Well-used, limber-pine-shaded campsites near the outlet will tempt late-starting backpackers, although clearings above the northeast shore

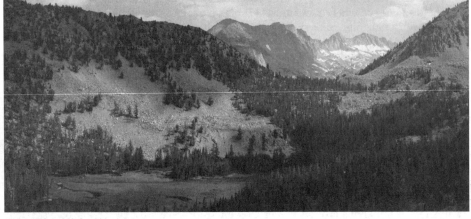

Grass Lake and the Sierra Crest

may offer more privacy. Anglers can test their skill on a resident population of brook and rainbow trout. Easy cross-country travel from Lower Lamarck Lake leads into the lovely backcountry around the Wonder Lakes.

Continue up the trail from the lower lake through the rock-strewn wash of Lamarck Creek. Following a series of short switchbacks, the trail drops to ford the creek and then follows the northwest bank through diminutive meadows dotted with pines. At 2.7 miles, reach the outlet of Upper Lamarck Lake (10,918′).

Tucked into a narrow, steep-walled canyon of rock, austere Upper Lamarck Lake is much longer than its lower counterpart. The stark surroundings create an inhospitable ambiance in comparison to the pine-shaded shores of Lower Lamarck Lake. Find campsites amid a copse of stunted pines clinging tenuously to a low rise above the southeast shore, or near some small tarns east of the lake. The upper lake also harbors brook and rainbow trout.

DAY 2 (Upper Lamarck Lake to North Lake Trailhead, 2.7 miles): Retrace your steps to the trailhead.

61 Darwin Lakes

Trip Data: 11S 350640 4116953; 14 miles; 3/1 days

Topos: *Mt. Darwin*

Highlights: Cradled in a hanging valley below 13,000-foot peaks, including the imposing north faces of Mt. Darwin and Mt. Mendel, the five Darwin Lakes offer an alpine setting that rivals any canyon in the Sierra for extraordinary mountain scenery.

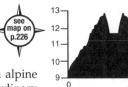

see map on p.226

HEADS UP! The route to 12,290-foot Lamarck Col is physically challenging, gaining 3600 feet in 5 miles; attempt this only if you are well acclimated. A short but steep ascent over a snowfield may be necessary to gain the col, and the cross-country route on the west side follows a steep descent over blocky talus all the way to the lakes. Avoid crossing Lamarck Col during thunderstorms.

DAY 1 (North Lake Trailhead to Upper Lamarck Lake, 2.7 miles): *(Recap: Trip 60, Day 1.)* From the true trailhead, go west and almost immediately reach the Piute Pass Trail junction; turn left (south). Now following the Lamarck Lakes Trail, make three bridged crossings of

North Fork Bishop Creek and climb moderately steeply past a junction with a lateral to Grass Lake. Go right (west) and continue climbing until you ford the outlet of and reach Lower Lamarck Lake at 2.2 miles (10,662´; 11S 354483 4120281). Climb another half mile along Lamarck Creek to Upper Lamarck Lake (10,918´) and locate a campsite on the low rise above the southeast shore or near tarns east of the lake.

DAY 2 (Upper Lamarck Lake to Darwin Lakes, 4.3 miles, cross-country): From Upper Lamarck Lake, retrace your steps down the trail several hundred yards to a use trail that crosses Lamarck Creek and then heads southeast up a rise. Take that path, beginning the cross-country section, and go past a small pond to a gurgling rivulet that bisects a meadow. Climb along this watercourse to its crossing and then follow a ducked route on a serpentine ascent of a boulder- and rock-strewn hillside. Nearing the crest, fine views open up of Grass Lake, Lamarck Lakes, North Lake, Lake Sabrina, and the Owens Valley, backdropped by the White Mountains.

The grade eases as the path follows the left-hand side of the ridge through widely scattered pines to a lush hillside well watered by seasonal brooks. Beyond this verdant oasis, the path zigzags more steeply across an arid hillside and then follows an ascending traverse before a stiff climb leads into a sloping valley below the Sierra Crest. Head up this valley toward the perennial snowfield just below the col. While crossing the snowfield may be straightforward under normal conditions, some parties might feel more comfortable ascending this potential obstacle with the aid of ice axes. Upon surmounting the snowfield, a very short rock scramble leads to 12,920-foot Lamarck Col (11S 351997 4117272), 5.5 miles from the trailhead. This lofty aerie offers an impressive view of Mt. Darwin and Mt. Mendel, Darwin Glacier, Darwin Lakes, and the deep cleft of Evolution Valley beyond Darwin Bench.

From the col, you will be forced to pick your way down a trailless, boulder- and talus-filled slope. Although the way to the lakes is clear and route finding is not particularly difficult, the actual descent can be quite tedious while carrying a full backpack, especially following the tiring climb to the col. The going becomes easier when you reach the faint use trail that runs along the north shore of the lakes. Proceed along this path to Lake 11592

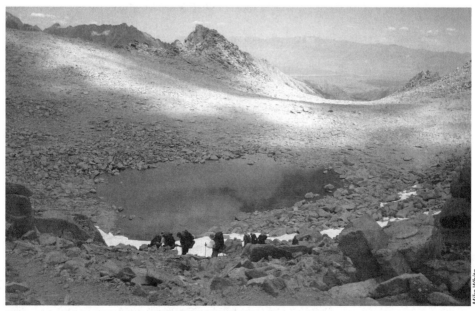

Mike White

Hikers descend a permanent snowfield on the east side of Lamarck Col.

(11,592´; 11S 349851 4116948), 7 miles from the trailhead, where a few decent campsites are scattered above the shoreline.

DAY 3 (Darwin Lakes to North Lake Trailhead, 7 miles, part cross-country): Retrace your steps to the trailhead.

62 Evolution Basin

Trip Data: 11S 349107 4115269; 39 miles; 6/1 days

see map on p.226

Topos: *Mt. Darwin, Mt. Henry, Mt. Hilgard, Mount Tom*

Highlights: Backpackers with off-trail skills can sample some of the High Sierra's most spectacular scenery on a mostly on-trail loop that visits such highlights as Darwin Canyon, Evolution Valley, Hutchinson Meadow, and Humphreys Basin.

HEADS UP! The route to 12,290-foot Lamarck Col is physically challenging, gaining 3600 feet in 5 miles; attempt it only if you are well acclimated. A short but steep ascent over a snowfield may be necessary to gain the col, and the cross-country route on the other side follows a steep descent over blocky talus all the way to the lakes. Avoid the crossing of Lamarck Col during thunderstorms.

DAY 1 (North Lake Trailhead to Upper Lamarck Lake, 2.7 miles): *(Recap: Trip 60, Day 1.)* From the true trailhead, go west and almost immediately reach the Piute Pass Trail junction; turn left (south). Now following the Lamarck Lakes Trail, make three bridged crossings of North Fork Bishop Creek and climb moderately steeply past a junction with a lateral to Grass Lake. Go right (west) and continue climbing until you ford the outlet of and reach Lower Lamarck Lake at 2.2 miles (10,662´). Climb another half mile along Lamarck Creek to Upper Lamarck Lake (10,918´) and locate a campsite on the low rise above the southeast shore or near tarns east of the lake.

DAY 2 (Upper Lamarck Lake to Evolution Lake, 6.7 miles, part cross-country): From Upper Lamarck Lake, retrace your steps down the trail several hundred yards to a use trail across Lamarck Creek and then head southeast up a rise. Proceed past a small pond, follow a rivulet to its crossing, and then make a serpentine ascent of a boulder- and rock-strewn hillside. Follow the left-hand side of the ridge through widely scattered pines to a lush hillside. Zigzag more steeply across an arid hillside, make an ascending traverse into a sloping valley, and proceed up this valley toward the snowfield below Lamarck Col. Above the snowfield, a very short rock scramble leads to the col at the boundary of Kings Canyon National Park, 5.5 miles from the trailhead.

From the col, pick your way cross-country down a boulder- and talus-filled slope toward the lakes below. The going becomes easier upon reaching the faint use trail that runs along the north shore of the lakes. Proceed along this path to Lake 11592 (11,592´; 11S 349851 4116948), 7 miles from the trailhead, where a few decent campsites are scattered above the shoreline.

Continue along the faint use trail as it parallels Darwin Creek toward lovely, tarn-dotted Darwin Bench. After the stark surroundings of Darwin Canyon, the alpine gardens of Darwin Bench combined with the stunning vistas across Evolution Valley create a picture-perfect scene. Eventually, you must bid farewell to lovely meadowlands of Darwin Bench and follow the use trail on a descent to the well-trod JMT. The goal is to meet the JMT near the top of the switchbacks (at approximately 10,700 feet) that climb out of Evolution Valley.

Once at the wide and well-maintained JMT, turn left (southeast) and stroll an easy 0.8-mile southeast to Evolution Lake. Splendidly scenic campsites can be found near the small peninsula on the northwest shore. While the dramatic scenery continues up the basin past Evolution Lake, campsites are at a premium and they become increasingly marginal the closer you get to Muir Pass. With an abundance of incredible scenery, spending additional layover days in Evolution Basin would be quite easy.

DAY 3 (Evolution Lake to Goddard Canyon Trail Junction, 9.8 miles): Retrace your steps 0.8 mile to where the cross-country route from Darwin Lakes intersected the JMT.

From there, go ahead on the JMT into a thickening forest of lodgepole pines. A zigzagging descent leads down the headwall of Evolution Valley, with periodic views through gaps in the trees of the deep cleft. Hop across a pair of flower-lined streams spilling across the trail and continue toward the floor of the canyon, passing below a thundering waterfall on Darwin Creek, and soon come to a crossing of this raucous stream.

Gradually graded trail winds down the valley through stands of scattered pines, across small pockets of meadow, and beside granite slabs and boulders to Colby Meadow. Lodgepole-shaded campsites near the fringe of the meadow will lure overnighters to this pastoral haven, where good views of the valley, the winding creek, and the surrounding peaks abound. Fishing in nearby Evolution Creek is reported to be decent for golden trout.

Continue the gentle descent downstream amid light forest, crossing a couple of streams on the way to McClure Meadow, the largest and probably most popular of Evolution Valley's meadows. Numerous campsites are spread around the edge of the meadow, some with fine views of the lazy creek sinuously coursing through the verdant clearing. The McClure Meadow Ranger Station (9671´; 11S 345298 4117174), summer home for the seasonal ranger who patrols the area, is found on a low rise just north of the trail.

Past the cabin, the gently graded trail continues to the end of the meadow. Away from McClure Meadow, the creek picks up speed again, and, over the next couple of miles, the trail travels in and out of lodgepole pine forest and crosses a trio of streams draining the north side of Glacier Divide. Breaks in the forest allow fine views of the surroundings, including a prominent avalanche swath and a picturesque waterfall below Emerald Peak.

Near the far end of Evolution Valley, skirt Evolution Meadow, passing by several lodgepole-shaded campsites, on the way to a crossing of a twin-channeled stream. From there, the trail curves south to ford Evolution Creek near the west end of Evolution Meadow, where the creek is wide and relatively slow moving. This is not the traditional JMT crossing, which is below Evolution Meadow; that crossing washed out years ago and is dangerous. Instead, look for a use trail across the meadow toward the creek; follow it and wade across (may be difficult in early season). Pick up another use trail on the south bank and follow it as it curves through campsites to meet the JMT on this side of the creek.

Back on the JMT, a stretch of nearly level trail along the south bank leads to a steep descent, where the creek suddenly begins a raucous plunge, tumbling over slabs and careering through boulders on the way to its convergence with South Fork San Joaquin River. The trail seems to match the fall of the plunging creek on a zigzagging drop across the exposed west wall of the canyon, with good views of the gorge and the river below. Nearing the floor of the canyon, enter the welcome shade of a mixed forest of aspens, lodgepole pines, and incense-cedars, and arrive at a wood bridge spanning South Fork San Joaquin River. On the far side of the bridge is a junction with the Goddard Canyon Trail (8485´; 11S 340686 4117757), 7.25 miles from where the cross-country route from Darwin Bench intersected the JMT. Find good campsites on either side of the bridge.

DAY 4 (Goddard Canyon Trail Junction to Hutchinson Meadow, 8 miles): Go north on the JMT from the junction, following the course of the river through mixed forest to a crossing of the stream draining the canyon east of Mt. Henry. A mixed bag of vegetation greets travelers over the next mile as they wander in and out of scattered forest and across open slopes covered with sagebrush, currant, and an assortment of wildflowers, including lupine, paintbrush, penstemon, pennyroyal, cinquefoil, and mariposa lily.

Just before another bridge across the river, a short spur trail leads above the south bank to good campsites amid a dense grove of pines. Downstream from the bridge, the canyon narrows to a slim gorge that powerfully propels the river through a rocky chasm. Walk alongside the raging waters to a more placid stretch of the river about a mile past the bridge. Just past the crossing of a side stream, arrive at Aspen Meadow, which is more an aspen-covered flat than a bona fide meadow. A few infrequently used campsites are nearby.

Past the meadow, continue downstream through mostly open, rocky terrain, following the trail as it bends around John Muir Rock. Veer away from the river and hike through widely scattered conifers to a lightly forested flat harboring a number of decent campsites. Just before reaching a steel bridge spanning Piute Creek, a sign indicates your imminent departure from Kings Canyon National Park.

Across the bridge is a junction with the Piute Pass Trail (8050´; 11S 337341 4121420), 3.5 miles from the Goddard Canyon Trail junction. Turn right (north) on rocky trail that climbs and then descends briefly to Piute Creek, which may provide the last easily accessible water late in the year until West Pinnacles Creek. The trail keeps to the west side and well above the briskly flowing creek as it ascends moderately and then steeply across a granite nose before reaching a ford of multibranched Tunnel Creek.

Follow switchbacks across hot, chaparral-covered slopes that reward hikers with excellent views of highly fractured Pavilion Dome and the surrounding, unnamed domes composing the west end of Glacier Divide. The trail then swings east through a narrowing canyon, crosses a couple of gullies on log bridges, fords tiny West Pinnacles Creek, pursues a steep, rocky course, and then enters moderate lodgepole forest cover on the way to the easy ford of East Pinnacles Creek. Views of the cascading tributary stream are frequent along this section of trail.

From the ford, the trail ascends gently to beautiful Hutchinson Meadow, where there are excellent campsites near the Pine Creek Pass Trail junction (9500´; 11S 342140 4125968). Fishing for golden and brook trout is reported to be good to excellent. The lovely meadow setting provides fine views of several granite peaks to the east and northwest, including Pilot Knob.

DAY 5 (Hutchinson Meadow to Humphreys Basin, 4.8 miles): Walk through Hutchinson Meadow, going ahead (east) at junctions with trails into French Canyon and crossing the braided distributaries of French Canyon Creek. Hike along Piute Creek through subalpine gardens and groves of shady lodgepole pine forest. The green meadowlands are rife with color from a wide array of seasonal wildflowers, including paintbrush, shooting star, fleabane, swamp onion, red mountain heather, buttercup, cinquefoil, penstemon, buckwheat, yarrow, senecio, and Douglas phlox. Labrador tea, lemon willow, and alpine willow shrubs complement the verdant grasses and flowers.

Eventually, the climb through Piute Canyon leads through progressively thinning forest into the stunningly beautiful environs of expansive Humphreys Basin, bordered by Glacier Divide to the south and towered over by the Sierra Crest to the east, with 13,986-foot Mt. Humphreys the dominant peak to the northeast.

The Piute Pass Trail continues to ascend to the cascading outlet of Desolation Lakes. Below, the Golden Trout Lakes gleam down in the cirque bottom. If headed for campsites on the knolls around Upper Golden Trout Lake (10,790´; 11S 347832 4123135), about a half mile south depending on the route, leave the main trail hereabouts and find little flats on the knolls around that lake. Lower Golden Trout Lake is closed to camping within 500 feet of the shoreline. Campsites in Humphreys Basin make fine base camps for exploring the area's wonders.

Farther up the Piute Pass Trail is the unsigned but highly visible use trail that heads north to the Desolation Lakes. Those intrigued by the Desolation Lakes' reputation for fishing and those fond of treeless, open camps will find some decent campsites above Lower Desolation Lake (11,200´) and on the wind-raked flats among the great white boulders surrounding aptly named Desolation Lake (11,375´), where anglers can ply the waters in search of golden trout. When searching for a campsite, seek a location well away from the trail, as those close to the trail have become grotesquely overused. Extra layover days could easily be spent exploring the various nooks and crannies of Humphreys Basin—use trails or cross-country routes provide easy access to many of the area's lakes.

DAY 6 (Humphreys Basin to North Lake Trailhead, 7 miles): (Recap in Reverse: Trip 59, Day 1.) Return to the main trail if necessary and follow it east across the gradually rising basin. Continue above austere Summit Lake to Piute Pass (11,423´; 11S 350613 4122714), 7.2 miles from the JMT junction.

Descending from Piute Pass, the trail weaves through granite terrain with widely scattered whitebark pines and past a handful of diminutive tarns to the northeast shore of Piute Lake (windy campsites). Leaving Piute Lake, make a winding, moderate descent past some small, unnamed lakes on the way to a bench holding Loch Leven. Switchbacks drop down the headwall and around the north side of North Fork Bishop Creek to a long, descending traverse below Piute Crags before another set of switchbacks leads to the floor of the canyon.

Cross the creek a couple of times and continue the descent on gently graded trail to a junction near the west end of North Lake Campground. Go ahead and almost immediately find the roadend (9344´; 11S 355642 4121338) in the campground, where there's a spot to park long enough to pick up or drop off people and packs. Remember, the shuttle car is 0.7 mile farther down the road and pack-station spur, past the pack station.

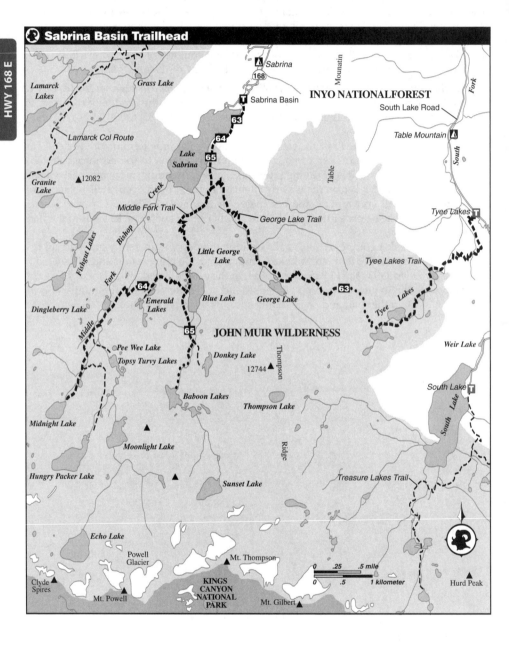

Sabrina Basin Trailhead

Sabrina

168

Sabrina Basin

INYO NATIONALFOREST

South Lake Road

Table Mountain

63

64

Lamarck
Lakes

Grass Lake

Lamarck Col Route

Lake
Sabrina

65

Middle Fork Trail

George Lake Trail

Tyee Lakes

Granite
Lake

▲12082

Little George
Lake

Tyee Lakes Trail

Dingleberry Lake

64

Emerald
Lakes

Blue Lake

George Lake

63

Tyee Lakes

Pee Wee Lake

65

JOHN MUIR WILDERNESS

Weir Lake

Topsy Turvy Lakes

Donkey Lake

12744 ▲

Thompson

South Lake

Baboon Lakes

Thompson Lake

Midnight Lake

Moonlight Lake

Ridge

Hungry Packer Lake

Sunset Lake

Treasure Lakes Trail

Echo Lake

Powell
Glacier

Mt. Thompson

0   .25   .5 mile

Clyde
Spires

Mt. Powell

KINGS
CANYON
NATIONAL
PARK

Mt. Gilbert

0   .5   1 kilometer

Hurd Peak

Mounatin

Fork

South

Table

Bishop

Creek

Fishgut Lakes

Fork

Middle

Sabrina Basin Trailhead   9078´; 11S 357136 4119777

DESTINATION/ UTM COORDINATES	TRIP TYPE	BEST SEASON	PACE (HIKING/ LAYOVER DAYS)	TOTAL MILEAGE
63 Tyee Lakes 11S 361138 4117763	Shuttle	Mid to late	2/0 Moderate, part cross-country	7.7
64 Midnight Lake 11S 353895 4114734	Out & back	Mid to late	2/1 Moderate	13
65 Baboon Lakes 11S 355871 4114911	Out & back	Mid to late	2/1 Moderate, part cross-country	9

Information and Permits: This trailhead is in Inyo National Forest: 351 Pacu Lane, Suite 200, Bishop, CA 93514, 760-873-2400, www.fs.fed.us/r5/inyo/. Quotas apply, and permits are required for overnight stays and are available at Inyo National Forest ranger stations in Lone Pine, Bishop, Mammoth Lakes, and Mono Basin Scenic Area Visitors Center.

Driving Directions: In the town of Bishop, turn west from Hwy. 395 onto West Line Street (Hwy. 168 East Side). Drive 18 miles southwest to backpackers' parking, just east of (below) the junction with the road to North Lake. You may want to drop off packs and most of your party at the actual trailhead, a half mile farther up this road on the left about 100 yards below Lake Sabrina's dam, and then have one of the party park the car and walk back to the trailhead.

63 Tyee Lakes

Trip Data: 11S 361138 4117763; 7.7 miles; 2/0 days

Topos: *Mt. Thompson*

Highlights: After a night at George Lake, which sees day users but few overnighters, this short but often steep trip climbs over

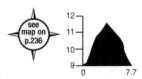

see map on p.236

Table Mountain, enjoying splendid, far-ranging views. Then it descends through the small and charming Tyee Lakes, where some will want to spend another night. Sturdy hikers can do this as a strenuous dayhike.

Shuttle Directions: In the town of Bishop, turn west from Hwy. 395 onto West Line Street (Hwy. 168 East Side). Drive 15.5 miles southwest to Hwy. 168's junction with signed South Lake Road. Turn left onto South Lake Road and drive 5 more miles to trailhead parking for the Tyee Lakes on the road's right side.

DAY 1 (Sabrina Basin Trailhead to George Lake, 3.2 miles): From the trailhead, the well-used trail climbs generally south above Sabrina Dam and begins a long traverse of the slope above the blue expanses of Lake Sabrina. The route is initially through lush greenery and over small streams, but it soon strikes out across the dry, sunny hillside above the lake, where there is a sparse cover of aspen, Jeffrey pine, juniper, lodgepole pine, western white pine, and mountain mahogany. Where the dusty trail crosses talus, the many aspens indicate a plentiful underground water supply. Views from here are excellent, extending all the way to the Sierra Crest.

The trail undulates gently until about halfway along the lake, and then it ascends steadily to a junction with the George Lake Trail, branching left (northeast, uphill; 9460´; 11S 356530 4118269). Take the George Lake Trail as it switchbacks up an open, exposed hillside for more than a half mile before reaching the first welcome clumps of whitebark pines. Cross the first stream and almost immediately recross it to continue on switchbacks up the steep hillside. As the forest cover grows thicker, the steep grade abates, becoming gradual.

Soon, the track reaches the level foot of a valley. At the head of a meadow, ford the stream and continue up the valley. Then the trail veers left to cross a sloping, willowed meadow. Beyond this meadow, the sandy trail rises steeply for about 100 vertical feet and then suddenly arrives at George Lake (10,738´; 11S 357785 4116560). There are good campsites near the trail on the east side of the lake, and fishing is good for brook and rainbow.

DAY 2 (George Lake to South Lake Road, 4.5 mile, part cross-country): Before reaching the far end of George Lake, the trail turns left (northeast) up slopes of granite sand dotted with whitebark pines. Although the tread is not always distinct on this slope, the route is not hard to follow.

Switchbacking some 500 feet up the increasingly steep trail, hikers enjoy increasingly good views of George Lake and the Sierra Crest beyond. Near the summit is a small stream where arnica blooms in midsummer. The trail becomes nearly level before reaching its high point (11,585´; 11S 358772 4116598), and many clumps of white phlox and lavender whorled penstemon grow on this seemingly barren, rocky plateau.

Next, the route drops down the trailless east side of a tributary of the Tyee Lakes and enters corn-lily country. This tall, flowering plant looks like a cornstalk and grows profusely in dozens of soggy hillside gardens here until late season. Where the little valley narrows and steepens, a trail becomes obvious on the right side of the creek. Just before the creek drops into a gorge, there is a beautiful lunch spot beside the stream with a commanding view of the fifth and largest Tyee Lake.

Then the trail winds down to that lake (11,015´), which has fair campsites on its north side in groves of whitebark pines. Cross the outlet stream to see that the trail is now more distinct. Circle the fourth lake, keeping some distance from its shore until the trail nears the outlet. Beside the outlet are some much-used but otherwise good campsites near a very picturesque, rock-dotted pond.

Beyond these campsites, the path again crosses the creek that connects the lakes and then winds down-canyon far from the third lake, seen in the east, to the shores of small, partly reed-filled Lake 2, whose campsites are poor. Lake 1 has practically no campsites, so skirt its swampy west edge and then veer away from its outlet past one or two possible campsites to begin a moderate descent through increasingly dense forest.

In a half mile, the trail fords the creek again and then switchbacks down in a generally eastward direction, crossing another stream soon after. The descent continues on dusty switchbacks down an often steep hillside, finally crossing a bridge over South Fork Bishop Creek to the Tyee Lakes Trailhead (9104´; 11S 361138 4117763), which is just downstream from the parking area on South Lake Road.

64 Midnight Lake

Trip Data: 11S 353895 4114734; 13 miles; 2/1 days

Topos: *Mt. Thompson, Mt. Darwin*

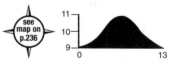

Highlights: This trip lets you explore a large number of beautiful lakes and creeks in unsurpassed surroundings. Their backdrop is the Sierra Crest, some 2500 feet above. You'll also delight in the many picturesque waterfalls and pools.

DAY 1 (Sabrina Basin Trailhead to Midnight Lake, 6.5 miles): From the trailhead, follow the trail generally south as it climbs above Lake Sabrina and skirts the lake, climbing gradually to the junction with the George Lake Trail.

Here, go ahead (southwest) to ford George Lake's vigorous outlet and begin ascending moderate-to-steep switchbacks through lodgepole forest above the lake, soon crossing another stream. Continue up onto a ridge as the trail curves south into a quiet ravine and climbs toward the north end of Blue Lake. Make a short descent through overused camp-sites to the outlet of picturesque Blue Lake (10,388´; no camping within 300 feet). This spot is a photographer's delight, with weather-beaten lodgepoles along the uneven shoreline and rugged Thompson Ridge towering above the lake's clear waters.

From the ford of the outlet, the trail winds through granite outcrops on the lake's west side. About midway along this side is a trail junction (10405´; 11S 356067 4116546), where going ahead (southwest and then south) leads to Donkey and Baboon lakes. This trip turns right (west-northwest) toward Dingleberry and Midnight lakes. The winding trail passes over a low saddle, down across a rocky slope, and back up granite ledges into a grassy valley spotted with lodgepole pines. Soon, it reaches the shaded outlet of the lowest of the Emerald Lakes. The trail then curves toward the Sierra Crest and reaches a junction with the use trail left (south) to Emerald Lakes (campsites).

Go right (generally southwest) toward Dingleberry Lake. The trail ascends gently to a saddle overlooking lovely Dingleberry Lake, to whose inlet and south side the trail shortly descends. The south side of Dingleberry Lake is swampy and buggy, but apart from the mosquitoes, there is excellent camping. Ford the broad inlet, walk through a forested area, cross a smaller stream, and continue southwest into a little valley (campsites).

The route to Midnight Lake continues southwest on the main trail. Soon, it bypasses an unsigned spur trail on the left that leads south-southeast to little Pee Wee and rockbound Topsy Turvy Lakes; go ahead (south-southwest) on the main trail here. A few moderate switchbacks take hikers past the signed trail to Hungry Packer Lake (campsites in the valley below Moonlight Lake and at Sailor Lake); go right (southwest) toward Midnight Lake.

Almost immediately, the trail fords the outflow creek from Hell Diver Lakes, 650 feet above to the west. Soon, the path comes to a tarn; from here, it climbs easily over granite shelves and quickly reaches Midnight Lake (10988´; 11S 353895 4114734). The lake lies at treeline in a granite bowl with sheer sides stretching upward to the Sierra Crest. A 300-foot waterfall courses down to its western shore. Excellent camping begins at the tarn and continues among the lodgepole pines that end at the lake's outlet.

"DRUNKEN SAILOR LAKE"

Peter Browning's book *Place Names of the Sierra Nevada* (Wilderness Press) is a wonderful source of information on this subject, and the following information comes from it. Browning writes that Art and John Schober ran a pack station on Bishop Creek, stocked the lakes, and mined in the eastern Sierra in the 1930s and 1940s. They were also responsible for most of the colorful names in this basin. As reported by Art Schober's wife: "There was an old sailor who hung out around the Lake Sabrina lodge. When the packers went up to this little lake [Sailor Lake] to stock it with fish, they found the sailor there sleeping off the effects of too much drink." Sailor Lake was labeled "Drunken Sailor Lake" on the 1983 7.5´ quad, but before and since then, it has been simply Sailor Lake. John Schober named Baboon Lakes for a group of Civilian Conservation Corps boys he saw there, looking "like a bunch of baboons" as they were waving their arms and going over the rocks. John also named Hungry Packer Lake, this time for an episode in the 1930s when he and his party, while stocking this lake and Midnight Lake, were caught by nightfall here and "had to spend the night without blankets or food." Guess for whom the Schober Lakes are named.

DAY 2 (Midnight Lake to Sabrina Basin Trailhead, 6.5 miles): Retrace your steps to return.

65 Baboon Lakes

Trip Data: 11S 355871 4114911; 9 miles; 2/1 days

Topos: *Mt. Thompson, Mt. Darwin*

Highlights: Sooner or later, everyone who returns to the High
Sierra will want to try a little cross-country hiking. This fairly
short trip is a fine choice for travelers who have reached that point.

HEADS UP! This trip requires some cross-country work.

DAY 1 (Sabrina Basin Trailhead to Baboon Lakes, 4.5 miles, part cross-country): From the
trailhead, follow the trail generally south as it climbs above Lake Sabrina and skirts the
lake, climbing gradually to the junction with the George Lake Trail.

Here, go ahead (southwest) to ford George Lake's vigorous outlet and begin ascending
moderate-to-steep switchbacks, soon crossing another stream. Continue up onto a ridge as
the trail curves south into a ravine and climbs toward the north end of Blue Lake. Make a
short descent through overused campsites to the outlet of Blue Lake (10,388´; no camping
within 300 feet). From the ford of the outlet, the trail winds through granite outcrops on
the lake's west side. About midway along this side is a trail junction (10405´; 11S 356067
4116546), where going ahead (southwest and then south) leads to Donkey and Baboon
lakes. This trip goes ahead.

Walk through granite-slab terrain under a forest of lodgepole pine, passing the south
end of Blue Lake (not visible) and crossing a seasonal tributary. From where the trail meets
the main stream, stay on the stream's west side, avoid the turnoff left (generally south-
southeast) to Donkey Lake (campsites), and continue south, more or less cross-country
from now on, to climb over slabs for 250 yards. The route climbs a steep, 20-foot-high slab,
at the top of which you turn right (generally west) and uphill. Climb over more slabs and
through a fissure before crossing the creek in a meadow. Beyond, head south up a ravine,
descend briefly, and turn right (generally west again) to climb a steep slope that heads to
a narrow ravine and Lower Baboon Lake (10,976´; 11S 355871 4114911; brook trout).

DAY 2 (Baboon Lakes to Sabrina Basin Trailhead, 4.5 miles, part cross-country): Retrace
your steps to the trailhead.

South Lake Trailhead   9837´; 11S 360986 4114804

DESTINATION/ UTM COORDINATES	TRIP TYPE	BEST SEASON	PACE (HIKING/ LAYOVER DAYS)	TOTAL MILEAGE
66 Treasure Lakes 11S 360017 4112243	Out & back	Mid to late	2/1 Leisurely	5
67 Chocolate Lakes 11S 362439 4112458	Semiloop	Mid to late	2/1 Leisurely	7.1
68 Dusy Basin 11S 362091 4107457	Out & back	Mid to late	2/1 Moderate	14
69 Palisade Basin 11S 366402 4104020	Semiloop	Mid to late	6/2 Strenuous, part cross-country	37.5
70 North Lake 11S 355653 4121354	Shuttle	Mid to late	8/1 Moderate	52.7

Information and Permits: This trailhead is in Inyo National Forest: 351 Pacu Lane, Suite 200, Bishop, CA 93514, 760-873-2400, www.fs.fed.us/r5/inyo/. Quotas apply, and permits are required for overnight stays and are available at Inyo National Forest ranger stations in Lone Pine, Bishop, Mammoth Lakes, and Mono Basin Scenic Area Visitors Center.

Driving Directions: In the town of Bishop, turn west from Hwy. 395 onto West Line Street (State Hwy. 168 East Side). Drive 15.5 miles southwest to the signed junction with South Lake Road. Turn left onto South Lake Road and drive 7 more miles to the roadend above South Lake (a reservoir). Overnighters may park in the lot above the day-users' parking nearer the restrooms. (If that lot is full, overnighters must park back down the road in spots reserved for overnighters and then walk up the road to the trailhead.) The signed trailhead is at the roadend, just slightly east of the restrooms.

66 Treasure Lakes

Trip Data: 11S 360017 4112243 (Lower Treasure Lake); 5 miles; 2/1 days

Topos: *Mt. Thompson*

see map on p.243

Highlights: Few trips offer so much High Sierra beauty for so little effort. Not only is there a wealth of dramatic scenery, there's also good camping and fishing. Sturdy hikers can easily do this as a dayhike.

DAY 1 (South Lake Trailhead to Lower Treasure Lake, 2.5 miles): Beyond the trailhead information signs, the trail dips briefly through a marshy, flowery area to a junction with the trail that comes up on the left from the pack station. Turn right (south) onto the main Bishop Pass Trail as it bottoms out and then climbs steadily under lodgepoles along the east side of South Lake. The views along this climb are splendid, and the trail presently reaches its junction with the Treasure Lakes Trail (10,255´; 11S 361013 4113789).

Turn right (south-southwest) toward the Treasure Lakes. Mostly over duff and sand, the trail descends to ford a stream, ascends briefly, and then descends again to a bridge over Bishop Creek's South Fork. This stretch affords good views of Hurd Peak and the glacier-topped peaks to the north. The trail then meanders over to the outlet from the Treasure Lakes, parallels it briefly downstream, and fords it.

Beyond this ford, the route begin a moderate-to-steep ascent on a duff-and-sand trail. As the elevation increases, the forest cover shows increasing whitebark pine mixed with the lodgepoles, and there is an abundance of wildflowers lining the trail and clustered in

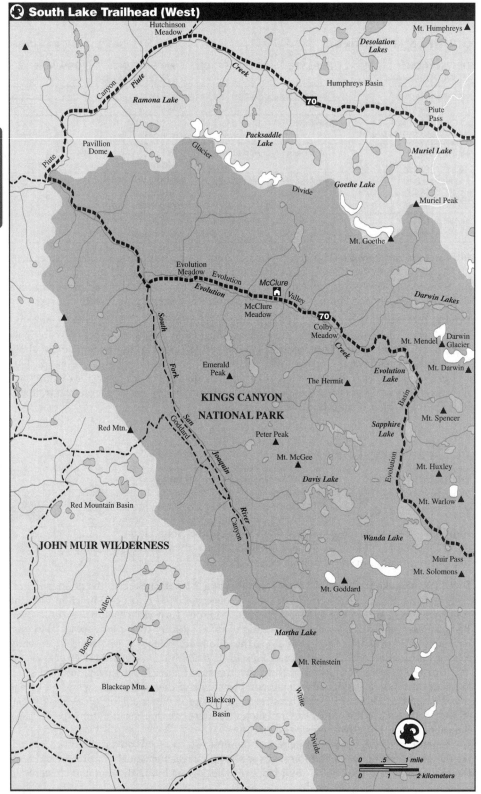

Mt. Humphreys ▲

Hutchinson Meadow

Desolation Lakes

Piute *Creek*

Canyon

Humphreys Basin

Piute

Ramona Lake

70

Piute Pass

Piute

Packsaddle Lake

Muriel Lake

Pavillion Dome ▲

Glacier

Divide

Goethe Lake

Muriel Peak ▲

Mt. Goethe ▲

Evolution Meadow

Evolution

Evolution

McClure

Darwin Lakes

Valley

70

McClure Meadow

Colby Meadow

Creek

Mt. Mendel ▲ Darwin Glacier

Evolution Lake

Mt. Darwin ▲

Emerald Peak ▲

The Hermit ▲

KINGS CANYON

NATIONAL PARK

South

Basin

Mt. Spencer ▲

Sapphire Lake

Fork

Red Mtn. ▲

Goddard

San

Peter Peak ▲

Mt. Huxley ▲

Joaquin

Mt. McGee ▲

Evolution

Red Mountain Basin

Davis Lake

Mt. Warlow ▲

River

JOHN MUIR WILDERNESS

Canyon

Wanda Lake

Muir Pass

Mt. Solomons ▲

Valley

Mt. Goddard ▲

Bench

Martha Lake

▲ Mt. Reinstein

White

Blackcap Mtn. ▲

Blackcap Basin

Divide

0	.5	1 mile

0	1	2 kilometers

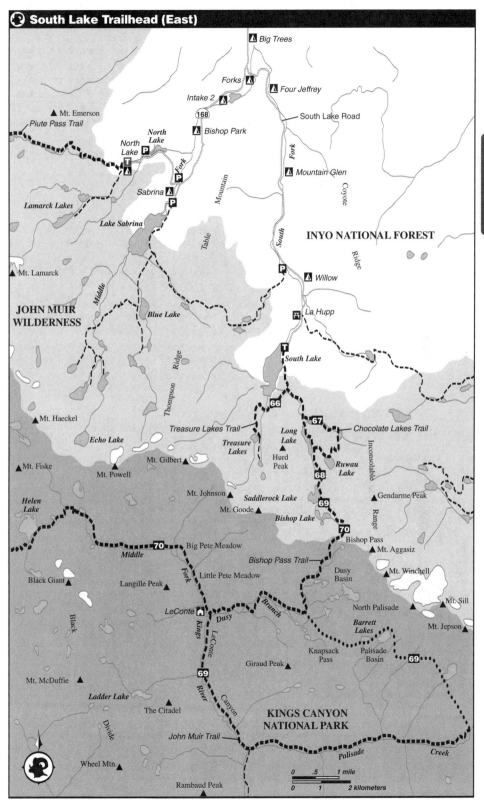

Big Trees

Forks

Four Jeffrey

Intake 2

168

South Lake Road

Bishop Park

North Lake

North Lake

Piute Pass Trail

Mt. Emerson

Mountain Glen

Sabrina

Lake Sabrina

Lamarck Lakes

Mt. Lamarck

Mountain Fork

North Fork

Middle Fork

South Fork

Coyote

INYO NATIONAL FOREST

Ridge

Table Ridge

JOHN MUIR WILDERNESS

Blue Lake

Thompson Ridge

Willow

La Hupp

South Lake

66

Treasure Lakes Trail

67

Chocolate Lakes Trail

Mt. Haeckel

Echo Lake

Treasure Lakes

Long Lake

Mt. Fiske

Mt. Powell

Mt. Gilbert

Hurd Peak

Ruwau Lake

68

Inconsolable

Helen Lake

Mt. Johnson

Saddlerock Lake

Mt. Goode

Bishop Lake

69

Gendarme Peak

Range

70

Bishop Pass

Big Pete Meadow

Bishop Pass Trail

Mt. Aggasiz

Black Giant

Middle Fork

Langille Peak

Little Pete Meadow

Dusy Basin

Mt. Winchell

Black Divide

LeConte

Dusy Branch

North Palisade

Mt. Sill

Kings

LeConte Canyon

Barrett Lakes

Mt. Jepson

Mt. McDuffie

69

Knapsack Pass

Palisade Basin

69

Ladder Lake

Giraud Peak

River

The Citadel

KINGS CANYON NATIONAL PARK

John Muir Trail

Palisade

Creek

Wheel Mtn.

Rambaud Peak

0   .5   1 mile
0   1   2 kilometers

the grassy patches that seam the granite. The ascent steepens, crosses an area of smoother granite slabs dotted with glacial erratic boulders, and fords the outlet stream from Lower Treasure Lake (difficult in early season). Then, in an easy half mile, the path arrives at the good campsites on the northeast side of that lake (10,682´; 11S 360017 4112243), directly under dramatic, pointed Peak 12047. This lake, the largest in the Treasure Lakes basin (12 acres), affords fair-to-good fishing for golden; the fishing is even better in the higher lakes, where there are other campsites.

DAY 2 (Lower Treasure Lake to South Lake Trailhead, 2.5 miles): Retrace your steps.

CROSS-COUNTRY SEMILOOP

Adventurous hikers can make a semiloop of this trip by adding a cross-country segment and returning on the main Bishop Pass Trail. This option adds a half mile to Day 2. Work your way into the Treasure Lakes' eastern, upper cirque to the northwest end of the first Upper Treasure Lake (11,171´; 11S 360112 4111450). Continue upward on the west side of the first two upper lakes, and then cross to the east side at the highest lake's outlet (Lake 11175). Skirt that lake until just beneath the obvious saddle 500 feet above; climb to that saddle (11,703´; 11S 360675 4110713), south of Peak 12192.

From the saddle, descend north-northeast about 100 yards and then veer over to a little stream, paralleling it momentarily beside a short waterfall. From there, work almost directly down to Margaret Lake's northwest side (10955´; 11S 361494 4111047) to find a use trail that leads northeast to the southernmost point of Long Lake. Ford the inlet, go east past campsites, and meet the Bishop Pass Trail; turn left (north) on it. Return to the trailhead, staying on the Bishop Pass Trail at all junctions.

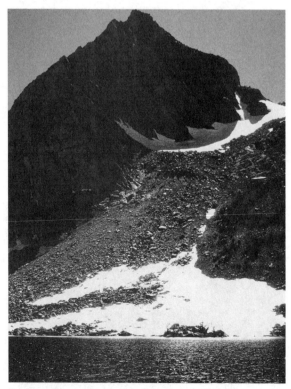

Peak 12047 over the lowest of the Treasure Lakes

67 Chocolate Lakes

Trip Data: 11S 362439 4112458 (Lower Chocolate Lake);
7.1 miles; 2/1 days

Topos: *Mt. Thompson*

Highlights: Like Trip 66, this trip also offers abundant, dramatic High Sierra scenery for relatively little effort—though it's a little more adventurous—and can be done as a dayhike. The lakes are named for the striking peak just west of them, Chocolate Peak, which looks from the north like a chocolate sundae.

DAY 1 (South Lake Trailhead to Lower Chocolate Lake, 3 miles): Begin by descending to meet the trail from the pack station and head south. After the trail bottoms out, climb steadily above South Lake. Go left (southeast) at the signed Treasure Lakes Trail junction. Climb past meadows and ford streams; presently, go right (south) at the sometimes signed Marie Louise Lakes use-trail junction.

At the signed Bull Lake/Chocolate Lakes trail junction, turn left, southeast and then east, away from the Bishop Pass Trail. Drop a little and then ascend to scenic Bull Lake (campsites), just beneath the north face of Chocolate Peak. Continuing, climb along and across Bull Lake's flowery inlet stream, ascending the narrow valley between Chocolate Peak and the rugged Inconsolable Range. Over-the-shoulder views are splendid.

The trail passes several good campsites at Lower Chocolate Lake (10,990´; 11S 362439 4112458). This lake and its two higher companions support a brook trout fishery. Take some time to explore the upper lakes on the increasingly faint trail. You may also find a campsite at the next higher one (11,060´), but the highest lake (11,100´), which sits in a very narrow, steep-sided cirque, is campsite-less.

DAY 2 (Lower Chocolate Lake to South Lake Trailhead, 4.1 miles): Continue up the increasingly faint trail toward the Upper Chocolate Lakes, fording the interconnecting stream between the lower and middle lakes and later between the middle and upper lakes. The track becomes more like a use trail as it rounds the upper lake's west side, almost vanishing in rockfall as it climbs toward a saddle on Chocolate Peak's southeast shoulder. You may notice a second route branching east and upward; this one also goes to the saddle. Snow may linger into mid-season on the north side of this saddle (11,344´). Views of the Inconsolable Range from here are breathtaking; the range's high point,

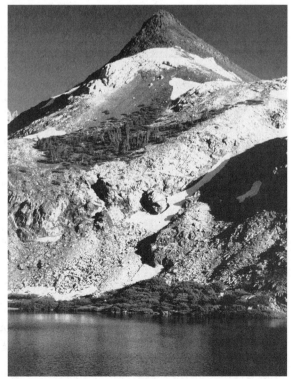

Chocolate Peak over Bull Lake

rugged, 13,525-foot Cloudripper, towers overhead. Chocolate Peak is a Class 2 scramble from here; the panorama from its summit is well worth the trouble.

On rough trail, descend from the saddle toward pretty Ruwau Lake (11,044´; poor campsites on its west side), a lake overseen from the south by Picture Puzzle Peak. Skirt the lake's north side before descending again, very steeply at the end, to meet the Bishop Pass Trail at beautiful Long Lake (10,763; poor campsites). Turn right (north) on the Bishop Pass Trail and trace Long Lake's east side; be sure to turn around occasionally and take in the amazing views southward toward Bishop Pass.

Shortly after leaving Long Lake's north end and fording its outlet, find the signed Bull Lake/Chocolate Lakes trail junction. Go ahead (north) here on the Bishop Pass Trail, retracing your steps to South Lake.

68 Dusy Basin

Trip Data: 11S 362091 4107457 (northernmost large lake); 14 miles; 2/1 days

Topos: *Mt. Thompson, North Palisade*

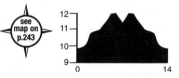

Highlights: Ascend the spectacular drainage of South Fork Bishop Creek on the popular Bishop Pass Trail to enter Kings Canyon National Park and find the high, granite country of Dusy Basin and its wonderland of alpine lakes, ponds, streams, and peaks.

DAY 1 (South Lake Trailhead to Dusy Basin, 7 miles): Begin by descending to meet the trail from the pack station and head south here. After the trail bottoms out, climb steadily above South Lake. Go left (southeast) at the signed Treasure Lakes Trail junction. Climb past meadows and ford streams; presently, go right (south) at the sometimes signed Marie Louise Lakes use-trail junction.

At the signed Bull Lake/Chocolate Lakes trail junction, go ahead (south) to stay on the Bishop Pass Trail as it levels off at the islet-dotted north end of Long Lake. After crossing this lake's outlet, the route undulates along the lake's east side (rainbow, brook, and brown). Near the lake's south end, find the junction with the trail left (east) to Ruwau Lake. Continue ahead (south) on the Bishop Pass Trail to ford Ruwau's outlet and then arrive at well-used campsites on the knolls above Long Lake.

Continue the ascent through occasional, subalpine, tarn-dotted meadows. Sometimes steep, this trail climbs steadily past one of the Timberline Tarns and then spectacular Saddlerock Lake (11,128´; overused campsites on the low bench to the east; rainbow). It's not long before the main trail meets the unmarked fisherman's spur trail right (south) to Bishop Lake (11,260´; exposed campsites; brook).

Beyond Bishop Lake, the trail fords one of that lake's inlets, passes treeline, and begins a series of well-engineered, moderate switchbacks at the head of this breathtaking cirque basin. (Note that a trail over Jigsaw Pass, shown on the topo as connecting with the Bishop Pass Trail, doesn't exist.) Breather stops offer unforgettable views. Occasional pockets of snow sometimes blanket the approach to Bishop Pass (11,972´; 11S 362714 4108733) late into the season. Views from the pass itself aren't memorable except for Mt. Agassiz to the east; walk a little north, from just below the pass, to overlooks above Bishop Lake for unforgettable scenery.

Near the pass, ignore a couple of use trails and stick to the more heavily used main trail—when in doubt, follow the horse dung. The main trail descends westward on a traverse interspersed with switchbacks, with expanding views over Dusy Basin and its surrounding peaks. From the traverse, the lakes are hidden by the basin's topography, and the basin may seem unappealingly barren and dry.

The sandy descent contours over rock-bench systems some distance north of the basin's northernmost large lake (11,347´; 11S 362091 4107457; not the small lake just west of Mt. Agassiz; golden and brook). Where the trail comes near the lake's inlet, branch left toward the lake, leaving the trail and crossing smooth granite and tundra to the fair campsites at the west end of this lake. Other fair campsites can be found a few yards to the southwest, along the outlet stream. A very sparse forest cover of gnarled whitebark pines dots the granite landscape on all sides, and the fractures in the granite are filled with grassy, heather-lined pockets. The setting at this upper lake is incomparable: The Palisades fill the northeastern skyline, while the southeastern horizon is defined by aptly named Isosceles Peak as well as Columbine Peak and Knapsack Pass. Giraud Peak towers in the south, catching the sunrise.

However, the area is very heavily used. Campsites farther afield may offer more peace and privacy. Find the splendid chain of eastern lakes by easy-to-moderate cross-country scrambling eastward over the ridge to the southeast that's topped by Peak 11603 (golden and brook). Find the beautiful, more forested lower lakes by staying on the main trail and descending another 1.7 miles to Lake 10742 at the northwestern end of that chain of lakes (golden); the chain extends southeastward for about a mile from there.

DAY 2 (Dusy Basin to South Lake Trailhead, 7 miles): Retrace your steps.

69 Palisade Basin

Trip Data: 11S 366402 4104020 (Lake 3559 east of Potluck Pass); 37.5 miles; 6/2 days

Topos: *Mt. Thompson, North Palisade, Split Mtn.*

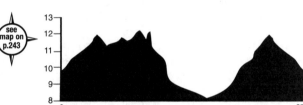

Highlights: For strong, adventurous hikers qualified to tackle this route, this semiloop's incomparable and widely varied scenery, especially on its remote, cross-country section, is a more than ample reward for its demands.

HEADS UP! This strenuous trip is only for backpackers experienced in cross-country navigation with map and compass (and perhaps GPS unit) at high altitudes and over Class 2 to 3 terrain with a full pack. The cross-country part requires cross three trailless Class 2 to 3 passes. If you can't find Knapsack Pass in order to begin the cross-country part, do not attempt to continue this trip.

DAY 1 (South Lake Trailhead to Dusy Basin, 7 miles): *(Recap: Trip 68, Day 1.)* Begin by descending to meet the trail from the pack station and head south here. After the trail bottoms out, climb steadily above South Lake. Go left (southeast) at the signed Treasure Lakes Trail junction. Climb past meadows and ford streams; presently, go right (south) at the sometimes signed Marie Louise Lakes use-trail junction.

At the signed Bull Lake/Chocolate Lakes trail junction, go ahead (south) to stay on the Bishop Pass Trail as it levels off at the north end of Long Lake. After crossing this lake's outlet, traverse the lake's east side to the junction with the trail to Ruwau Lake. Continue ahead (south), ford Ruwau's outlet, and then ascend through occasional, subalpine, tarn-dotted meadows. Pass one of the Timberline Tarns and then spectacular Saddlerock Lake and presently meet the unmarked fisherman's spur trail right (south) to Bishop Lake

Beyond Bishop Lake, pass treeline and begin a series of switchbacks up to Bishop Pass (11,972´; 11S 362714 4108733; snow patches possible late into the season). Near the pass, ignore a couple of use trails and stick to the more heavily used main trail—when in doubt, follow the horse dung. Descend westward on a traverse interspersed with switchbacks, contouring over rock-bench systems some distance north of the basin's northernmost large lake (11,347′; 11S 362091 4107457; not the small lake just west of Mt. Agassiz; golden and brook). Where the trail comes near the lake's inlet, branch left toward the lake, leaving the trail and crossing smooth granite and tundra to the fair campsites at the west end of this lake and a few yards to the southwest, along the outlet stream.

DAY 2: (Dusy Basin to Lake 11672, 6 miles, cross-country): You can cross into Palisade Basin via any one of three climbers' passes: Knapsack Pass, the unnamed pass between Columbine Peak and Isosceles Peak, and what has come to be known as "Thunderbolt Pass," just southwest of Thunderbolt Peak. The route we describe here uses Knapsack Pass (11,673′), the prominent saddle just south of Columbine Peak. Whichever route you choose, don't expect to find ducks or use trails.

Hikers have a choice of cross-country routes through Dusy Basin to the base of Knapsack Pass, which is just east of the marshy area that's west of and below the pass, at about 10,980′ and 11S 362244 4105508: 1. Return to the main trail and descend generally southwest as far as a pronounced east-pointing switchback, from which an obvious eastward use trail begins. The use trail soon peters out, but you can keep working your way east. 2. From Dusy Basin's chain of lower lakes, follow the chain's north side southeast for a while, but be sure to climb about 200 feet well before reaching the easternmost lake in order to avoid a large talus field at that lake. 3. This is probably the most difficult and beautiful way. Go over the ridge southeast of the northernmost large lake that was Day 1's destination and work your way down the eastern chain of lakes to the pass's base, possibly cutting over to the pass above its base. There are one or two Spartan campsites on an outcrop west of the marshy area.

Cross-country routes through Dusy Basin converge as beaten paths at Knapsack Pass's base, where a use trail leads into large boulders to begin the climb. The path soon gives way to a steady, trackless ascent over heavily fractured rock. It requires a little route-finding skill and becomes steeper on the final climb to the pass (11,704′; 11S 362818 4105262). Impossible as it may seem, there are recorded visits to Palisade Basin via this pass with stock!

THE VIEW FROM KNAPSACK PASS

Views from the pass include Black Giant, Mt. Powell, and Mt. Thompson to the northwest, and the Palisade Basin and crest to the east. These peaks look, as one climber expressed it, "like mountain peaks are supposed to look." Precipitous faces composed of relatively unfractured rock, couloirs, buttresses, and glaciers combine to make this crest one of the finer climbing areas in the Sierra Nevada. From this vantage point, the vast, convoluted expanses of Palisade Basin appear totally barren of life except for an isolated whitebark pine or a golden snag stretching toward the deep blue sky.

The secret to descending from Knapsack Pass into Palisade Basin is to keep to the left at first, climbing a little before descending moderately to steeply over talus and then a ledge system to the westernmost large lake in the Barrett chain (Lake 11468). After passing around the south end of this rockbound lake, this boulder-hopping route crosses the rocky saddle east of that lake to the largest lake of the chain (Lake 11523) and follows a fisherman's track around the north end. From this lake, the sheer cliffs of the west face of North Palisade dominate the skyline. Your route continues east, climbing past several tiny, rockbound lakelets. Those preferring a less strenuous trip will enjoy an overnight in Palisade Basin.

Climb the ridge east of Lake 11523 to the saddle just northeast of Point 12005. Keeping to the left, descend a little into the shallow bowl west of Potluck Pass and pass a pond, west

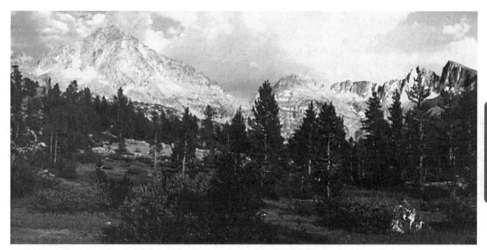

From lower Dusy Basin: Columbine Peak is at left; Knapsack Pass is the saddle to its right.

of which there's a possible campsite. Continuing, ascend the easier west side of Potluck Pass (12,148′; 11S 365949 4104759), the definite saddle between Point 12698 and Polemonium Peak. Along with the continuing views of the Palisades, this vantage point also looks across the Palisade Creek watershed to Amphitheater Lake. To the southwest, the terrain seems swirled into peaks like meringue topping on a pie.

The descent from Potluck Pass is a scramble over a steep, smoothed granite ledge system, keeping to the right. This downgrade continues over scree and then levels out near an unnamed small lake. From here, scramble over a slabby ridge separating that lake from rockbound Lake 11672 (Lake 3559 on the metric *Split Mtn.* topo). At this lake, there are good campsites on the west shore and just below the lake around the outlet (11,690′; 11S 366402 4104020; golden), which becomes Glacier Creek. Grassy sections around the sandy-bottomed lake provide a foothold for colorful alpine wildflowers, including yellow columbine, sturdy white heather, and blue sky pilot.

DAY 3 (Lake 11672 to Deer Meadow, 5 miles, part cross-country): An early start is in order, for the cross-country ascent is followed by a 3200-foot descent whose first 1300 feet are trailless and challenging.

After fording Lake 11672's outlet—Glacier Creek—ascend steep granite ledges up the slope southeast of the creek to the saddle called Cirque Pass (12,075′; 11S 366658 4103793). Cirque Pass is the most difficult of the three climbers' passes on this route. The ascent is relatively short, however, and views from this saddle are good of Devils Crags and Mt. McDuffie to the west, North Palisade to the north, and Middle Palisade to the east.

Sometimes over snow, the long, steep descent heads generally south-southeastward on talus and ledges past several tiny tarns in the fractured granite. Partway down, Palisade Lakes and the glacially smoothed, bowl-like cirque surrounding the lakes comes into view. The route levels out briefly as it crosses a bench and veers westward past a pair of lakelets. Beyond the bench, the descent becomes steeper and more exposed as it nears the little lake west of Palisade Lakes. Class 3 slabs separated by steep, wet, grassy sections are found if descending directly (almost southward) toward the little lake; reportedly, a Class 2 to 3 route can be worked out by staying more to the west as you approach the lake, where there's a possible campsite. From the little lake, the descent becomes much easier as it curves east for the final 200 feet, meeting the JMT just west of the Palisade Lakes (campsites; no wood fires). Make this day less strenuous day by camping in this area.

However, today's leg continues westward on the JMT. The route descends by seemingly endless, zigzagging switchbacks along the north side of Palisade Creek.

THE GOLDEN STAIRCASE

This section of the JMT is known as the "Golden Staircase" and was one of the last links in the JMT. The top of these switchbacks is an excellent vantage point from which to see the crest of Middle Palisade peak to the northeast, and in the west beyond Deer Meadow, lying immediately below, Devils Crags, Wheel Mountain, and Mt. McDuffie. Slopes on both sides of this steep descent are dramatically glacially smoothed.

As the trail reaches the head of the flats above Deer Meadow, it enters a moderate stand of lodgepole and western white pine. Abundant wildflowers, including western mountain aster, Douglas phlox, pennyroyal, red columbine and tiger lily, appear as the trail comes close to the creek, and red fir, juniper, and aspen occasionally mingle with the predominantly lodgepole forest cover. At the foot of the Golden Staircase, the path begins winding through patchy but extensive fire damage (from a lightning-caused fire in 2002) that has limited the available campsites. However, beyond its fords of the several branches of Glacier Creek, the trail intersects an obvious use trail down onto an unscarred, low ridge whose far end is at the creek—Palisade Creek (golden and brook). There are numerous, well-used campsites under lodgepoles on this ridge (about 8878´; 11S 364431 4102153), which is part of the "Deer Meadow" area, a now misnamed area that has long been more forest than meadow.

DAY 4 (Deer Meadow to Grouse Meadows, 5 miles): Continue westward on the JMT, descending gradually and soon fording the unnamed, multibranched outlet of Palisade Basin. Look for Cataract Creek's showy cascades across Palisade Creek; however, the trail that once ascended Cataract Creek as shown on the topo no longer exists. The now moderate descent passes through many burned-over areas with few if any safe campsites due to the threat of fire-killed trees that might fall. Concentrations of wildflowers here include Indian paintbrush, penstemon, white cinquefoil, mariposa lily, and goldenrod. The underfooting is mostly duff and sand, through alternating forest and meadow. In places, a kind of wiry grass grows right in the trail, testifying to the relatively light use of the JMT in this area.

Then the trail veers away from Palisade Creek, only to return, and, keeping to the north side of the creek, it descends steadily over morainal debris to the confluence of Palisade Creek and the Middle Fork Kings River. A bridge used to connect the Middle Fork Kings River Trail with the JMT here, but high water destroyed it in the early 1980s, and there are no plans to replace it. There are a few campsites on the flat between the trail and this confluence.

This trip, however, doesn't need the absent bridge, as its route bears right (west and then northwest) to begin ascending moderately up LeConte Canyon along the roaring Middle Fork Kings River. There's a campsite on a small flat on the river side of the trail a couple of switchbacks north of the confluence and another site a little below Grouse Meadows on a flat uphill from the trail and just north of a dashing cascade. If you haven't camped yet, continue to the damp, overused campsites on the north edge of scenic, peaceful Grouse Meadows (8247´; 11S 358703 4103087), where the river temporarily flows in placid meanders. There are a few campsites farther upriver on Day 5's route, too.

DAY 5 (Grouse Meadows to Dusy Basin, 7.5 miles): Leaving the pleasant grasslands of Grouse Meadows behind, the trail continues its gradual but steady ascent. To the west, the Citadel's granite face stands guard over an obvious hanging valley and the cascades from Ladder Lake. Early-morning travelers are often treated to a burst of reflected sunlight from glacially polished surfaces high on the canyon's west wall north of that valley.

The trail undulates on the east wall, sometimes 80 to 100 feet above the river, sometimes right alongside it. The thin lodgepole forest cover occurs mostly in stands, with intermittent stretches of grassy pockets, and the underfooting is mostly rocky. There are a few overused campsites along the way, on the river side of the trail. Ahead, the canyon narrows, and the trail crosses Dusy Branch creek via a substantial steel footbridge to meet the Bishop Pass Trail. A few yards north of this junction is a signed junction with a lateral to the LeConte Ranger Station (emergency services perhaps available).

This trip turns right (east) onto the Bishop Pass Trail and begins a steep, switchbacking ascent of the east canyon wall. This ascent is broken into two distinct steps that gain a total of 2000 feet in about 2 miles. The steepness of the slopes is tamed by switchbacks, though their condition is sometimes poor. Touching the creek at strategic intervals, the trail offers magnificent views. Near the creek, lush shooting star, fireweed, penstemon, pennyroyal, and some yellow columbine nest next to damp, moss-covered rocky grottos. Along the switchbacks, occasional lodgepole and juniper break the monotony of the slab granite, and there are rewarding views of Dusy Branch as it plunges down the steep slabs in sparkling cascades. Near the top of the first climb, one particular juniper with a near-record girth stands out, like a beetle-browed sentinel. There are possible campsites on the bench where the climb briefly eases and the route fords Dusy Branch.

Continue up swithbacks, some forested, to cross the creek on a bridge, and then resume switchbacking up through a sparse cover of aspen. This ascent levels out near the outlet of the lowest of the Dusy Basin lake chain (campsites) and emerges to open, breathtaking views of Mt. Winchell, Mt. Agassiz, Thunderbolt Peak, and Columbine Peak.

After rounding the north side of the lower Dusy Basin lake chain (campsites), the trail turns north and climbs a series of grass-topped ledges.The route veers up and away from the creek, climbing moderately into upper Dusy Basin and to the vicinity of the basin's northernmost large lake, which was also Day 1's destination (11,347´; 11S 362091 4107457).

DAY 6 (Dusy Basin to South Lake Trailhead, 7 miles): Reverse the steps of Day 1 to the trailhead.

70 North Lake

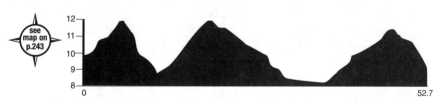

Trip Data: 11S 355653 4121354; 52.7 miles; 8/1 days

Topos: *Mt. Abbot; Mt. Thompson, North Palisade, Mt. Goddard, Mt. Darwin, Mt. Hilgard, Mount Tom, Mt. Henry*

Highlights: This trip is the quintessential High Sierra hike. In between two crossings of the Sierra Crest, it visits beautiful and famous Evolution Basin and Evolution Valley. There's even an optional layover-day trip to a wilderness hot spring. Unlike Trip 69, this adventure is on trail. This trip's trailheads—both out of Bishop—are close enough together that it's relatively easy to set up the shuttle.

Shuttle Directions: In the town of Bishop, turn west from Hwy. 395 onto West Line Street (Hwy. 168 East Side). Drive 18 miles southwest past the signed junction with South Lake Road and almost to Lake Sabrina. At the signed junction with dirt North Lake Road, turn right, cross the creek on a bridge, and continue 2 airy miles past little North Lake to a junction with the signed spur road to the pack station. Turn right here, pass the pack station's entrance, and shortly find the overnighters' parking lot. Alas, this lot is 0.7 mile from the true trailhead, which is farther up the road at the roadend and at the west end of North Lake Campground.

DAY 1 (South Lake Trailhead to Dusy Basin, 7 miles): *(Recap: Trip 68, Day 1.)* Begin by descending to meet the trail from the pack station and head south here. After the trail bottoms out, climb steadily above South Lake. Go left (southeast) at the signed Treasure Lakes Trail junction. Climb past meadows and ford streams; presently, go right (south) at the sometimes signed Marie Louise Lakes use-trail junction.

At the signed Bull Lake/Chocolate Lakes trail junction, go ahead (left, south) to stay on the Bishop Pass Trail as it levels off at the north end of Long Lake. After crossing this lake's outlet, traverse the lake's east side to the junction with the trail to Ruwau Lake. Continue ahead (south), ford Ruwau's outlet, and then ascend through occasional subalpine, tarn-dotted meadows. Pass one of the Timberline Tarns and then spectacular Saddlerock Lake and presently meet the unmarked fisherman's spur trail right (south) to Bishop Lake. Stay on the Bishop Pass Trail.

Beyond Bishop Lake, pass treeline and begin a series of switchbacks up to Bishop Pass (11,972´; 11S 362714 4108733; snow patches possible late into the season). Near the pass, ignore a couple of use trails and stick to the more heavily used main trail—when in doubt, follow the horse dung. Descend westward on a traverse interspersed with switchbacks, contouring over rock-bench systems some distance north of the basin's northernmost large lake (11,347´; 11S 362091 4107457; not the small lake just west of Mt. Agassiz; golden and brook). Where the trail comes near the lake's inlet, branch left toward the lake, leaving the trail and crossing smooth granite and tundra to the fair campsites at the west end of this lake and a few yards to the southwest, along the outlet stream.

DAY 2 (Dusy Basin to Big Pete Meadow, 6 miles): The trail from the northernmost large lake (11,350´) of Dusy Basin descends over smooth granite ledges and tundra sections.

VIEWS THROUGH DUSY BASIN

Occasional clumps of the flaky-barked, five-needled whitebark pine dot the glacially scoured basin, and impressive Mt. Agassiz, Mt. Winchell, and Thunderbolt Peak dominate the eastern skyline. To the south, the heavily fractured and less well-defined summits of Columbine and Giraud peaks occupy the skyline. Look for the prominent gap of Knapsack Pass, just south of Columbine Peak.

This moderate descent swings westward above the lowest lakes of Dusy Basin (10,742´), leaves the basin, and begins a series of steady switchbacks along the north side of Dusy Branch creek. Colorful wildflowers along this descent include Indian paintbrush, pennyroyal, lupine, white cinquefoil, penstemon, shooting star, and some yellow columbine. Just below a waterfall, a wooden bridge crosses to the creek's east side. Enjoying views of the U-shaped Middle Fork Kings River canyon, zigzag downhill, and, on the far side of the valley, notice the major peaks of the Black Divide, foregrounded by the Citadel and Langille Peak.

As the trail descends, the very sparse forest cover of stunted whitebark seen in most of Dusy Basin gives way to the trees of lower altitudes, including western white pine, juniper, lodgepole, aspen, and some red fir near the foot of the switchbacks. The trail recrosses Dusy Branch creek on a forested bench (actually a series of little benches; campsites), and then makes the final 1.5-mile switchbacking descent, much of it overlooking the sparkling creek as it dashes down 700 feet of near-vertical granite.

At the descent's foot, reach a signed junction with the JMT in LeConte Canyon (8650´). A few yards northwest on the JMT, there's a signed junction with a spur trail west (riverward) to a summer ranger station; you may find help here in an emergency if the ranger is in. There are campsites south of and below the granite outcrop on which the ranger station sits.

This trip turns right (north) onto the famous JMT and ascends moderately over duff through moderate-to-dense stands of lodgepole. Campsites dot the route between the ranger station junction and Big Pete Meadow.

VIEWS IN LECONTE CANYON

Langille Peak dominates the views to the left (west), and its striking white, fractured granite face is a constant reminder of the massive forces exerted by the river of ice that once filled this canyon. Abundant fields of wildflowers color the trailside, including corn lily, tiger lily, fireweed, larkspur, red heather, shooting star, monkeyflower, pennyroyal, penstemon, goldenrod, and wallflower.

As the trail approaches the south end of Little Pete Meadow, look for the occasional mountain hemlock mixed with the lodgepole. The view north at the edge of the meadow includes Mt. Powell and Mt. Thompson. There are good but heavily used campsites at Little Pete Meadow (8879´; 11S 357946 4107412; rainbow, golden, and brook).

The trail from Little Pete to Big Pete Meadow climbs moderately on rock and sand through a sparse-to-moderate forest cover of lodgepole and occasional hemlock. There are fine over-the-shoulder views of LeConte Canyon, while ahead the granite walls where the canyon veers west show glacially smoothed, unfractured faces. Look for quaking aspen as the trail climbs through Big Pete Meadow (more forest than meadow) and reaches a large area of campsites (9249´; 11S 357352 4108578).

DAY 3 (Big Pete Meadow to Wanda Lake, 8.5 miles): This is a long, strenuous day on rough trail with a 2750-foot elevation gain.

Leaving Big Pete Meadow, the trail turns westward, and there are excellent views of the darker rock of Black Giant. A few yards beyond the turn, the trail fords the stream draining the slopes of Mt. Johnson and Mt. Gilbert and passes more campsites. The path continues west on an easy-to-moderate climb through grassy extensions of Big Pete Meadow. Most of the rock underfooting encountered to this point has been of the rounded morainal variety, but as soon as the trail leaves the westernmost fringes of Big Pete Meadow, the rock exhibits sharp, fractured edges. Over this talus, the trail ascends more steeply through a partial forest cover of western white, lodgepole, whitebark pine, and some hemlock. Loose rock and sand make poor footing, while the dashing cascades of Middle Fork Kings River offer visual relief on this steep, rugged ascent.

There are excellent campsites near the lake southwest of the trail at 10,560 feet, and the route passes occasional campsites from here to the lake at about 10,884 feet (11S 354146 4109810), which is the last chance to camp before Wanda Lake.

The final ascent to Muir Pass starts with a steady climb over sand and rock through a sparse whitebark pine. That timber cover soon disappears, giving way to low-lying heather. At the talus-bound, round, unnamed lake at about 11,327 feet (11S 353042 4109671) and east of Helen Lake, cross and recross the river's trickling headwaters on rocks, often losing sight of the trail. Hikers heading west up to Muir Pass should approach this lake on the outlet stream's north side and then, just below the lake, cross the stream and trace the lake's south shore. Hikers descending from Muir Pass must trace the lake's south shore before crossing its outlet just below the lake to the outlet's north side, against the rock face on the northeast corner of the lake.

Excellent views to the southeast of the Palisades and Langille, Giraud, and Columbine peaks make breather stops welcome occasions. The trail becomes rocky and the slope more moderate as it winds up the terminal shoulder of the Black Divide to Helen Lake (11,617´). Nearing Helen's outlet stream, you may think, especially if you're descending from Muir

Pass, that the trail on the south side of the outlet stream looks as good as the one on the north side, which is the one shown on the topo. Don't take the south-side "trail," which dead-ends in snow and boulders.

Rocks in the colorful reds, yellows, blacks, and whites that characterize this metamorphic divide are on every hand. The trail rounds the loose-rocked south end of barren Helen Lake and ascends steadily over a rocky slope that is often covered with snow throughout the summer. Looking back, you can see the striking meeting of the black metamorphic rock of the Black Divide and the white granite just east of Helen Lake.

Muir Pass (11,964´; 11S 351580 4108596) is marked by a sign and a unique stone shelter, Muir Hut, erected by the Sierra Club in 1931 in memory of John Muir. Camping in the vicinity of Muir Hut, including staying inside the hut, is prohibited except in emergencies, principally because of human-waste problems in this very fragile environment, where waste products may take years to decompose. Leave nothing but your boot tracks.

VIEWS FROM MUIR PASS

From this pass, the views are magnificent. In the morning light, the somber crags to the north and south relieve the intense whites of the lighter granite to the east. Situated in a gigantic rock bowl to the west, Wanda Lake's emerald-blue waters contrast sharply with its lower white edges, which on the south side merge into the darker rock of the Goddard Divide.

The descent from the pass is moderate to gradual over fragmented rock, and then it levels out, passing the southeast end of talus-bound Lake McDermand. Skirting the east side of Wanda Lake, the trail affords excellent views of snow-and-ice-necklaced Mt. Goddard, and then arrives at the barren campsites near the lake's outlet (11,426´; 11S 349158 4110532). The expansive views from these campsites include Mt. Goddard and the Goddard Divide to the south, and Mt. Huxley, Mt. Spencer, Mt. Darwin, and Mt. Mendel to the north.

DAY 4 (Wanda Lake to Colby Meadow, 6.5 miles): As it leaves Wanda Lake behind, the descending trail soon finds occasional wildflowers, including heather, wallflower, and penstemon. Below Wanda Lake, the trail crosses Evolution Creek and stays on the west

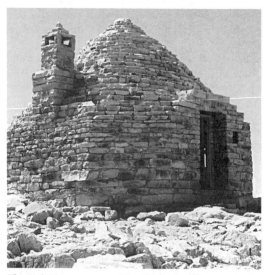

bank on a moderate descent that becomes switchbacks above Sapphire Lake. Fine views of the Sierra Crest to the east make watching your footing a difficult task. Between Wanda and Evolution lakes, there are almost no campsites. Sapphire Lake (10,966´; trout) is indeed a high-country gem, fringed with green, marshy grass, and situated on a large glacial step.

The route traverses the lake's steeper west side and, after a steady drop on good trail, refords Evolution Creek just above Evolution Lake (10,852´) on a long series of large boulders. The trail stays above Evolution's meadowed shoreline until it reaches the lake's north end, where there are a few fair-to-poor campsites. Glacial

The Muir Hut was erected by the Sierra Club in 1931.

smoothing and some polish can be seen in the granite surrounding the lake and on the abrupt walls on either side of the lake.

"EVOLUTION" RAMBLING

A layover day at Evolution Lake allows time to explore the glorious lakes on Darwin Bench or the lakes cupped beneath the peaks to the east on the Sierra Crest, which are named for 19th century naturalists instrumental in developing the theory of evolution by natural selection. At these lakes, you can swim with only deer for company.

After passing several campsites just below the lake, the trail makes a brief northward swing before switchbacking down to Evolution Valley. This northward swing passes the trail ascending to Darwin Canyon and the route to the Darwin Glacier. The zigzagging downgrade over morainal debris re-enters forest cover and passes clumps of seasonal wildflowers that include penstemon, paintbrush, swamp onion, lupine, forget-me-not, cinquefoil, buckwheat, and tiger lily. At the foot of the grade, where the trail fords the stream emptying Darwin Canyon, the route passes more campsites, and then continues down a series of small benches through moderate stands of lodgepole to the good campsites at Colby Meadow (9840´; 11S 346546 4116611; golden in nearby Evolution Creek).

Hikers with energy left may want to continue to campsites at McClure or Evolution Meadow, as described in the first part of Day 5. This would shorten the long Day 5, too.

DAY 5 (Colby Meadow to Bridge over Piute Creek, 8.7 miles): From Colby Meadow, the route continues westward, passing severely overused McClure and Evolution meadows (campsites at both). The trail joining these meadows is a pathway that winds through moderate and dense stands of lodgepole and, midway down McClure Meadow, passes a ranger station (emergency services may be available here). As the route winds past the campsites in McClure Meadow—Evolution's Valley's largest—travelers can see the toll taken by the heavy traffic, both human and stock.

Below McClure Meadow, the path makes a moderate-to-steady descent that fords several tributaries draining the Glacier Divide. The next "official" ford of Evolution Creek used to be below Evolution Meadow, but that ford has been washed out, leaving deep holes around large boulders in the creekbed. Find a safer ford by following an angler's trail from near the meadow's east end, across the meadow, and to a crossing where the stream is broad and relatively placid, though it may be knee deep. Pick up a use trail on the other side, and follow its westward curve through the meadow and then some campsites. Soon, it rejoins the main trail just west of the old ford.

Now back on the PCT/JMT, continue west to the head of the switchbacks that drop down to South Fork San Joaquin River. Views before the dropoff are excellent of the cascades of the stream draining Emerald Peak, the falls and cascades of Evolution Creek below the ford, and the South Fork San Joaquin River drainage. Midway down the switchbacks, there are impressive views of Goddard Canyon. The forest cover along the zigzags is sparse-to-moderate lodgepole, juniper, and some aspen. Mountain flowers seen along the trail include pennyroyal, larkspur, penstemon, cinquefoil, currant, monkeyflower, buckwheat, and paintbrush. At the bottom, the trail passes several good campsites as it leads through a heavy stand of lodgepoles. Just beyond these campsites, this trip crosses a footbridge and meets the Goddard Canyon/Hell-for-Sure Pass Trail branching left (south).

This trip turns right (north-northwest) to stay on the JMT, soon crossing the river again to its east bank. Continue northwest through Aspen Meadow to a fine footbridge across Piute Creek at the boundary of Kings Canyon National Park and John Muir Wilderness and at the junction of the JMT and the Piute Pass Trail (8078´; 11S 337341 4121412). Just before the footbridge and still within the park, there's a large, Jeffrey pine-shaded flat with an understory of scattered manzanita shrubs. Among these shrubs are several shady, flat spots for campsites; nearby Piute Creek's music is your lullaby.

SIDE TRIP: BLAYNEY HOT SPRINGS

About 3.8 miles northwest of this flat, along the Florence Lake Trail, is Blayney Hot Springs, more fully described in Trip 14, Day 1. To make the 7.6-mile out-and-back detour from this trip, cross Piute Creek to the PCT/JMT-Piute Creek Trail junction. Turn left (west) and follow the PCT/JMT to its junction with the Florence Lake Trail. Here, turn left (northwest) onto the Florence Lake Trail and continue to heavily used campsites near Blayney Hot Springs (7664'; 11S 332993 4122555) and Muir Trail Ranch, a wilderness resort. The resort uses the hot pools on the river's north side; the public must ford the river (possibly dangerous in early season) to a meadowed pool and a nearby cool lake on the south side, where there are more, well-used campsites. Look for well-trod use trails to help find the pool.

We recommend you visit Blayney Hot Springs from this trip on a layover day from your campsite near the Piute Creek bridge. Retrace your steps to return.

DAY 6 (Bridge over Piute Creek to Hutchinson Meadow, 4.2 miles): Turn right (north) on the rocky Piute Pass Trail as it climbs and then descends briefly to Piute Creek (possibly the last easily accessible water late in the year until West Pinnacles Creek). The trail keeps to the creek's west side and well above it as the route ascends a granite nose before fording multibranched Turret Creek.

Follow switchbacks across hot chaparral-covered slopes and then swing east through a narrowing canyon, crossing a couple of gullies on log bridges, fording tiny West Pinnacles Creek, and then entering moderate lodgepole forest cover on the way to the easy ford of East Pinnacles Creek. From the ford, the trail ascends gently to beautiful Hutchinson Meadow, with excellent campsites near the Pine Creek Pass Trail junction (9500', 11S 342140 4125968; golden and brook).

DAY 7 (Hutchinson Meadow to Humphreys Basin, 4.8 miles): *(Recap: Trip 62, Day 5.)* From the Pine Creek Pass junction, go ahead (east) through Hutchinson Meadow, fording French Canyon Creek's distributaries. (The "second junction" shown on the topo with a trail part-way up French Canyon Creek may not exist.) Climb along Piute Creek, eventually into thinning forest and large Humphreys Basin. The Piute Pass Trail continues to ascend to the cascading outlet of the Desolation Lakes; there are good campsites on the knolls around Upper Golden Trout Lake (10,790'; 11S 347743 4123129), about a half mile south, depending on the route. When searching for a campsite, seek a location well away from the Piute Pass Trail, as those close to that trail have become grotesquely overused.

Farther up the Piute Pass Trail is the unsigned but highly visible use trail that heads north to the Desolation Lakes (golden) and their windy, Spartan campsites.

DAY 8 (Humphreys Basin to North Lake Trailhead, 7 miles): *(Recap in Reverse: Trip 59, Day 1.)* Follow the main trail across the gradually rising basin and continue above Summit Lake to view-rich Piute Pass (11,423'; 11S 350613 4122714). Descending from Piute Pass, the trail passes diminutive tarns and presently reaches the northeast shore of Piute Lake (windy campsites; brook and rainbow).

Leaving Piute Lake, the path skirts some small, unnamed lakes on the way to a bench holding Loch Leven (campsite; brook and rainbow). Switchbacks drop down a headwall and around the north side of North Fork Bishop Creek to a long, descending traverse below Piute Crags and then more switchbacks to the canyon floor. Cross the creek a couple of times and continue the descent on gently graded trail to a junction near the west end of North Lake Campground. From there, go ahead (northeast), almost immediately reaching the trailhead (9344'; 11S 355642 4121338); remember, the car is another 0.7 mile down the road.

Big Pine Creek Trailhead
7710´; 11S 373187 411066

DESTINATION/ UTM COORDINATES	TRIP TYPE	BEST SEASON	PACE (HIKING/ LAYOVER DAYS)	TOTAL MILEAGE
71 Big Pine Lakes 11S 365667 4111231 (Sixth Lake)	Semiloop	Mid to late	3/2 Moderate	15.4
72 Brainerd Lake 11S 370422 4106015	Out & back	Mid to late	2/1 Moderate	8.5

Information and Permits: This trailhead is in Inyo National Forest: 351 Pacu Lane, Suite 200, Bishop, CA 93514, 760-873-2400, www.fs.fed.us/r5/inyo/. Quotas apply, and permits are required for overnight stays and are available at Inyo National Forest ranger stations in Lone Pine, Bishop, Mammoth Lakes, and Mono Basin Scenic Area Visitors Center.

Driving Directions: From Hwy. 395 in Big Pine, turn west on Crocker Street, which becomes Glacier Lodge Road. The true trailhead is at the road's end at 10 miles, but the parking there is only for day users. Overnight parking and an undesirable, secondary backpackers' trailhead are 0.7 mile back down the road. This backpackers' trailhead serves only North Fork—Big Pine Lakes and the free walk-in campground, First Falls Campground—and is not recommended: It is not only 0.7 mile east of and away from where you want to start, it also requires a long, climbing traverse on a scorching, shadeless, south-facing slope. Recommended for starting both trips: Drop your party and all your packs at the roadend, which is the true trailhead, and then elect one person to drive the car back to overnight parking and carefully walk back to the trailhead on the shady, creekside road.

71 Big Pine Lakes

Trip Data: 11S 365667 4111231 (field); 15.4 miles; 3/2 days

Topos: *Split Mountain, Coyote Flat, Mount Thompson, North Palisade*

see map on p.258

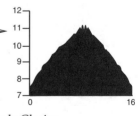

Highlights: At least 10 named, beautiful lakes (with fish!) and numerous ponds and streams await visitors to this very popular area, the watershed of North Fork Big Pine Creek, which also offers the easiest access to the Sierra's largest glacier, Palisade Glacier.

HEADS UP! *There is a free, backpack-in campground, First Falls Campground, on the way to Big Pine Lakes (North Fork Big Pine Creek) near a connector to the trail to Brainerd Lake (up South Fork Big Pine Creek). It's worth considering staying there the night before your trip.*

DAY 1 (Big Pine Creek Trailhead to the Flat between First and Second Lakes, 4.5 miles): From the true trailhead at the roadend (not the overnight parking lot), skirt a gate and walk along a creekside road past summer cabins. The road bobs up and down, crosses a wide spot, and soon reaches a second wide spot where the hiker's trail turns right (north) uphill a few paces before abruptly veering left (north-northwest) onto a footpath. This track soon makes a switchback above the cabins to a bridge over First Falls, a series of cascades on North Fork Big Pine Creek. Across the bridge, it's a short way to a junction with the trail

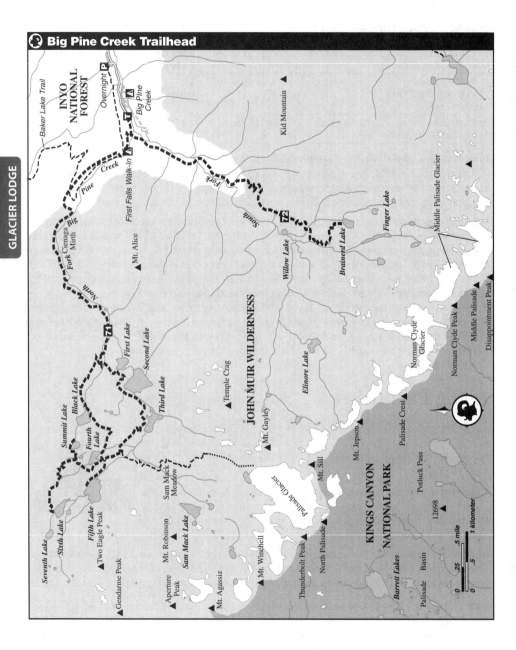

Big Pine Creek Trailhead

up South Fork Big Pine Creek (left, ahead, south). Turn hard right (north-northwest) along North Fork Big Pine Creek and begin climbing sandy, sometimes steep but often shady switchbacks along First Falls.

At the top of First Falls, the trail straightens out and meets an old road; the road system in this area was largely destroyed by floods in the 1980s and never rebuilt. Left here (south) descends to a junction with the trail up South Fork Big Pine Creek.

However, for this trip, the correct path makes a gentle right, crosses North Fork on another bridge, and comes to a confusing junction. The old road, which goes left and right here, is called Lower Trail. Going right (south) here will take you to the free, walk-in First Falls Campground. Going left (north, curving gradually west) takes you along broad Lower Trail, along North Fork, and toward Second Falls. Ahead is a short connector trail to sandy Upper Trail, a footpath that roughly parallels Lower Trail but traverses the scrubby hillside well above Lower Trail; Upper Trail has little shade but fine views, especially of Second Falls.

Hikers can take Lower Trail or Upper Trail; as it nears Second Falls, Lower Trail switchbacks up to meet Upper Trail. If you take Lower Trail, make a hard left (west-northwest) at the top of the switchbacks, onto Upper Trail and toward Second Falls; ahead, the apparent continuation of Lower Trail becomes the rough, steep trail east toward Baker Lake. If you take Upper Trail, continue ahead (west-northwest) at its junction with Lower Trail and the Baker Lake Trail, and head toward Second Falls.

From the junction where Upper and Lower trails rejoin, the open, rocky-sandy trail climbs steadily to the top of Second Falls, where it enters John Muir Wilderness, curves northwest along the rollicking creek, and then curves west toward Cienaga Mirth. In season, Cienaga Mirth is a moist, meadowy strip full of wildflowers like leopard lilies, Indian paintbrush, groundsel, rein orchids, fireweed, and monkshood. Actor Lon Chaney built the handsome stone cabin here in the 1920s, and now it's a backcountry Forest Service building. The area offers a welcome rest stop.

Beyond Cienaga Mirth, the trail repeatedly climbs above the creek, traverses spring-fed gardens, and then meets the creek again. Hikers running out of energy, daylight, or good weather can stop for the night at a couple of spots. At 11S 369164 4110364 (field), a very obvious, sandy use trail takes off left (southeast) to a forested flat near the creek (9601´). Farther on, at 11S 368786 4110153 (field) and 9769´, look for an orange-painted, metal, California Snow Survey sign nailed to a tree across the creek; from here, a steep, rocky use trail leads about 20 feet down to the creek, which the use trail crosses on a bridge of cabled-together logs. The forested campsite across the creek is probably too near the water, but a use trail from the back of the campsite leads out to a sandy flat.

Continuing, the main trail climbs through more meadows, crosses the north fork of the North Fork once, switchbacks up again, and, just before it crosses the outlet of Black Lake, reaches a junction with the trail to Black Lake, where the loop part of this trip begins (9969´; 11S 368158 4110275 (field)) at 4.2 miles. Black Lake is many hot, dusty, rocky switchbacks above if you make a hard right turn (northeast) here. Ahead (southwest), the trail crosses Black Lake's outlet and makes a switchback as it climbs to First Lake, which is much closer than Black Lake.

Go ahead, make the switchback, and then follow the trail as it straightens out in forest and at about 4.4 miles passes a draw with a hard-to-spot use trail down to First Lake (10,067´; 11S 368027 4110141 (field)) and a campsite on a flat near the lake. The lake itself is hard to see from the main trail. All these lakes have brook trout; there may also be rainbow and brown. As the path continues to a viewpoint, the sight of First Lake is apt to take your breath away: First, Second, and Third lakes are a beautiful, milky, turquoise-green from the "glacial flour" (extremely fine, glacier-ground particles of granite) in their waters.

At just under 4.5 miles, the main trail meets a spur trail (10,076´; 11S 367977 4109938 (field)) leading left (south) to a forested flat and a very large camping area near the stream

GLACIER LODGE

between First and Second lakes. While not very scenic, this roomy flat makes a good base for exploring those lakes.

DAY 2 (Flat between First and Second Lakes to Sixth Lake, 3.5 miles): On this day, you'll find plenty of camping options along the way. You may wind up at Third, Fourth, Fifth, Sixth, or Summit Lake, or somewhere in between! Arbitrarily, we've picked Sixth Lake for its remoteness; a base at Fourth or Fifth Lake is probably best for exploring the rest of the basin.

Return to the main trail and go left (south-southwest) to continue around Second Lake to Third Lake. The trail remains high above the water as it curves around Second Lake; only a few tiny campsites cling to the steep slopes that lead down to the water.

As the path leaves Second Lake behind, hikers can hear the roar of Third Lake's outlet making its final fall into Second Lake. Between Second and Third lakes, the trail winds between that connecting creek on the trail's downhill side (campsites) and imposing granite faces on its uphill side, from which springs emerge and nurture flower gardens. At one point, the trail travels high above the creek on a rock "causeway."

The nearer (east) end of Third Lake has a broad, stubby peninsula with two knolls (roughly 11S 367331 4109462; 10,271´) at about 5.2 miles, and, in this area, there are a number of scenic, very overused, and extremely popular campsites. Third Lake has the best view of Temple Crag, the fascinating, formidable, convoluted peak across the water. At least 20 named climbing routes exist on Temple Crag (see Steve Roper's *Climbers' Guide to the High Sierra*, from Sierra Club Books).

Beyond Third Lake's peninsula, the trail climbs toward Fourth Lake on long switchbacks, and the number of campsites on the slopes above Third Lake dwindles quickly as the vertical distance from water rapidly increases. As the switchbacks end, the trail parallels a lovely meadow with, alas, few if any campsites; however, where a bridge crosses Fourth Lake's outlet, there's a campsite on the low knoll just beyond. At the next junction, with the trail left (west) toward Palisade Glacier (signed GLACIER TRAIL; 10,641´; 11S 366642 4109957 (field)), a use trail about 50 yards down that trail leads left (southeast) to a campsite. (The Glacier Trail peters out long before it reaches the glacier, leaving you to work your way across talus and possibly snowfields, but the sight is worth the trouble.)

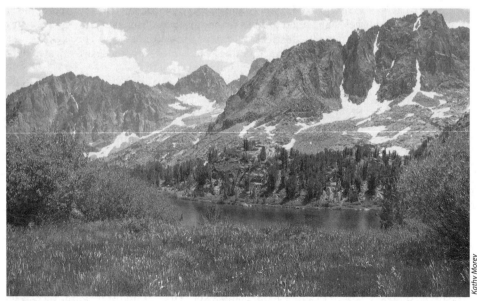

Kathy Morey

Sixth Lake

Today's route continues on the main trail, which presently reaches a junction (10,769´; 11S 366512 4110257 (field)) about a mile from Third Lake's peninsula, where it's left (southwest) for 0.4 mile on a spur trail to Fifth Lake, straight ahead (north) for 0.1 mile to visible Fourth Lake and beyond it to Sixth and Seventh lakes, and right (northeast) for 0.8 mile to Black Lake. For peace and quiet, we recommend Sixth Lake, but here's an overview of the many options at this junction:

Fifth Lake: Below Mt. Robinson and Two Eagle Peak, this lake has perhaps the loveliest setting but relatively poor camping. A cluster of beat-out sites at its outlet, crowded between the trail and the stream, are surely illegal now. The spur trail leads high above the lake to a saddle where a use trail takes off to Fourth Lake, and there are campsites on this saddle.

Fourth Lake: There are a few campsites off the trail that curves around Fourth Lake's west and north sides; its long, slender peninsula, however, is too narrow to permit legal camping. The use trail from the saddle above Fifth Lake meets the trail around Fourth Lake in a meadowy draw a little past a fine Fourth Lake camping area (below the trail). Just before the trail crosses Fourth Lake's major inlet, a use trail leads left and upstream (generally north) along the base of a low ridge on which there may be campsites. Across the inlet, the trail quickly climbs to a large, well-used camping area on the right (south) that was once the site of a walk-in lodge built in the 1920s and demolished after the area became part of John Muir Wilderness.

Sixth Lake: Continue on the trail around Fourth Lake from the camping area that was once the walk-in lodge. The path continues climbing above Fourth Lake and the little pond north of it. Soon, the track reaches an unsigned junction (10,888´; 11S 366496 4110773 (field)) with the trail left (north-northeast) to Sixth Lake, perhaps the most remote and therefore peaceful lake in this busy area, and also to Seventh Lake (closed to camping). Ahead (northeast), the trail leads to Summit Lake.

Summit Lake: This 0.4-mile, one-way trip leaves from the junction above Fourth Lake. Go ahead on the rocky-sandy path, passing a little spring-fed garden and topping a ridge among stunted trees and high above Summit. The trail plunges east toward Summit and then curves around it, passing an obvious campsite and a use trail to the lakeshore. Abruptly, the track grows very faint and rocky as it wanders up the northeast side of this rocky bowl to a ridgetop overlooking Black Lake, 330 feet below. There is no trail between Black and Summit lakes; hikers at home on Class 2 terrain may wish to hike cross-country between them. Or retrace your steps to Fourth Lake.

To continue to Sixth Lake from here, walk to the unsigned junction with the trail to Sixth and Seventh lakes. Turn north-northeast (left if you are coming from Fourth, right if you are returning from Summit Lake) and switchback up to a beautiful little meadow with an idyllic pond and stream (the inlet to the pond north of Fourth Lake). The meadow is cupped by low ridges, on which you may find campsites quieter than those at Fourth Lake. The path traces the meadow's west side and, at its end, climbs switchbacks over the ridge west of this first meadow. Next, the path descends the ridge's west side to a smaller second meadow, crosses the meadow and a tributary to Fourth Lake's inlet, and ascends this second meadow's west side. At the upper end of the meadow, the stony trail climbs to and crosses a rocky saddle, dips generally west through a sandy-grassy bowl, and climbs out, finally reaching its high point above Sixth Lake (11,264´). There are brief views of Sixth and Seventh lakes and stunning views of the peaks around them. Then the track pitches down on rocky-dusty, moderate-to-steep switchbacks to Sixth Lake, ending abruptly near the lake's northeast end (11,164´; 11S 365667 4111231 (field)). Note this point for your return so that you can find the trail.

From here, use trails lead to campsites under clusters of whitebark pines; at this point, the sites are fairly high above the lake. Reportedly, sites are better nearer the outlet (left, southeast). Use trails also lead from here to Seventh Lake (right, northwest; no camping).

DAY 3 (Sixth Lake to Big Pine Creek Trailhead, 7.4 miles): Return to the junction between the trails from Third, Fourth, Fifth, and Black lakes, and resume the loop part of this trip by going northeast toward Black Lake—right if you have just come from Third Lake; left if you're returning from Fourth Lake (or Sixth Lake via Fourth Lake); or ahead if you're coming back from Fifth Lake. The trail crosses Fourth Lake's outlet before ascending a low ridge and then making a short descent to Black Lake's south shore 0.8 mile from the previous junction. Black Lake offers a few campsites.

Continuing downward, the path crosses a trickle and soon leaves forest for a scrubby slope high above North Fork Big Pine Creek. Black Lake's outlet runs under the rocks where the trail goes through a rockfall, and then the trail briefly follows the outlet. Soon the track drops down the exposed slope on rocky-dusty, moderate-to-steep switchbacks that nevertheless boast some fine wildflowers (in season), spectacular views, and occasional shade from tall mountain-mahogany shrubs.

In a long-seeming 0.9 mile, the trail reaches the junction where hikers originally turned toward First Lake and crossed Black Lake's outlet. End the loop part of this trip by retracing your steps to the trailhead.

Or, if you wish to take the more gradual trail back to the overnighters' parking lot, retrace your steps, staying on Upper Trail, to the junction with the unsigned connector leading down to Lower Trail. Don't go to Lower Trail. Instead, continue ahead (southeast and then east), climbing a little above the walk-in campground before beginning your long but usually gentle, sandy, sun-struck descent past two turnoffs downhill to the pack station and—finally!—to the parking lot.

72 Brainerd Lake

Trip Data: 11S 370422 4106015 (field); 8.5 miles; 2/1 days

Topos: *Split Mountain*

Highlights: A very demanding climb on trail that's sometimes hard to follow leads to a beautiful high lake with fine Class 2 to 3 cross-country rambling around the watershed of South Fork Big Pine Creek. You may have Brainerd Lake all to yourself!

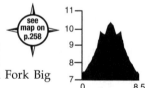

HEADS UP! This trip is not recommended for beginners and large parties. Do not take the trail from the backpackers' parking lot; it goes far out of your way, unless you want to spend the night at First Falls Campground. Brainerd Lake has few (all but one very small) campsites.

DAY 1 (Big Pine Creek Trailhead to Brainerd Lake, 4.25 miles): From the true trailhead at the road's end, skirt a gate and walk along a creekside road past summer cabins. The road bobs up and down, crosses a wide spot, and soon reaches a second wide spot where the hiker's trail turns right (north) uphill a few paces before abruptly veering left (north-northwest) onto a footpath. This track soon makes a switchback above the cabins to a bridge over First Falls on North Fork Big Pine Creek. Across the bridge, it's a short way to a junction with the trail up South Fork Big Pine Creek (left, ahead, south).

Turn left toward South Fork, visible in the valley below, and begin traversing the base of Mt. Alice above the creek, with little shade but fine views up the creek. Wildflowers along this leg are seasonally splendid and include a pink Indian paintbrush, yellow (aging to brick red) sulfur blossom, creambush, western thoroughwort, currant, red penstemon, and bitter cherry; fragrant sagebrush is abundant, too. The rocky-sandy trail climbs gradually toward distant peaks.

At a flat spot, the trail meets the old road coming down from North Fork Big Pine Creek (right, north). The trail up South Fork continues southward from the south side of the road, still climbing gradually.

Presently, the trail switchbacks through boulders and then curves southwest before passing between clumps of willow and cottonwood to cross a seasonal trickle. At this point, the main creek is only a few yards downhill to the left for a while, and rough use trails lead to it. Ahead, outliers of Kid Mountain rise to the south. Farther on, the trail passes some shady rest spots under mountain mahoganies.

The path's grade increases a little as it passes cottonwoods and splashes through a tributary before winding up, steeply at times, through the next boulder field. After leveling and passing a use trail left to the creek, the main trail almost immediately crosses the creek on a wide, flattened-log bridge. Top up on water here; many dry switchbacks lie ahead.

The track is still level for a while as it curves south again, away from the creek, and across the head of the valley, down whose west side the South Fork plunges in showy cascades. About halfway across the valley, the trail climbs stony switchbacks to a low bench, enters John Muir Wilderness, and soon begins a series of long, moderate-to-steep switchbacks up the valley's head. The rough, rocky route yields spectacular views north down the valley.

The grade eases and the tread improves as the trail ascends through occasional patches of water birch and alder that offer bits of shade, while wildflowers like columbine and larkspur brighten the way. Soon, the path enters a zone of scattered western white pines and passes a NO FIRES sign on one of them. Subsequent switchbacks grow steeper and rougher, and here, almost at the headwall, snow may linger and force tricky detours on the steep, loose slope.

Now the route crosses a tiny hillside meadow and then resumes ascending very steeply, at first over rocks. Soon, the trail's surface gets better, but it continues winding up steeply and tightly next to a deep vertical notch in the headwall.

Among rounded outcrops and whitebark pines, the trail at last straightens out and the grade temporarily eases. Far ahead there are breathtaking views of the Palisade Crest and its glaciers. Soon, the path crests and begins descending through narrow, lodgepole-fringed meadows, crossing four streams (some seasonal) on its way down to a signed junction with the use trail heading west and down to Willow Lake. The meadows and trees offer no decent campsites, but tired hikers will find fair-to-poor sites in the vicinity of buggy Willow Lake. The use trail to that lake begins as a well-beaten track but soon becomes very hard to follow; ducks may help.

From the junction with the use trail to Willow Lake (9704´; 11S 370524 4106740 (field)), go south toward Brainerd Lake (ahead on the main trail, right if coming from Willow

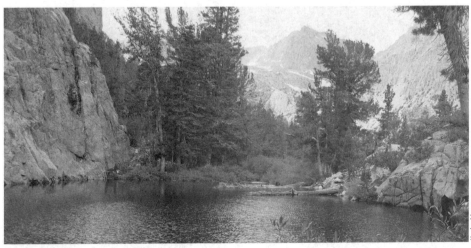

Idyllic tarn on the way to Brainerd Lake

GLACIER LODGE

Kathy Morey

Lake). Climb steeply before descending slightly to ford Brainerd's outlet (difficult in early season) in a meadow. Leave the meadow behind and begin climbing steeply again, occasionally leveling out at points where bivouacs may be possible. Ford a small stream and climb moderately to yet another easy ford, and then climb moderately to very steeply through forest with dense undergrowth.

The rocky trail winds up, up, up, first within sound and then within sight of Finger Lake's noisy outlet far below. Turning away from the outlet, the path climbs to a handsome, year-round pond, hooks left (east) to follow ducks over an outcrop bordering the pond, and returns to the pond. A bivouac may be possible around this pond.

Now the trail descends to squish across a lush meadow and its streams. On the meadow's other side, the climb resumes, sometimes faint and sometimes steep. Ducks may help here, too. Passing a seasonal pond, the route climbs a granite outcrop on the pond's other side, passes through a notch in the outcrop, and, curving right (south) leads shortly to the shore of Brainerd Lake.

First-time visitors may be puzzled by the lack of campsites at this point. The best bet is to turn right (west) on a use trail, pass through a small flat area too close to water for camping, and reach the foot of a tall outcrop. Climb this first outcrop on one of its use trails and descend into a little gully between that first outcrop and a second outcrop to the west. Ascend this second outcrop to the best campsite around Brainerd Lake, under a large lodgepole (10,289′; 11S 370422 4106015 (field)). There are three tent sites here; water is a scramble away down the gully between the first and second outcrops. (There are smaller campsites on other outcrops around the lake, including the first one you climbed.)

The views here include Peak 3994T and Kid Mountain on the east; on the west are peaks 3401T and 3862T. Lovely Brainerd Lake is largely hemmed in by cliffs; cross-country scrambling to the higher lakes, such as Finger Lake, is rewarding.

DAY 2 (Brainerd Lake to Big Pine Creek Trailhead, 4.25 miles): Retrace your steps to the trailhead.

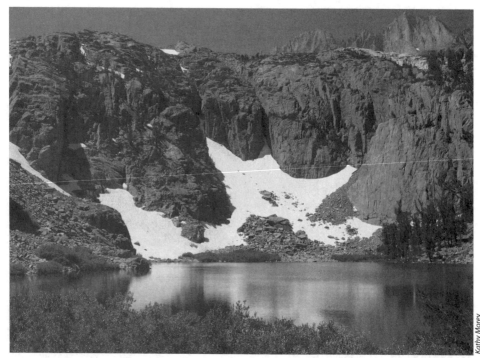

Brainerd Lake

Kathy Morey

Sawmill Pass Trailhead

4700´; 11S 385170 4088862

DESTINATION/ UTM COORDINATES	TRIP TYPE	BEST SEASON	PACE (HIKING/ LAYOVER DAYS)	TOTAL MILEAGE
73 Sawmill Lake 11S 379909 4083246	Out & back	Early	2/0 Strenuous	16
74 Bench Lake 11S 369475 4090412	Out & back	Mid to late	6/1 Strenuous	46

Information and Permits: This trailhead is in Inyo National Forest: 351 Pacu Lane, Suite 200, Bishop, CA 93514, 760-873-2400, www.fs.fed.us/r5/inyo/. Quotas apply, and permits are required for overnight stays and are available at Inyo National Forest ranger stations in Lone Pine, Bishop, Mammoth Lakes, and Mono Basin Scenic Area Visitors Center.

Driving Directions: From the town of Big Pine, take Hwy. 395 south 17.5 miles and turn right (west) on a dirt road signed BLACK ROCK SPRING ROAD. Go 0.8 mile to a junction and turn right (north) to follow old Hwy. 395 1.2 miles to Division Creek Road, leading west. Turn left and follow this road 2.1 miles to the Sawmill Pass Trailhead.

73 Sawmill Lake

Trip Data: 11S 379909 4083246; 16 miles; 2/0 days

Topos: *Aberdeen*

Highlights: This extremely strenuous trip climbs steeply from the sweltering Owens Valley at 4700 feet to a refreshing, beautiful alpine lake at 10,000 feet. After the long, steep, exposed climb, you'll arrive weary but with a mountaineer's "high" from the hard work. Expect solitude here: Few dare tackle this grueling climb.

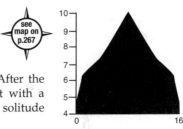

HEADS UP! *Only strong hikers in top condition should undertake this long, hot slog.*

DAY 1 (Sawmill Pass Trailhead to Sawmill Lake, 8 miles): The route leaves the trailhead, heading south, and climbs a hot, dry, sage-covered slope. In early season, this dry slope is dotted with flowering shrubs and blossoms of bright blue woolly gilia and yellow and white buckwheat. As the trail gains elevation, views of the Big Pine volcanic field appear to the north. The lava field is spotted with reddish cinder cones and black lava flows that erupted from the west side of Owens Valley.

Once the path climbs out of the sage, a line of trees appears on a crest. Upon gaining this crest, the trail suddenly enters completely different terrain. Molded rocks appear to rise, and Sawmill Canyon opens to the southwest. The waters of Sawmill Creek appear as a white ribbon 1000 feet below. The path descends slightly, then contours, and finally climbs along the precipitous north wall of Sawmill Creek's canyon.

As the path nears the sloping ridge called the Hogsback, Jeffrey pines, oaks, and white firs make a most welcome appearance. A careful look at the lower end of the Hogsback may reveal the remains of the Blackrock sawmill and flume (dating from the 1860s), after which Sawmill Creek and Sawmill Pass are named. For some distance above the

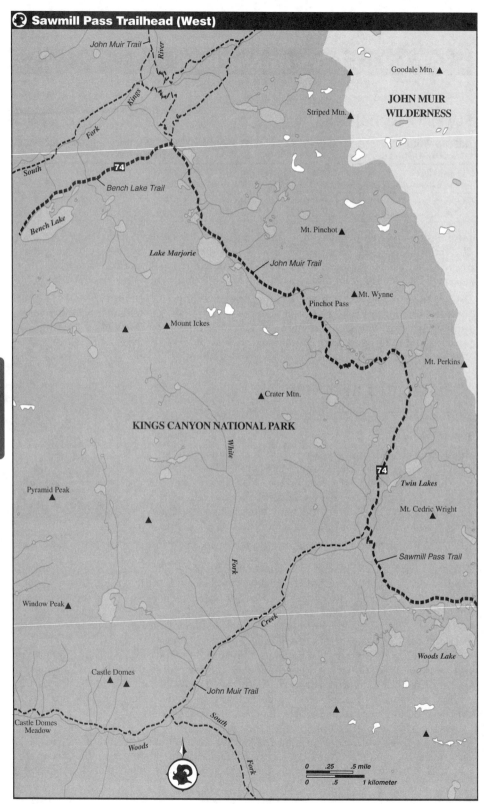

John Muir Trail

Kings Fork River

South Fork

74

Bench Lake Trail

Bench Lake

Lake Marjorie

John Muir Trail

Goodale Mtn. ▲

JOHN MUIR
WILDERNESS

Striped Mtn. ▲

Mt. Pinchot ▲

▲ Mt. Wynne

Pinchot Pass

Mt. Perkins ▲

▲ Mount Ickes

▲ Crater Mtn.

KINGS CANYON NATIONAL PARK

White Fork

74

Twin Lakes

Mt. Cedric Wright ▲

Sawmill Pass Trail

Pyramid Peak ▲

▲

Window Peak ▲

Creek

Woods Lake

Castle Domes ▲ ▲

John Muir Trail

Castle Domes
Meadow

Woods

South Fork

▲

▲

0   .25   .5 mile
0   .5   1 kilometer

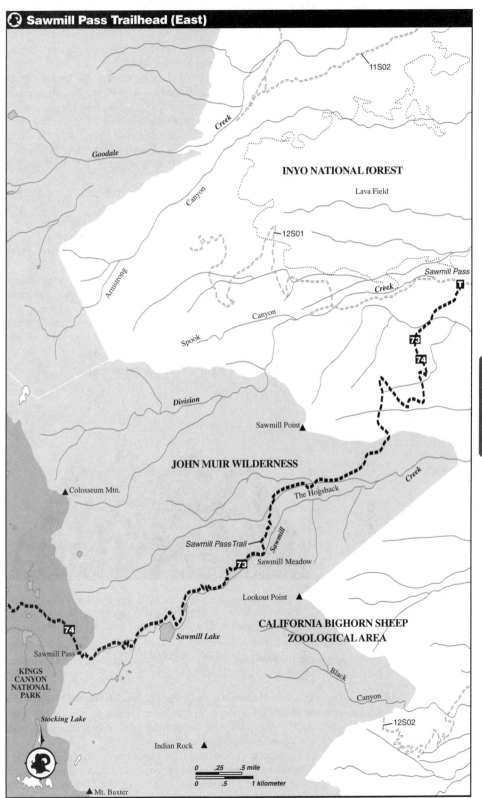

SAWMILL CR

Hogsback, you can occasionally see stumps, felled trees, and logs used as "gliders" in this long-gone operation to supply Owens Valley miners with lumber.

The trail climbs to meet a tributary stream north of the Hogsback—the first water to appear on this hot climb (7300´; 11S 382596 4085562). There's a flat next to the stream that provides a fine rest stop but is illegal for camping. The path fords this creek three times as it heads east before ascending to a long, rounded ridge. About a mile after the water stop, the track veers south, contouring and climbing on a moderate grade back into the main canyon. It passes a pine-shaded bench just below Sawmill Meadow that offers fair campsites with water from the creek being a steep 50 to 60 feet below (8415´; 11S 381467 4084390).

Sawmill Meadow itself is boggy and lush green in early season but dries considerably as the months progress; there are a few poor campsites on the north side of the trail through this meadow. Beyond, the track follows the creek southwest before zigzagging steeply up and west through Jeffrey pine and red fir. The trail briefly brushes the creek and then passes a sandy, Jeffrey-shaded flat (9400´; 11S 380556 4083730), where there are a few poor campsites (get water back down the trail at the creek).

The remaining climb to Sawmill Lake is steep, except where it skirts campsite-less Mule Lake, precariously perched on a small bench high up the canyon. Then the path climbs through a jumbled mass of metamorphic rocks, home to a large colony of grass-harvesting conies. After crossing a creek, the trail finally arrives at the northeast shore of beautiful Sawmill Lake. There are a couple of good campsites under clumps of foxtail pine here, and fishing for rainbow trout is fair to good (10,023´; 11S 379909 4083246).

DAY 2 (Sawmill Lake to Sawmill Pass Trailhead, 8 miles): Retrace your steps.

74 Bench Lake

Trip Data: 11S 369475 4090412; 46 miles; 6/1 days

see map on p.267

Topos: *Aberdeen, Mt. Pinchot, Fish Springs*

Highlights: The price of admission to the incredible scenery beyond Sawmill Lake is the

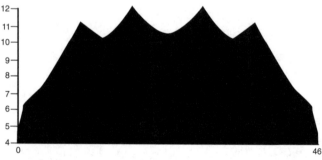

extremely strenuous climb to that lake on Day 1. Once that price has been paid, however, the next few days traverse highly varied and endlessly beautiful terrain, with expansive views into vast cirques and majestic peaks.

HEADS UP! *Only strong hikers in top condition should undertake this long, hot slog. Bears are serious problems on the west side of Sawmill Pass.*

DAY 1 (Sawmill Pass Trailhead to Sawmill Lake, 8 miles): *(Recap: Trip 73, Day 1.)* Head south to climb a hot, dry, sage-covered slope. Once the path climbs out of the sage, a line of trees appears on a crest. After gaining the crest, the path descends slightly, contours, and finally climbs the precipitous north wall of Sawmill Creek's canyon.

The trail climbs north of the Hogsback to meet the first water on this hot climb (7300´; 11S 382596 4085562). There's a flat next to the stream that provides a fine lunch stop but is illegal for camping. The path fords this creek three times as it heads east before traversing a long, rounded ridge. About a mile after the water stop, the trail veers south, contouring and climbing on a moderate grade back into the main canyon before passing a pine-shaded bench just below Sawmill Meadow. Beyond, the track follows the creek southwest and then zigzags steeply up to the west.

The remaining climb to Sawmill Lake is steep, except where it skirts campsite-less Mule Lake. After crossing a creek, the trail finally arrives Sawmill Lake (10,023´; 11S 379909 4083246).

DAY 2 (Sawmill Lake to Twin Lakes, 6 miles): The trail leaves Sawmill Lake heading southwest and winds gently up through a thinning forest of foxtail and whitebark pine. The path passes a lakelet, crosses a small treeline basin, and then climbs steeply up switchbacks to reach Sawmill Pass (11,347´; 11S 378430 4082746), on the border of Kings Canyon National Park.

From the pass, the trail heads northwest across nearly level talus and sand, and then drops into the lake-dotted headwaters of Woods Creek. Unfortunately, the basin's steep, convoluted topography and its lakes' marshy shorelines mean that it has very few pleasant, legal campsites. The path becomes quite faint at times as it winds westward through the meadows (you may have to rely on bootprints, hoofprints, or dung for clues). In general, the track heads west and descends, passing just north of several small, nameless lakes. The largest body of water in the basin, Woods Lake, is a short cross-country jaunt south of the trail, and there are a couple of fair-to-good campsites on the knolls above it to the northwest (10,722´; 11S 376450 4083198).

The faint trail continues to descend until it reaches the lower end of the basin and turns abruptly north to climb and contour along the lower slopes of Mt. Cedric Wright. Spectacular views unfold southward down Woods Creek's canyon. Here, very rough trail alternates with sections showing recent trailwork.

Finally, the route drops to North Fork Woods Creek, crosses a bench with one or two exposed campsites, fords the multistranded outlet of Twin Lakes, meets the JMT 100 feet west of the creek at an unsigned junction (10,369´), and joins the JMT by turning right (north). The trail then veers away from the creek into an avalanche area. A short half mile up, the forest clears and a use trail veers right (northeast) toward the as-yet-unseen Twin Lakes. Follow this faint trail to the good campsites on the west shore of Lower Twin Lake (10,565´; 11S 375651 4085742; serious bear problems).

DAY 3 (Twin Lakes to Bench Lake, 9 miles): Return to the JMT and turn right (north) on it. In about a mile, the trail angles west, now heading directly toward Pinchot Pass. It leaves expansive meadows to switchback up over granite to the pass (12,110´; 11S 374213 4088757), where Mt. Wynne nudges your elbow on the east. Mt. Pinchot itself is north of Mt. Wynne, and, to the northeast, a valley of lakes shimmers below.

The JMT turns northwest and follows switchbacks downhill to cross an icy rivulet. It continues descending over granite benches and boulder fields toward magnificent but almost campsite-less Lake Marjorie, passing two stark lakelets. The path enters a stand of stunted whitebark before passing along the verdant east shore of that lake. This setting is as richly colorful as any in the Sierra: To the left, ramparts of steel-gray granite rise abruptly from the lake; south, above the lake's head, are slopes of black and ruddy brown; just visible on the southeast skyline is the dark notch of Pinchot Pass. There is an exposed campsite near Lake Marjorie's outflow, below the trail, and another in the rocks above the trail (11,150´; 11S 372473 4089928).

The trail continues to descend lazily, passing several smaller lakes with idyllic camping at each. Whitebarks soon give way to clumps of lodgepole pine as the track winds through rocky meadows. Past a large lake below the trail's east side, you may see a large tent: A ranger often camps there at intervals during the summer months. Shortly beyond this lake, the trail comes to a faint, unsigned junction (10,800´; 11S 371932 4091481) some

20 yards before the JMT fords the stream connecting the lakes. A good path to Bench Lake turns left (west-southwest) from the junction, and the lake grows more visible as the trail heads through a meadow.

The trail is easy as it traverses a flowery meadow west, descends a short distance, and then contours southwest along a granite bench under a canopy of lodgepole pines. After fording a shallow stream, the track passes two small tarns, and in 1.5 miles from the JMT, it reaches the northeast shore of Bench Lake. For its absolutely clear waters and splendid setting amid granite peaks and spurs, this sparkling jewel has few peers in the High Sierra. Fine campsites abound among the lodgepoles lining the north shore (10,550′; 11S 369475 4090412). This is an idyllic spot for a well-earned layover day.

DAYS 4–6 (Bench Lake to Sawmill Pass Trailhead, 23 miles): Retrace your steps.

Kearsarge Pass Trailhead
9139´; 11S 380345 4070458

DESTINATION/ UTM COORDINATES	TRIP TYPE	BEST SEASON	PACE (HIKING/ LAYOVER DAYS)	TOTAL MILEAGE
75 Flower Lake 11S 378624 4070102	Out & back	Early to mid	2/0 Leisurely	5
76 Rae Lakes 11S 375226 4074684	Out & back	Mid to late	6/0 Leisurely	27
77 Sixty Lake Basin 11S 373184 4075273	Out & back	Mid to late	6/1 Leisurely	33

Information and Permits: This trailhead is in Inyo National Forest: 351 Pacu Lane, Suite 200, Bishop, CA 93514, 760-873-2400, www.fs.fed.us/r5/inyo/. Quotas apply, and permits are required for overnight stays and are available at Inyo National Forest ranger stations in Lone Pine, Bishop, Mammoth Lakes, and Mono Basin Scenic Area Visitors Center.

Driving Directions: From Hwy. 395 in Independence, turn west on Market Street, which becomes Onion Valley Road. Follow this road to its end in Onion Valley. There are toilets, a campground, and three trailheads here. The Kearsarge Pass Trail, which you want for these trips, is the middle one, to the west past the toilets and the campground entrance.

75 Flower Lake

Trip Data: 11S 378624 4070102; 5 miles; 2/0 days

Topos: *Kearsarge Peak*

Highlights: A short hike over well-graded trail and a 1300-foot elevation gain (the equivalent of 130 flights of stairs) bring you to the justly popular lakes that compose the headwaters of Independence Creek. The angling is good and the scenery grand. This trip also makes an excellent dayhike.

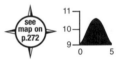

see map on p.272

ONION VALLEY

DAY 1 (Kearsarge Pass Trailhead to Flower Lake, 2.5 miles): From the trailhead, a few steps north and west of the campground, ascend the dry, manzanita-covered switchbacks of the Kearsarge Pass Trail, enjoying the views and the flowers as you head west along Independence Creek.

FOXTAIL PINES
    About a third of a mile up the trail to Flower Lake, notice the distinctive shapes of the large foxtail pines nearby. Found only at high altitudes in the mountains of California, foxtail pines have distinctive dark purple cones that take two years to mature. The densely needled (in clusters of five) branches look like tails and look inviting to touch—but you'll probably get sticky fingers if you do.

The trail enters John Muir Wilderness, and, after a mile, it comes close enough to tumbling Independence Creek that only a few steps are needed to reach the wildflower-lined stream bank. The path crosses many runoff rills in early and mid-season. At the top of this gentle grade is Little Pothole Lake, with a beautiful pair of cascades dashing into it.

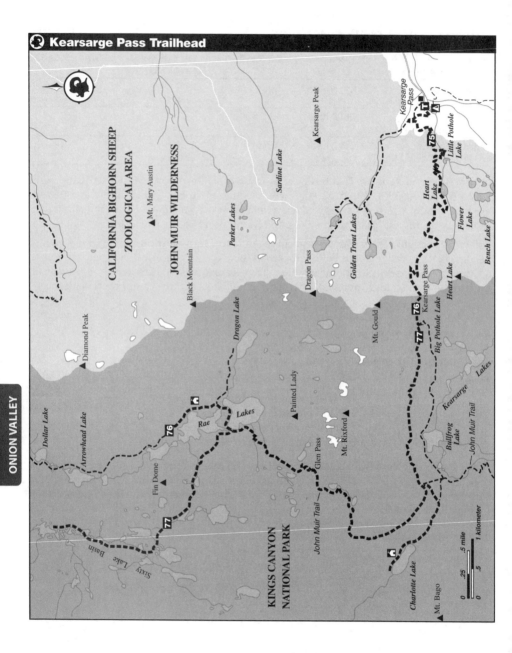

ONION VALLEY

Kearsarge Pass Trailhead

After another set of rocky switchbacks, the trail levels off in a slightly ascending groove across a glacial moraine and then reaches small, round Gilbert Lake (10,417′). Campsites that are poor from overuse dot the shores of this fine swimming lake, and fishing for rainbow and brook trout is good in early season. This small lake absorbs much of the dayhiking impact from people camping at Onion Valley, as does Flower Lake, which you reach at the top of the next set of switchbacks (10,531′; 11S 378624 4070102). There are many highly used campsites along the north and east sides of this shallow lake.

CAMPING FARTHER AFIELD

Slightly less visited and more scenic are nearby Matlock and Bench lakes. Reach Matlock by a fairly obvious trail that leads south from the east side of Flower Lake and goes over the ridge south of Flower. From there, it's a cross-country route west to Bench Lake. Fishing for rainbow and some brook trout is fair in Flower Lake, but serious anglers will hike to the more distant lakes in the timbered cirque basin to the south.

DAY 2 (Flower Lake to Kearsarge Pass Trailhead, 2.5 miles): Retrace your steps.

76 Rae Lakes

Trip Data: 11S 375226 4074684; 27 miles; 6/0 days

see map on p.272

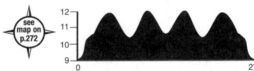

Topos: *Kearsarge Peak, Mt. Clarence King*

Highlights: This trip ascends to the alpine "moonscape" of rugged Kearsarge Pass, descends to the forested shores of bright blue Charlotte Lake, and then joins the PCT/JMT to climb over Glen Pass and visit the rightfully famous—and consequently well-visited—Rae Lakes. It's an exciting mix of grand and varied scenery and good angling.

HEADS UP! Due to heavy use, camping at Charlotte Lake, Arrowhead Lake, Dollar Lake, and at the end of the Rae Lakes is restricted to a maximum of two nights. In Paradise Valley, camping is limited to designated sites at three camps (two-night limit). Crafty bears have made the use of bear canisters mandatory. Along the Rae Lakes, the permanent metal food-storage boxes are for use by through-hikers on the PCT or JMT only. Campfires are not permitted above 10,000 feet.

DAY 1 (Kearsarge Pass Trailhead to Flower Lake, 2.5 miles): *(Recap: Trip 75, Day 1.)* From the trailhead, a few steps north and west of the campground, ascend the dry, manzanita-covered switchbacks of the Kearsarge Pass Trail, enjoying the views and the flowers as you head generally west along Independence Creek. As the trail levels off, pass Gilbert Lake. After a few more switchbacks, reach Flower Lake (10,531′; 378624 4070102). Many heavily used campsites line the shore; for a little more peace and different scenery, try Matlock and Bench lakes in a sub-basin to the south, accessed by a trail with which there's a junction on the east shore of Flower Lake. Sturdy hikers may want to continue as described in Day 2.

DAY 2 (Flower Lake to Charlotte Lake, 5.5 miles): From Flower Lake, the Kearsarge Pass Trail turns north and ascends steeply to a viewpoint above Heart Lake. Now the trail switchbacks up to another overlook, this time above the nearly perfect blue oval of Big Pothole Lake. Continuing, the trail rises above treeline, except for a few hardy whitebark specimens, and then makes two long-legged traverses across an exposed shaley slope to the low saddle of Kearsarge Pass (11,823′; 11S 377167 4070609). To the west, the impressive view encompasses the Kearsarge Lakes, Bullfrog Lake, and the serrated spires of the Kearsarge Pinnacles.

ONION VALLEY

On the west side of the pass, your route descends very steeply at first, then more gently, on a traverse high above the basin holding the Kearsarge and Bullfrog lakes. After passing a spur trail branching left (south) to the Kearsarge Lakes and Bullfrog Lake, the route continues westward on a gentle descent into sparse timber. On this view-rich slope you reach a fork (10,860´; 11S 373987 4070617) whose branches both go to the JMT. You take the left fork southwest. The route descends gently onto a sandy flat in a broad saddle overlooking Charlotte Lake, where you meet another trail junction (10,750´; 11S 373702 4070326): left (southeast) to stay on the JMT; right (west) to Charlotte Lake (10,400´; 11S 372843 4070985). Take the right turn to Charlotte, where there is a ranger station and good (though heavily used) camping on the lake's north side.

DAY 3 (Charlotte Lake to Rae Lakes, 5.5 miles): Retrace your steps to the junction with the JMT and turn left (north) to begin your climb over Glen Pass. The trail makes a long, steady, rocky ascent that rounds a granite promontory with fine views of Charlotte Lake, Charlotte Creek's canyon, Charlotte Dome, and Mt. Brewer. The track descends slightly and veers east. As the headwall of Glen Pass comes into view, it is hard to see where a passable trail could go up it. And, indeed, the last 500 feet up to the top are steeply switchbacking. At the knife's-edge pass (11,978´; 11S 374208 4072466), look down on the unnamed glacial lakes immediately north, and to several of the Rae Lakes below, after taking in the awesome views of the high peaks to the south and southwest.

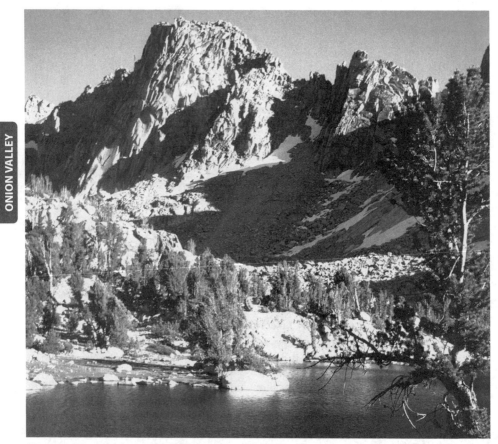

Kearsarge Pinnacles over one of the Kearsarge Lakes, just a short trip from Day 2's route

The descent from the pass is all zigzagging, rocky switchbacks to the granite bench holding the unnamed lakes seen from the pass. Loose footing here requires care, and the upper part of this side of the pass may be snow covered until late season. After crossing the outlet stream of the lakes on the bench, the trail resumes its switchbacking descent, re-enters a sparse pine forest cover, and skirts the west shore of Upper Rae Lake. Just before the trail crosses the narrow "isthmus" separating the upper lake from the rest of the chain, bypass a signed spur trail branching left (northwest) to Sixty Lake Basin (see Trip 77).

Stay on the PCT/JMT by curving right (east) here to cross the "isthmus" and the stream (difficult in early season) connecting rockbound Upper Rae Lake with Middle Rae Lake. The route swings north, passes the unmarked, unmaintained lateral to Dragon Lake, and arrives at the many good but overused campsites near the east shore of Middle Rae Lake (10,560´; 11S 375226 4074684, at the bay on Middle Rae Lake's east side). Fishing is good for brook trout and some rainbow. Views from these campsites across the beryl-green lake waters to dramatically exfoliating Fin Dome and the King Spur beyond are among the best and longest remembered of the trip, along with morning views of Painted Lady in the south. A summer ranger is stationed on the east shore of the middle lake.

Campsites at Middle Rae Lake may be very crowded. There are other campsites at Lower Rae Lake and still-lower Arrowhead Lake; mileage to them isn't included in this trip.

DAYS 4–6 (Rae Lakes to Kearsarge Pass Trailhead, 13.5 miles): Retrace your steps.

77 Sixty Lake Basin

Trip Data: 11S 373184 4075273;
33 miles; 6/1 days

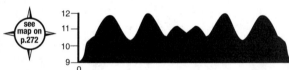

Topos: *Kearsarge Peak, Mt. Clarence King*

Highlights: Sixty Lake Basin is a worthy companion to the nearby Rae Lakes. Its convoluted landscape leads to generally smaller lakes and a more intimate feel than does the open landscape of the Rae Lakes. Each hollow in the granite holds a pleasant surprise: a meadow, a small campsite, a bubbling stream, or maybe your own private lake. And, happily, there is no camping limit for backpackers, as there is at the Rae Lakes (but stock users are limited).

HEADS UP! On the way to Sixty Lake Basin, camping is limited to two nights at the Kearsarge Lakes and Charlotte Lake, and to two nights per lake at the Rae Lakes. Bears are serious problems in this area. The permanent metal food-storage boxes along the PCT/JMT are reserved for through-hikers on the PCT and JMT only. Campfires are prohibited above 10,000 feet.

DAY 1 (Kearsarge Pass Trailhead to Flower Lakes, 2.5 miles): *(Recap: Trip 75, Day 1.)* Find the Kearsarge Pass Trail just past the campground's north end and follow it 2.5 scenic miles generally west up to pretty Flower Lake.

DAY 2 (Flower Lake to Charlotte Lake, 5.5 miles): *(Recap: Trip 76, Day 2.)* From Flower Lake, the Kearsarge Pass Trail turns north and ascends to Heart Lake. Switchback up to an overlook of Big Pothole Lake. Continuing, the trail rises above treeline and traverses to Kearsarge Pass (11,823´; 11S 377167 4070609) and its impressive views.

On the west side of the pass, traverse high above the Kearsarge (camping) and Bullfrog (no camping) lakes. Pass a spur trail branching left to those lakes as the route continues west on a gentle descent. At a fork (10,860´; 11S 373987 4070617) whose branches both go to the PCT/JMT, take the left fork southwest and descend to a sandy flat in a broad saddle overlooking Charlotte Lake. Here is another trail junction (10,750´; 11S 373702 4070326);

you go right to Charlotte, where there is a ranger station and good but heavily used camping on the lake's north side.

DAY 3 (Charlotte Lake to Sixty Lake Basin, 8.5 miles): This is a big hiking day. Spend a restful night at one of the Rae Lakes if you don't feel up to the mileage. See *HEADS UP!* for camping information (page 275).

Retrace your steps to the PCT/JMT. Turn left (north) on the PCT/JMT, switchback over Glen Pass, and zigzag down into the Rae Lakes basin. At a junction (10,550′; 11S 374883 4073915) near the "isthmus" between the first two Rae Lakes, turn left to leave the PCT/JMT and bear northwest toward Sixty Lake Basin. Cross a marshy area and then climb west on switchbacks offering superb views of Rae Lakes. A northwest traverse and some switchbacks end at the lakelet just below the unnamed saddle that is the "pass" into Sixty Lakes Basin. Round the lakelet on its north side, traverse to the saddle (11,200′), and take in the fine view to the west of stark, sharp-peaked Mt. Cotter and Mt. Clarence King before descending on steep, rocky switchbacks to the shore of a lake at almost 11,000 feet with a sandy campsite near its outlet.

Beyond the outlet, round the ridge that separates upper Sixty Lake Basin into east and west sub-basins, and pause to get your bearings near a good campsite (10,762′; 11S 373184 4075273) that overlooks the lake at 10,720 feet, north of the nose of this ridge. Fin Dome serves as a reference point from most of the high, sparsely forested basin.

SIDE TRIPS FROM SIXTY LAKE BASIN

It's a pleasure simply to explore all the nooks and crannies of this basin. Or pay a cross-country visit to remote upper Gardiner Basin and its large, alpine lakes by scrambling west over the low point (col) south of Mt. Cotter from the long, slender lake in western Sixty Lake Basin (locally called "Finger Lake"). Stay high around Finger Lake's north end. Crossing the col at its south end (about 11,656′; 11S 371423 4074123) may be easier than at its north end, but let the land tell you where to go. Once served by a trail and pass on its south side, west of Charlotte Lake, Gardiner Basin is now trailless and seldom visited.

Peakbaggers can try adding Mt. Clarence King and Mt. Cotter to their "trophies" from Sixty Lake Basin, too. Clarence King's autobiographical account of his and Richard Cotter's adventures in the Sierra in the 1860s, *Mountaineering in the Sierra Nevada*, as part of the Whitney Survey party, is still a thrilling and worthwhile read, though it has been said that King tended to embellish things. These noble peaks are named for—surprise—King and Cotter.

DAYS 4–6 (Sixty Lake Basin to Kearsarge Pass Trailhead, 16.5 miles): Retrace your steps.

Mt. Whitney Trailhead

8360′; 11S 389083 4049779

DESTINATION/ UTM COORDINATES	TRIP TYPE	BEST SEASON	PACE (HIKING/ LAYOVER DAYS)	TOTAL MILEAGE
78 Mt. Whitney Summit 11S 384337 4048894	Out & back	Mid to late	5/0 Leisurely	22

Information and Permits: This trailhead is in Inyo National Forest: 351 Pacu Lane, Suite 200, Bishop, CA 93514, 760-873-2400, www.fs.fed.us/r5/inyo/. Quotas apply, and permits are required for overnight stays and are available at Inyo National Forest ranger stations in Lone Pine, Bishop, Mammoth Lakes, and Mono Basin Scenic Area Visitors Center. Wilderness permits are required on the Mt. Whitney Trail. To get a permit to start any trip from Whitney Portal, follow the instructions below.

Reserved Permits: Any hiker intending to enter the wilderness via the Mt. Whitney Trail between May 1 and November 1 should apply during the lottery. There are 60 overnight permits and 100 dayhike permits ($15 per person) awarded for each day of the quota season. Get permit applications online at www.r5.fs.fed.us/inyo/. Applications are accepted only during February. Mail applications to the address above or fax them to 760-873-2484. If you get a place in the lottery, you will receive your trip confirmation by the end of March.

On–Demand Permits: Inyo National Forest will issue on-demand permits beginning the day before your trip starts. Visit the Mt. Whitney Ranger Station (open spring through fall, 8:30 A.M. to 4:30 P.M.) at the south end of Lone Pine on the east side of Hwy. 395. Call the office in Lone Pine on the unlikely chance that the quota for that day is not full: 760-876-6200. If you're planning a trip during the non-quota season, November 2 through April 30, you can self issue a permit at the Mt. Whitney Ranger Station or the Lone Pine InterAgency Visitors Center, about a mile farther south near the southeast corner of the junction of Hwy. 395 and Hwy. 136.

Driving Directions: From the intersection of Hwy. 395 and Whitney Portal Road in the town of Lone Pine—at the town's only traffic light—go 12 miles west on Whitney Portal Road to its end at Whitney Portal (toilets, water, store, café).

78 Mt. Whitney Summit

Trip Data: 11S 384337 4048894; 22 miles; 5/0 days

Topos: *Mt. Langley, Mount Whitney*

Highlights: At 14,491 feet, Mt. Whitney is the highest peak in the contiguous 48 states. Because of that claim—and the fact that the mountain is accessible and offers unparalleled views over the southern Sierra and the Owens Valley—Whitney is also the Sierra's most popular peak. This trip describes the easiest way to backpack the Mt. Whitney Trail.

see map on p.278

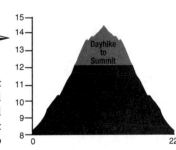

HEADS UP! *Expect to be part of a crowd everywhere along the Mt. Whitney Trail. The Forest Service asks that hikers on Mt. Whitney pack out their solid wastes. Too many people use the trail, and the climate is*

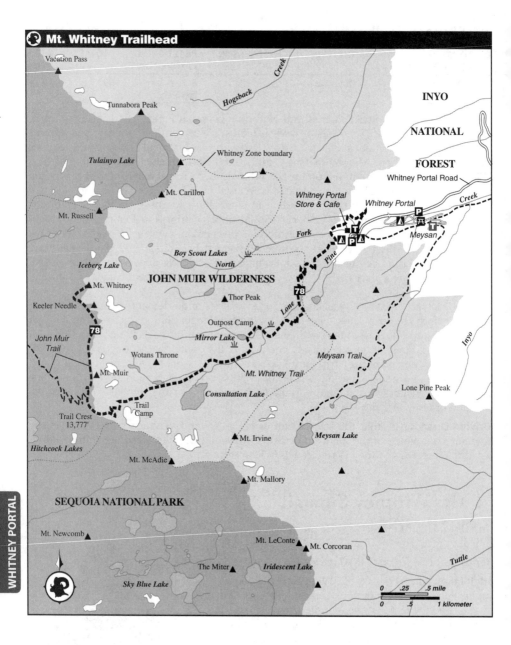

too unfriendly, for burial and biological degradation to dispose of these wastes. Composting toilets, tried for decades, have not proved to be a solution. See www.fs.fed.us/r5/inyo/recreation/wild/ packitout.shtml for how to get the ingenious pack-out kits, use them, and dispose of them.

DAY 1 (Mt. Whitney Trailhead to Outpost Camp, 3.5 miles): From just east of the small store at road's end (8360´), the trail climbs steadily, at first north but soon generally southwest, on seemingly endless, dusty switchbacks through a moderate forest cover of Jeffrey pine and red fir. After a half mile, the trail crosses North Fork Lone Pine Creek and shortly enters John Muir Wilderness. Soon the forest cover thins, and the slope is covered with a chaparral that includes mountain mahogany, Sierra chinquapin, and sagebrush.

Another ford provides a cool nook, a welcome rest stop because this steep slope can get scorching by mid-morning (the trip is best begun as early as possible). Breather stops on this trail section provide a view down the canyon framing the Alabama Hills, the background for hundreds of television shows and movies (including *Tarzan, Superman,* and countless westerns). Then the trail levels off somewhat through willow-clad pockets with a moderate forest cover of lodgepole and foxtail pines. It passes fields of corn lilies, delphinium, and lupine, and, in 1.5 miles, it approaches a ford of Lone Pine Creek.

Beyond this ford is a junction with the signed lateral that leads left (east) to sparkling Lone Pine Lake (campsites), visible from the junction (10,050´). This trip goes ahead on the Mt. Whitney Trail and leads up a barren, rocky wash to switchback up another slope to Outpost Camp (10,365´; 11S 387322 4048144), a lovely, willow-covered meadow that was once a lake. This is the first legal camping area on the Mt. Whitney Trail, and there are several pleasant campsites.

DAY 2 (Outpost Camp to Trail Camp, 3 miles): The trail veers away from the waterfall that tumbles down into Outpost Camp from the southwest, fords Lone Pine Creek, and makes a few switchbacks beside the cascading creek past blossoming creambush, mountain pride,

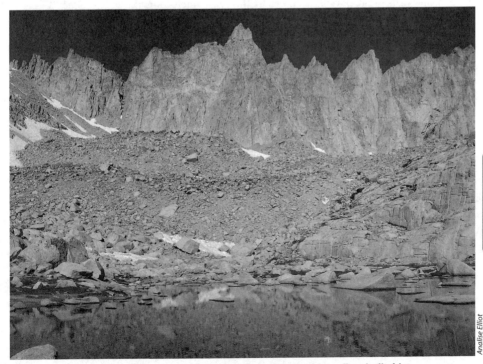

WHITNEY PORTAL

Analise Elliot

To the south of Mt. Whitney are a series of "needles" offering fine big-wall rock climbing.

Indian paintbrush, Sierra chinquapin, currant, pennyroyal, fireweed, and senecio. Just after the trail crosses the outlet stream on rocks, it arrives at Mirror Lake (10,650′), cradled in its cirque beneath the south face of Thor Peak. This cold lake has fair fishing for rainbow and brook trout, but camping is prohibited here.

Leaving Mirror Lake, the trail climbs the south wall of the cirque via rocky switchbacks. Ascending steeply under the north flanks of Mt. Irvine, the rocky trail crosses the south fork of Middle Fork Lone Pine Creek and winds up past giant blocks and granite outcroppings. Looking across the canyon, you'll see the cascading outlet of Consultation Lake.

After ascending again, the trail arrives at the second and last legal camping area on the Mt. Whitney Trail, Trail Camp (12,025′; 11S 385538 4047137). This is the last reliable water on the trail as well as a fine jumping-off point for summiting Mt. Whitney on the layover day. Campsites are very Spartan and crowded together on the stony ground.

Day 3 (Dayhike from Trail Camp to Mt. Whitney Summit and Back, 9 miles): Because of the high elevation and changeable weather of Mt. Whitney's summit, this is not an ordinary dayhike. Be sure your daypack includes survival gear like extra food, water, clothing, rain gear, and a map and compass. Allow plenty of time and don't try to hurry; in air this thin, even the fittest will be gasping. There is no water or shelter at the summit.

Leave Trail Camp behind and head west-southwest to begin the seemingly endless switchbacks to Trail Crest. On this climb, Mt. Whitney disappears behind its needles. The steep, rocky slope up to the crest is not entirely barren, for, in season, hikers may see a dozen species of flowering plants, climaxed by the blue flower clusters of polemonium—the "sky pilot." The building of this trail involved much blasting with dynamite, and the natural fracture planes of the granite are evident in the blasted slabs.

Finally, the 1800-foot ascent from Trail Camp ends at Trail Crest (13,777′), on the boundary between John Muir Wilderness and Sequoia National Park. Hikers suddenly have vistas of a great part of Sequoia to the west, including the entire Great Western Divide. To the east, far below, are several small, unnamed lakes, lying close under the steep faces of Mt. Whitney and Mt. Muir. These lakes may be covered in ice well into summer.

From Trail Crest, the main Mt. Whitney Trail enters Sequoia National Park (no pets or firearms) and descends 100 yards to a junction (13,600′) with the 2-mile lateral to Mt. Whitney's summit. This is the beginning (or end, depending on which way you're traveling it) of the JMT.

The JMT turns right (north) toward the summit and climbs along a barren, exposed ridge past Mt. Muir and Keeler Needle. The going is rocky and rough, but the views are spectacular. Near the summit plateau, multiple use trails zigzag up toward the stone summit hut, east of which is a pit toilet.

The official summit benchmark is a little southeast of the hut (not open to visitors), hammered into a flat boulder. If a storm breaks, stay out of the summit hut and get off the peak! There have been fatalities in the hut due to its metal roof conducting lightning strikes to those who took refuge inside it from storms. Sign the register outside the hut, and then walk around the surprisingly flat plateau and take in the breathtaking views.

The peak was named in 1864 for Josiah D. Whitney, California state geologist and chief of the famed "Whitney Survey" of 1860–74. However, European Americans didn't actually climb it until August 18, 1873, when three fishermen from Lone Pine ascended the southwest slope. They named the mountain "Fisherman's Peak," but it was "Mt. Whitney" that stuck.

Retrace your steps to Trail Camp.

DAY 4–5 (Trail Camp to Mt. Whitney Trailhead, 6.5 miles): Retrace your steps to Whitney Portal.

Cottonwood Lakes Trailhead

10,040´; 11S 395183 4034876

DESTINATION/ UTM COORDINATES	TRIP TYPE	BEST SEASON	PACE (HIKING/ LAYOVER DAYS)	TOTAL MILEAGE
79 South Fork Lakes 11S 390560 4038358	Semiloop	Mid to late	2/2 Leisurely, part cross-country	10.3
80 Upper Rock Creek 11S 385119 4039866	Loop	Mid to late	4/3 Leisurely	23.3

Information and Permits: This trailhead is in Inyo National Forest: 351 Pacu Lane, Suite 200, Bishop, CA 93514, 760-873-2400, www.fs.fed.us/r5/inyo/. Quotas apply, and permits are required for overnight stays and are available at Inyo National Forest ranger stations in Lone Pine, Bishop, Mammoth Lakes, and Mono Basin Scenic Area Visitors Center.

Driving Directions: From the intersection of Hwy. 395 and Whitney Portal Road in the town of Lone Pine—at the town's only traffic light—go 3.5 miles west on Whitney Portal Road to its intersection with Horseshoe Meadows Road. Turn left (south) and head 20 more miles, eventually curving west into Cottonwood Creek's drainage and then curving south again. Turn right at the signed turnoff northward for Cottonwood Lakes and drive another half mile to trailhead parking (one-overnight campground, toilets, and water).

79 South Fork Lakes

Trip Data: 11S 390560 4038358; 10.3 miles; 2/2 days

Topos: *Cirque Peak*

Highlights: With relatively little effort, hikers on this route enter the true High Sierra to find a rugged cirque sur-

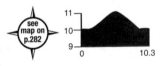

rounded by peaks up to 14,000 feet and filled with lakes, meadows, and streams. The South Fork Lakes, immediately adjacent to the extremely popular Cottonwood Lakes, offer a little more privacy than, yet ready access to, the latter. An easy cross-country section adds excitement to the return route.

HEADS UP! *The first 1.5 miles of trail are not shown on the topo. Don't expect solitude: Large group trips are regularly scheduled here during the summer months. There are no wood fires in the Cottonwood Lakes Basin or at South Fork Lakes. Read and observe regulations for this well-used area. The Mt. Langley topo is helpful for dayhiking old Army Pass to Mt. Langley.*

DAY 1 (Cottonwood Lakes Trailhead to South Fork Lakes, 5.3 miles): From the trailhead, the trail leads west and then north on a gentle and brief ascent through an open stand of lodgepole and foxtail pine. It passes a spur to the equestrian area and soon enters Golden Trout Wilderness. The sandy trail soon begins to descend gently and then levels out. In about 1 mile, cross South Fork Cottonwood Creek. It's often willow-choked, but the more open stretches are ideal for fly-rod casting.

In another half mile, pick up the trail as it's shown on the topo; the junction is imperceptible, the old trail south of it abandoned and overgrown. Skirt the west side of the meadows along Cottonwood Creek and ascend steadily, passing privately operated Golden Trout Camp (10,210´).

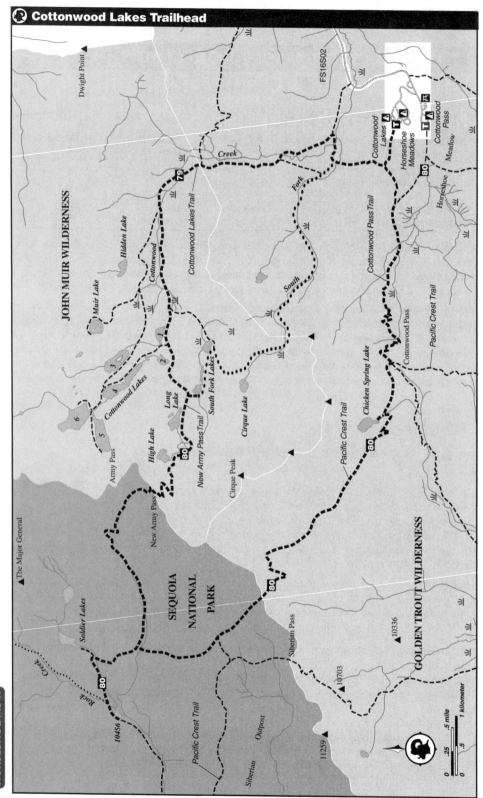

The trail shortly enters John Muir Wilderness and soon crosses Cottonwood Creek (10,260′). Beyond the crossing, the trail swings west, with the creek and its meadows to the southwest. The ascent levels during these stretches.

At the next junction (10,500′), take the left fork south and cross Cottonwood Creek before curving west again. (The right fork is the Cottonwood Lakes Trail.) Now the trail climbs moderately above the creek. Beside a large meadow, reach another junction (10,980′). Here, take the right fork ahead (west) and ascend a forested moraine to a junction at the meadowed west end of the lowest Cottonwood Lake, Cottonwood Lake 1, and to a fine view of Cottonwood Basin and Mt. Langley. Go left (west) here to stay on the New Army Pass Trail.

On the New Army Pass Trail, pass Cottonwood Lakes 1 and 2 (unlabeled on the *Cirque Peak* 7.5′ topo but just west of Lake 1), and then veer southwest through a jumbled area of near-white granite blocks. From the point where the trail turns west-northwest, a short spur trail descends a few yards to the good campsites at the west end of the westernmost South Fork Lake (11,073′; 11S 390560 4038358) in a sparse grove of foxtail pines with fine views of Cirque Peak to the southwest. Oddly, this lake is labeled "Lake 2" on the 7.5′ *Cirque Peak* topo, as if it were Cottonwood Lake 2. It's not; as noted earlier, the real Cottonwood Lake 2 is the lake just west of the labeled "Lake 1."

DAYHIKING AND CAMPING AROUND SOUTH FORK AND COTTONWOOD LAKES

The westernmost South Fork Lake, although the most convenient to New Army Pass, is far from the only place to camp, and, from there, there are numerous places to visit on layover days. There's good fishing at most of them. Here are a few suggestions:

Cottonwood Lakes: Established trails lead to or near all of the nearby Cottonwood Lakes, which are crowded and offer many campsites. Also check out Muir Lake (camping), accessible via a lateral from the Cottonwood Lakes Trail. Peakbaggers may want to attempt Mt. Langley (14,023′; 11S 389032 4042734) from old Army Pass (above the head of Cottonwood Lake #5). The high-altitude meadows in this area are more fragile than they look, so avoid cutting through them; stay on established trail.

Long and High Lakes, Cirque Peak: From the westernmost South Fork Lake, return up the spur trail to the New Army Pass Trail and turn generally west (left). This trail passes Long and then High lakes; there's good camping at Long Lake and a little Spartan camping around fragile High Lake. If you continue to New Army Pass (great views), from there it is a straightforward, 4-mile, out-and-back, Class 2, cross-country detour to bag Cirque Peak, which commands panoramic views. Work southeast and then southwest around the cirque holding Long and High lakes to reach the broad peak (12,805′; 11S 389193 4037546).

Down South Fork Cottonwood Creek: Work your way east-southeast down South Fork Lakes to the largest, easternmost one (fine camping and fishing, more privacy than the westernmost lake), and then follow its outlet creek, South Fork Cottonwood Creek, through meadows and forest as far as you wish for good angling, more solitude, and beautiful scenery. (This is actually part of Day 2's route.)

DAY 2 (South Fork Lakes to Cottonwood Lakes Trailhead, 5 miles, part cross-country):

Although official, mapped, maintained trails don't exist for much of this day's route, the network of use trails pounded out by anglers make for easy cross-country hiking on this day.

From the west side of the westernmost South Fork Lake, the now cross-country route heads south and then east toward the easternmost lake South Fork Lake, skirting the large talus area between the two lakes. Round the south side of the easternmost lake (golden) and pick up a use trail (not shown on the topo) that leads downstream from its outlet.

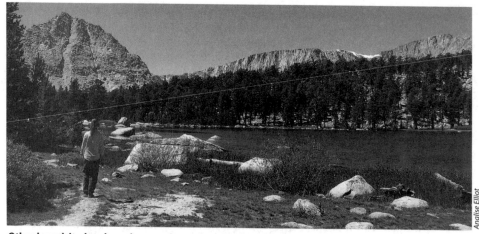

Analise Elliot

Other less visited and scenic campsite options are found at Muir Lake.

Keeping on the north and then the east side of the outlet stream, this route descends over heavily fractured granite past foxtail and lodgepole pines on a slope where the dashing stream cascades and falls from one rocky grotto to the next. Clumps of shooting star, topped by showy yellow columbine and orange tiger lily, line the stream.

The trail levels off in a meadow and then descends into a larger meadow, where the outlet of Cirque Lake joins South Fork Cottonwood Creek. Following the creek's course, swing east and descend steeply in lodgepole forest to traverse another meadow.

Beyond this meadow, the use trail drops steeply again, veers away from South Fork Cottonwood Creek, and rounds the moraine between this fork and the main fork. Then the track goes north up the west side of the main fork of Cottonwood Creek for 0.3 mile to join the trail described in Day 1. Turn right (southwest), ford Cottonwood Creek, and curve south to retrace in reverse the steps of the first part of Day 1.

80 Upper Rock Creek

Trip Data: 11S 385119 4039866; 23.3 miles; 4/3 days

Topos: *Cirque Peak, Mount Whitney, Johnson Peak*

see map on p.282

Highlights: One of the finest circuits in the Sierra, this route travels up an elegant cirque past spectacular peaks, visits lonely alpine lakes and meadowed ponds, and climbs past treeline into desolate moonscapes. The scenery and dayhiking opportunities are spectacular.

HEADS UP! *The first 1.5 miles of trail are not shown on the topo but are shown on the map in this book. Don't expect solitude: Large group trips are regularly scheduled here during the summer months. There are no wood fires in the Cottonwood Lakes Basin, at South Fork Lakes, and within 0.3 mile of Chicken Spring Lake. Read and observe regulations for this well-used area. The Mt. Langley topo is helpful for dayhiking. Away from the trail, especially when exploring Miter Basin, map-and-compass skills and some boulder-scrambling experience are needed. Finally, you can cut almost a mile off Day 4 by setting up a shuttle car at the nearby Cottonwood Pass Trailhead (follow the same driving directions, but instead of turning onto the road to the Cottonwood Lakes Trailhead, continue about a half mile west to the roadend and trailhead parking).*

DAY 1 (Cottonwood Lakes Trailhead to South Fork Lakes, 5.3 miles): *(Recap: Trip 79, Day 1.)* From the trailhead, the trail ascends west and then north , passes a spur to the equestrian area, and soon enters Golden Trout Wilderness. Descend a little, level out, and, in about 1 mile, cross South Fork Cottonwood Creek. In another half mile, pick up the trail as it's shown on the topo. Skirt the west side of Cottonwood Creek's meadows and ascend steadily, passing Golden Trout Camp (10,210'). Enter John Muir Wilderness, cross Cottonwood Creek, and then swing west, with the creek to the southwest.

At the next junction, take the left fork south and cross Cottonwood Creek before curving west again. Climb moderately to reach another junction by a meadow. Take the right fork west, ascend a moraine to a junction at the west end of Cottonwood Lake 1, and find a great view of Cottonwood Basin and Mt. Langley.

Take the left fork west past Cottonwood Lake 2, veer southwest through granite blocks, and, from the point where the trail turns west-northwest, take a short spur a few yards down to at the west end of the westernmost South Fork Lake (11,073'; 11S 390560 4038358).

DAY 2 (South Fork Lakes to Upper Rock Creek, 6.5 miles): From the westernmost South Fork Lake, the trail ascends westward through thinning timber to Long Lake. After skirting the south shore, the route begins a long traverse above the campsites at the west end of the lake. Views of the lake are photographers' favorites, but save some film for the panoramic shots farther up. This traverse takes hikers above treeline as the trail skirts a wet area covered with grass, willows, and wildflowers. Where the trail touches the south edge of High Lake, a pause will brace travelers for the upcoming rocky switchbacks.

The trail soon begins a series of long, gently graded zigzags that climb the cirque wall to New Army Pass (12,300'). The higher the track climbs, the better are the views east to the lakes immediately below and to the Cottonwood Creek drainage.

BAGGING CIRQUE PEAK

From New Army Pass, you can bag Cirque Peak (12,900') with just a little scrambling by following the gently ascending, boulder-strewn plateau to the west in a cross-country arc west and then east to splendid views from the peak's summit. This is about 4 miles out and back.

Descending from New Army Pass into Sequoia National Park, the trail crosses a long, barren slope of coarse granite sand sprinkled with exfoliating granite boulders. A half mile north of the pass, the route passes an unmaintained trail (not shown on the topo map) that branches right to old Army Pass, the original pass built by the army in the 1890s. Beyond this junction, the route swings west and descends steeply over rocky tread to level off on a more gentle descent in a barren cirque. The trail crosses to the north side of the unnamed stream in the cirque and re-enters moderate forest cover.

About 2 miles from New Army Pass, the trail meets a trail to Siberian Pass, and there are good campsites on the south side of the stream just south of this junction. This trip's route turns right (north), continuing to descend through denser lodgepole pine. When the forest gives way to the open spaces of a lovely meadow, the trail fords a little tributary of Rock Creek and turns left (southwest) on the Rock Creek Trail. (If you turned right, in 0.3 level mile you'd reach campsites on both sides of the lower of the unnamed Soldier Lakes—10,794', just southwest of the Major General.)

The trail descends steeply alongside a willow-infested tributary of Rock Creek until the rocky slope gives way to a meadow just above the almost heart-shaped lake on Rock Creek (10,456'; 11S 385119 4039866; golden). There are fair campsites at the head of this meadow, others are located at the lake's outlet, and more primitive ones are to be found on the south side of the lake. Fishing for golden in the lake and adjoining stream is good.

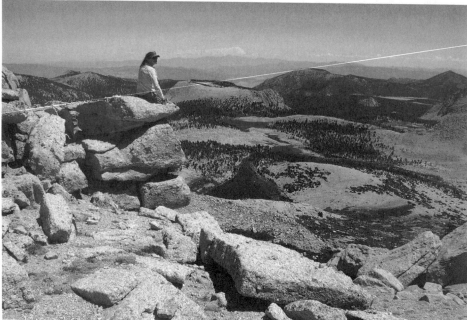

Atop New Army Pass, look east for wide-ranging views of the numerous barren lakes of the Cottonwood Creek drainage.

DAYHIKING FROM UPPER ROCK CREEK LAKE

This marshy-meadowed lake makes a fine base camp for side trips to rugged Miter Basin and adjoining, unnamed Soldier Lakes. A use trail to Miter Basin makes a hard-to-spot exit along the north side of the large, overused campsite just east of Upper Rock Creek Lake's meadow. This trail is easy to follow to the place where Rock Creek cascades out of the basin; from there, it's cross-country. Vast, barren Siberian Outpost, with its fascinating soil colors, is nearby, too; return to the Siberian Pass junction and go right (west) to the next junction, and then head cross-country west into this huge meadow.

DAY 3 (Upper Rock Creek to Chicken Spring Lake, 6 miles): Begin this hiking day by retracing your steps for 1 mile to the meadowed Siberian Pass Trail junction passed during Day 2. Fill your canteens here; this is the last reliable water source before Chicken Spring Lake. From the junction, turn right and ascend gradually southward over a moderately to densely forested slope of foxtail and lodgepole pine. The route crosses a barren area, climbs over an easy ridge and, 1 mile south of the last junction, turns left (southeast) onto the PCT.

Traversing Cirque Peak's southern slopes, the ascending PCT skims the forested eastern fringe of Siberian Outpost before leaving Sequoia National Park for Golden Trout Wilderness at an unsigned boundary on a ridge west of Cirque Peak. The trail soon curves around a meadow below the trail before resuming its southeastward course over a blunt ridge, today's high point at about 11,430 feet.

Beyond, the sandy PCT begins a gradual, view-filled, descending traverse toward the west wall of Chicken Spring Lake's cirque. Follow switchbacks down the wall, and reach that lake (11,258´; 11S 390100 4035262). There's fair camping on its west side and good camping on its east end. This foxtail pine-ringed lake is a very popular stop; you're sure to have company.

DAY 4 (Chicken Spring Lake to Cottonwood Lakes Trailhead, 5.5 miles): Today, you'll come out of the wilderness near the Cottonwood Pass Trailhead (Horseshoe Meadow) and then walk a little less than a mile on roads to close the loop at the Cottonwood Lakes Trailhead.

Return to the PCT and soon curve east toward Cottonwood Pass. Just before the pass, there's a junction where today's route leaves the PCT, going left (west) over the 11,100-foot pass. Descend moderate switchbacks while enjoying views eastward to the Inyo and Panamint ranges.

At the foot of the switchbacks, the eastbound trail skirts north of a small meadow full of willows, paintbrush, columbine, and penstemon. Presently, the path makes two quick stream crossings and then, as it grows quite sandy, begins skirting the north side of large Horseshoe Meadow. Breaks in the lodgepole and foxtail pine forest permit southward and eastward views of Mulkey Pass, Trail Pass, Trail Peak, and over the shoulder to Cottonwood Pass.

At all junctions along this stretch, keep going ahead (generally east) toward the trailhead. By the time the trail passes the signed boundary of Golden Trout Wilderness, only 150 yards remain to the paved Cottonwood Pass Trailhead parking lot (11S 395115 4034251).

Walk eastward through the parking lot and then eastward down the paved road, altogether a little less than a half mile, to the signed junction for the Cottonwood Lakes Trailhead. Turn left (north) here and walk a little over a half mile north and then west to the neighboring Cottonwood Lakes Trailhead (11S 395183 4034876) and your car.

Cottonwood Pass Trailhead
9937'; 11S 395115 4034251

DESTINATION/ UTM COORDINATES	TRIP TYPE	BEST SEASON	PACE (HIKING/ LAYOVER DAYS)	TOTAL MILEAGE
81 Whitney Portal 11S 389095 4049781	Shuttle	Mid to late	7/2 Leisurely to moderate	34.7
82 Milestone Basin 11S 370482 4056261	Shuttle	Mid to late	9/3 Moderate	54.5
83 Rocky Basin Lakes 11S 381814 4034184	Out & back	Mid to late	4/1 Moderate	27

Information and Permits: This trailhead is in Inyo National Forest: 351 Pacu Lane, Suite 200, Bishop, CA 93514, 760-873-2400, www.fs.fed.us/r5/inyo/. Quotas apply, and permits are required for overnight stays and are available at Inyo National Forest ranger stations in Lone Pine, Bishop, Mammoth Lakes, and Mono Basin Scenic Area Visitors Center.

Driving Directions: From the intersection of Hwy. 395 and Whitney Portal Road in the town of Lone Pine—at the town's only traffic light—go 3.5 miles west on Whitney Portal Road to its intersection with Horseshoe Meadows Road. Turn left (south) and head 20 more miles, eventually curving west into Cottonwood Creek's drainage and then veering south again. Don't turn right at the signed turnoff northward for Cottonwood Lakes. Instead, continue ahead about a half mile west to a large parking area for a trailhead on the northeast edge of large Horseshoe Meadow. This is the Cottonwood Pass Trailhead for the Kern Plateau and Golden Trout Wilderness (one-overnight campground, toilets, and water).

81 Whitney Portal

Trip Data: 11S 389095 4049781; 34.7 miles; 7/2 days

see map on p.291

Topos: *Cirque Peak, Johnson Peak, Mount Whitney, Mt. Langley*

Highlights: This adventure is a superb alternative to the straightforward hike up and down Mt. Whitney's east face (Trip 78). This trip, instead, makes a leisurely swing through some of the most memorable scenery in the southeastern Sierra and climbs Whitney by its gentler west face.

HEADS UP! *This trip enters the Mt. Whitney Zone (as far as the JMT and Mt. Whitney Trail are concerned, roughly from Timberline Lake on the west to Lone Pine Lake on the east). Entering the Mt. Whitney Zone requires an additional permit reservation and per-person fee, which you must apply for at the same time you apply for your trailhead permit reservation. See www.fs.fed.us/r5/inyo/recreation/wild/mtwhitney.shtml. Bear canisters are required on the Mt. Whitney Trail.*

The Forest Service asks that hikers on Mt. Whitney pack out their solid wastes. Too many people use the trail, and the climate is too unfriendly, for burial and biological degradation to dispose of these wastes. Composting toilets, tried for decades, have not proved to be a solution. See www.fs.fed.us/r5/inyo/recreation/wild/packitout.shtml for how to get the ingenious pack-out kits, use them, and dispose of them.

Shuttle Directions: From the intersection of Hwy. 395 and Whitney Portal Road in the town of Lone Pine—at the town's only traffic light—go 12 miles west on Whitney Portal Road to its end at Whitney Portal (toilets, water, store, café).

DAY 1 (Cottonwood Pass Trailhead to Chicken Spring Lake, 4.5 miles): The trail heads west, skirting Horseshoe Meadow's north edge, and, in 150 yards, it enters Golden Trout Wilderness. At the head of Horseshoe Meadow, the trail makes two quick stream crossings and climbs gradually to a small meadow. From there, about a dozen switchbacks lead to Cottonwood Pass (11,100′). Views eastward include the Inyo and Panamint ranges, and to the west the more Sierra-like Great Western Divide.

A few feet west of the pass, you come to the famous PCT, and from this junction, turn right (northwest) to stay on the PCT. Follow the PCT for an easy 0.6 mile on level, dynamited footing to the outlet (often dry by late season) of Chicken Spring Lake. Follow the outlet upstream toward good campsites east of and fair campsites west of foxtail-pine-rimmed Chicken Spring Lake (11,258′; 11S 390100 4035262).

DAY 2 (Chicken Spring Lake to Rock Creek Lake, 6 miles): *(Recap in Reverse: Trip 80, Day 3.)* There's no reliable water until Rock Creek, so fill water bottles here. The PCT switchbacks westward up and away from Chicken Spring Lake before it levels off over sandy slopes at Golden Trout Creek's headwaters.

The route presently enters Sequoia National Park on a ridge west of Cirque Peak. At the next junction, turn left (west), staying on the PCT. As the trail descends, there are good views of Mt. Kaweah and the Great Western Divide, as well as large, bleak Siberian Outpost.

The trail descends steadily to a junction where the PCT turns left. Leave the PCT for now by continuing ahead (north) about one more mile to ford a tributary of Rock Creek and then find a junction with the trail that descends from New Army Pass. This trip continues ahead (north) for about another half mile to another junction. Going ahead (north) at this junction leads in a quarter mile to the lower of the Soldier Lakes, southwest of the peak called the Major General, at 10,801 feet (11S 386237 4040491).

But for this trip, turn left (west) and descend steeply and then more gradually along willow-infested Rock Creek toward a lovely lake that's presently visible ahead as a gleaming blue disk in a large meadow. Just before the lake, ford Rock Creek well below its exit from Miter Basin. The lake itself looks almost heart shaped on the topo and offers fair campsites with fine scenery (10,456′; 11S 385119 4039866; golden).

DAY 3 (Rock Creek Lake to Guyot Creek, 4.8 miles): Continue generally west down Rock Creek, fording it in about 1.3 miles. Over the next 1.25 miles, leave the creek, skim a long, patchy meadow while descending a forested slope, and, at a shady junction, meet the PCT again. Go ahead (west) on the PCT to another ford of Rock Creek in another mile. On the south side of the ford, pass through an unattractive, overused camping area.

On the north side of the ford, pass east of an equestrian camping area as the trail begins its long climb northwest and then north to the saddle east of Mt. Guyot known as Guyot Pass. Ascend steeply via forested, rocky switchbacks that afford occasional, spectacular views west over the canyon of the Kern River to the jagged peaks of the Great Western Divide. The PCT levels briefly as it reaches its ford of Guyot Creek, where there are campsites (10,373′; 11S 379725 4040980), here, and upstream, where there's a sizeable meadow.

DAY 4 (Guyot Creek to Guitar Lake, 8.5 miles): Return to the PCT. There's no reliable water between Guyot Creek and Crabtree Meadow, but there's a steep climb, a moderate descent, and a long traverse, all normally dry, so top up on water here.

The jumbled, symmetrical crest of Mt. Guyot takes up the skyline to the west, and highly fractured Joe Devel Peak looms to the east as the PCT begins another steep ascent through lodgepole and foxtail pine. This bouldery climb culminates at Guyot Pass (10,921′; 11S 379139 4042257). From the saddle, the trail descends moderately to the large, sandy basin of Guyot Flat and then traverses the forest east of the flat.

Beyond Guyot Flat, the trail undulates through moderate forest, bobbing over a pair of sandy ridges, before dropping steeply on very rocky switchbacks into the Whitney Creek

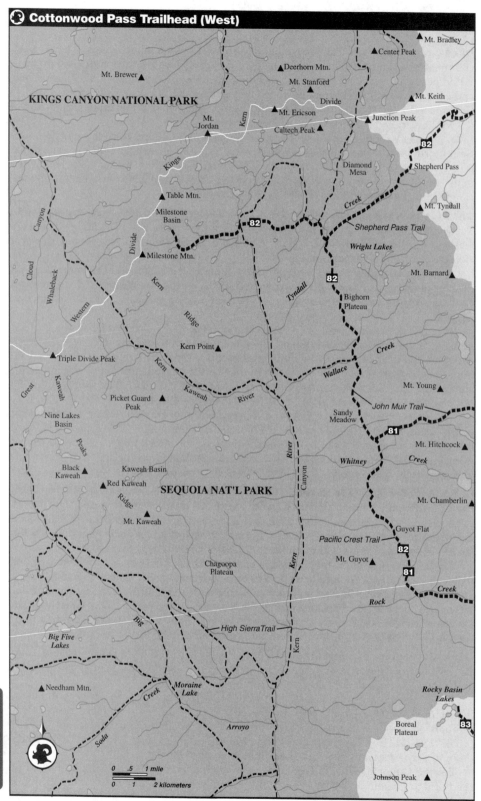

▲ Mt. Bradley

▲ Center Peak

KINGS CANYON NATIONAL PARK

Mt. Brewer ▲

▲ Deerhorn Mtn.

Mt. Stanford ▲

Divide

▲ Mt. Keith

Mt. Ericson ▲

Junction Peak ▲

82

Mt. Jordan ▲

Caltech Peak ▲

Shepherd Pass

Kern

Kings

Diamond Mesa

▲ Table Mtn.

Milestone Basin

Creek

▲ Mt. Tyndall

82

Shepherd Pass Trail

Canyon

Divide

▲ Milestone Mtn.

Wright Lakes

Cloud

Whaleback

Western

Kern

Ridge

Tyndall

82

Mt. Barnard ▲

Bighorn Plateau

Triple Divide Peak ▲

Kern Point ▲

Creek

Wallace

Mt. Young ▲

Great

Kaweah

Peaks

Picket Guard Peak ▲

Kaweah

River

Sandy Meadow

John Muir Trail

81

Nine Lakes Basin

Black Kaweah ▲

Kaweah Basin

Red Kaweah ▲

SEQUOIA NAT'L PARK

River

Canyon

Kern

Whitney

Creek

Mt. Hitchcock ▲

Mt. Chamberlin ▲

Ridge

▲ Mt. Kaweah

Guyot Flat

Pacific Crest Trail

82

Chagoopa Plateau

Mt. Guyot ▲

81

Creek

Rock

Big

High Sierra Trail

Kern

Big Five Lakes

Rocky Basin Lakes

▲ Needham Mtn.

Moraine Lake

Creek

83

Soda

Arroyo

Boreal Plateau

0 .5 1 mile

0 1 2 kilometers

Johnson Peak ▲

HORSESHOE MDW

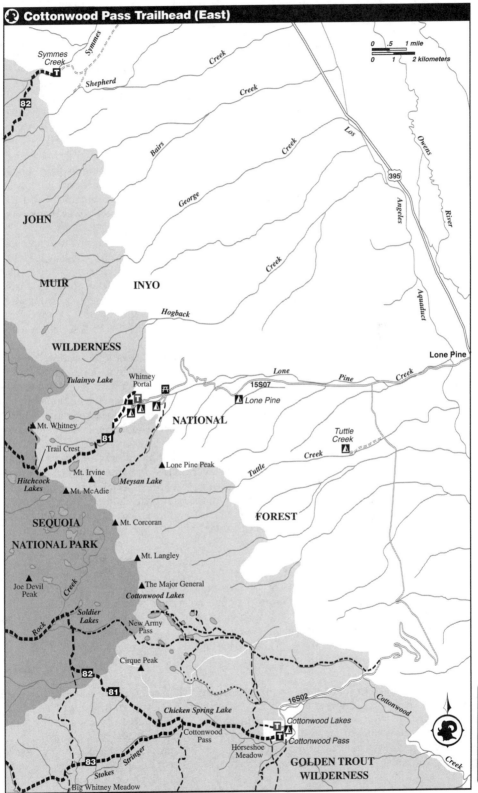

Symmes Creek

Symmes

Creek

Shepherd

Creek

82

Bairs

Creek

Creek

George

Creek

Los

395

Angeles

Owens

River

Aqueduct

JOHN

MUIR

INYO

Hogback

Creek

WILDERNESS

Lone Pine

Tulainyo Lake

Whitney Portal

Lone

Pine

Creek

15S07

Lone Pine

Mt. Whitney

NATIONAL

81

Tuttle Creek

Trail Crest

Lone Pine Peak

Tuttle

Creek

Mt. Irvine

Hitchcock Lakes

Meysan Lake

Mt. McAdie

FOREST

SEQUOIA

Mt. Corcoran

NATIONAL PARK

Mt. Langley

Joe Devil Peak

The Major General

Cottonwood Lakes

Rock

Creek

Soldier Lakes

New Army Pass

82

Cirque Peak

81

16S02

Cottonwood

Chicken Spring Lake

Cottonwood Lakes

83

Stringer

Cottonwood Pass

Horseshoe Meadow

Cottonwood Pass

Stokes

Big Whitney Meadow

GOLDEN TROUT WILDERNESS

Creek

0   .5   1 mile
0   1   2 kilometers

HORSESHOE MDW

GUYOT VIEWS AND GEOLOGY

From Guyot Pass there are good views north across Kern Canyon to the Kern-Kaweah drainage and of Red Spur, Kern Ridge, and the Great Western Divide. Like the Chagoopa Plateau across the canyon, this flat and the subsequent "shelf" traversed later in this hiking day were part of an immense valley floor in preglacial times. However, much of the granular sand deposits are a result of later weathering and erosion of the granite peaks to the east.

drainage. The descent into this drainage affords views eastward to Mt. Whitney—the long, flat-topped, avalanche-chuted mountain that towers over the nearer, granite-spired shoulder of Mt. Hitchcock. After a barren, rocky stretch to lower Crabtree Meadow, the route passes good campsites and then fords Whitney Creek to arrive at a junction. The PCT branches left here, while this trip turns right (east) along Whitney Creek's west bank on a lateral to the JMT/High Sierra Trail, leaving the PCT for good.

A half mile of easy climbing ends at upper Crabtree Meadow, where the route passes the unsigned, almost invisible use trail heading east to the Crabtree Lakes (golden). Continuing northeast beside Whitney Creek, the trail ascends gradually, fords the creek, and climbs to yet another ford. Just before the ford, find a junction with a spur to Crabtree Ranger Station (10,640´; emergency services may be available); there are good campsites along the spur. After crossing the ford, you arrive at a junction with the JMT/High Sierra Trail near good campsites on a rise above the creek (10,646´; 11S 379225 4047359; golden trout).

In order to ease tomorrow's climb of Mt. Whitney, this trip turns right (northeast) at the JMT junction and follows the JMT up Whitney Creek toward Guitar Lake, another 3.8 miles away. Contrary to what's shown on the 7.5´ topo, the JMT stays on Whitney Creek's north side as it ascends through a pretty meadow in another half mile. It's not long before the trail reaches one of the JMT's most popular photo spots, Timberline Lake (golden), with its stunning view and reflection of Mt. Whitney's west face. Timberline Lake is closed to camping and grazing.

Pressing on, hikers continue up the JMT beyond timberline to find campsites around barren Guitar Lake, enormously popular as an overnight stop before tackling Whitney. Because the trail traces Guitar's peninsula, campsites there are especially overused by late season. You may find better sites farther afield: on the rise above Guitar's "neck" (11,488´; 11S 382255 4048082) or on the bench above the lake. Or go cross-country to the Hitchcock Lakes, about 0.6 mile south and southeast of Guitar Lake, where there may be a few campsites.

PRIVACY IN GUITAR LAKE'S VICINITY

The area around and above Guitar Lake is open and barren, with no trees and few large rocks to provide privacy for elimination. In one of the co-authors' personal experience, that means that solid wastes tend to accumulate unpleasantly and unsanitarily in the few nooks and around the few rocks that do provide some privacy. Consider getting and using a pack-out kit in this area; see the information about packing out solid wastes under **HEADS UP!** on page 288.

DAY 6 (Guitar Lake to Trail Camp, 4.4 miles): Get an early start, for even without bagging Mt. Whitney's summit, this is a tough day because of the elevation. If you wish to climb 14,491-foot Mt. Whitney, albeit with a daypack, it is a 4-mile, out-and-back side trip. Top off water supplies; there's no reliable water between Guitar Lake and Trail Camp.

Leaving Guitar Lake, the trail crosses a couple of streams; the first is one Arctic Lake's outlet. The route skirts a large, marshy bench overlooking Guitar Lake as it curves east-southeastward on a gradual-to-moderate ascent to begin climbing Mt. Whitney's west

SUMMIT PREPARATION

It's a good idea to prepare for this day by being ready to drop your backpack at the junction south of the summit and making the summit with a daypack. Take plenty of food and water, extra warm clothes, and wind- and raingear. Avoid the summit if a storm is brewing. If a storm catches you at the summit, stay out of the summit hut, whose metal roof can conduct fatal electrical jolts from lightning strikes to anyone inside.

face. The long, rocky, barren switchbacks begin at a little over 12,300 feet, and while the grade is moderate, the increasing altitude leads to frequent rest stops from which the views just get better and better—reward enough for your labor.

GEOLOGY AND BOTANY ON THE CLIMB

Particularly striking are the views of the Hitchcock Lakes, gemlike and blue-green in a cirque basin that has changed little since its glacier melted. The parallel avalanche chutes on the northeast wall of Mt. Hitchcock, towering above the lakes, all terminate at the upper limit of glacial erosion. Along the switchbacks, the most prominent flower is the yellow, daisy-like hulsea, or alpine gold. No matter how lifeless all this granite gravel appears at first glance, closer inspection always reveals dwarf plants and busy bugs—a bustling world in miniature.

About 2 miles south of the summit, the JMT reaches a junction where it turns left (north) to climb to the summit itself. As described more fully in Trip 78 drop the backpacks, grab the prepared daypacks, and follow this moderate but sometimes rough trail north to the summit. The view-filled route culminates in some messy, indistinct switchbacks, and soon hikers stand on the highest peak in the US outside of Alaska.

AT THE TOP OF WHITNEY

Surprise, Whitney's summit is more like a broad, gently sloping plateau than a point, and the official benchmark is hammered into a large, flat boulder that's a few yards southeast of the summit hut. This is an extraordinary popular spot, and the crowd on Whitney on a summer day may seem unsettling compared the relative solitude of the preceding five days. The summit hut is not open for visitors' use; the register is outside the hut; and there's a pit toilet on the plateau's northern edge. Ignore the crowd and enjoy the 360-degree views, including the abrupt drop on the east past small, high, jewel-like lakes, down almost 11,000 feet to the town of Lone Pine in the Owens Valley. Mt. Whitney's summit is the southern terminus of the JMT.

Retrace your steps to the junction, bid the JMT farewell, put away the daypacks, hoist the backpacks, and turn left (east) on the Mt. Whitney Trail. Ascend about 100 yards to Trail Crest (13,700´), the pass where Sequoia National Park ends and John Muir Wilderness begins.

Begin descending past the crowd ascending the seemingly endless switchbacks, blasted into the granite, that lead 1600 feet down to Trail Camp. Ice and snow can linger all summer on some of these switchbacks, but there are still a surprising number of flowers, especially the fragrant blue "sky pilot" (polemonium) of high altitudes.

The switchbacks finally cease near Trail Camp (12,028´; 11S 385533 4047132), the higher of the two areas where camping is permitted on this trail. There are numerous, crowded, barren, level campsites; dozens of campers; and the first reliable water since Guitar Lake. Wotan's Throne towers on the north, and Mt. Irvine is on the south.

DAY 7 (Trail Camp to Whitney Portal, 6.5 miles): *(Recap: Trip 31, Day 9.)* The Mt. Whitney Trail leaves Trail Camp on an eastward descent carved out of the granite ridge above Consultation Lake, to the south, crossing a small stream and winding through giant boulders. The route presently fords, curves away from, and then curves back to parallel Lone Pine Creek. After a while, the path veers north down the south wall of Mirror Lake's cirque to that lake (10,640´; closed to camping).

Leaving Mirror Lake, the trail crosses the outlet and descends eastward again. It's not long before the path fords Lone Pine Creek again and arrives at Outpost Camp (10,365´) at Bighorn Park, the other area where camping is permitted on this heavily used trail. Quickly skirting this pretty meadow, into which Lone Pine Creek cascades on the west, the trail heads through a rocky wash to a junction with the lateral to Lone Pine Lake (campsites).

Go left (northeast) at this junction, cross Lone Pine Creek again, and soon begin steady switchbacks down the creek's canyon through moderate lodgepole forest. The trail presently breaks out into chaparral and offers views that frame the Alabama Hills. The switchbacks end and the grade eases shortly after the route leaves John Muir Wilderness.

Cross North Fork Lone Pine Creek on a long, descending traverse, returning to forest before angling east and then south to Whitney Portal with its parking lot, café, and small store (8296´; 11S 389095 4049781).

82 Milestone Basin

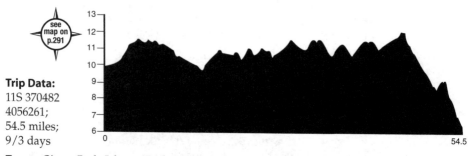

Trip Data:
11S 370482
4056261;
54.5 miles;
9/3 days

Topos: *Cirque Peak, Johnson Peak, Mount Whitney, Mt. Langley*

Highlights: Visit some of the most beautiful and sought-after alpine cirques and lakes in the southern Sierra on this multiday adventure that includes famed Milestone Basin. There's no easy way to reach any of these destinations, so that even if the busy PCT/JMT passes nearby, you'll find relative solitude while exploring them.

Shuttle Directions: From Hwy. 395, take Market Street, which becomes Onion Valley Road, west 4.5 miles from Independence and turn left on signed Foothill Road. Go 1.3 miles to a fork and take the right-hand fork . Go past an old corral on the left, and then immediately cross Symmes Creek. In a half mile, take the right fork, and take the right fork again at the next two forks (they are usually signed; when in doubt, follow the signs to the trailhead). From the last fork, proceed a half mile to the trailhead near Symmes Creek (6423´; 11S 385588 4065119).

DAY 1 (Cottonwood Pass Trailhead to Chicken Spring Lake, 4.5 miles): *(Recap in Reverse: Trip 80, Day 4.)* The trail heads west, skirting Horseshoe Meadow's north edge, and, in 150 yards, it enters Golden Trout Wilderness. At the head of Horseshoe Meadow, the trail makes two quick stream crossings and climbs gradually to a small meadow. About a dozen switchbacks lead to Cottonwood Pass (11,200´). Views eastward include the Inyo and Panamint ranges, and to the west the more Sierra-like Great Western Divide.

A few feet west of the pass, you cross the famous PCT, and from this junction, turn right (northwest) to stay on the PCT. Follow the PCT for an easy 0.6 mile on level, dynamited footing to the outlet (often dry by late season) of Chicken Spring Lake. Follow the outlet upstream toward good campsites east of and fair campsites west of foxtail-pine-rimmed Chicken Spring Lake (11,258´; 11S 390100 4035262).

DAY 2 (Chicken Spring Lake to Lower Rock Creek Lake, 6 miles): *(Recap in Reverse: Trip 80, Day 2.)* There's no reliable water until Rock Creek, so fill water bottles here. The PCT switchbacks westward up and away from Chicken Spring Lake before it levels off over sandy slopes at Golden Trout Creek's headwaters.

The route presently enters Sequoia National Park on a ridge west of Cirque Peak. At the next junction, turn left (west), staying on the PCT. As the trail descends, there are good views of Mt. Kaweah and the Great Western Divide, as well as large, bleak Siberian Outpost.

The trail descends steadily to a junction where the PCT turns left. Leave the PCT for now by continuing ahead (north) about one more mile to ford a tributary of Rock Creek and then find a junction with the trail that descends from New Army Pass. This trip continues ahead (north) for about a half mile to another junction. Going ahead (north) at this junction leads in a quarter mile to the lower of the Soldier Lakes, southwest of the peak called the Major General, at 10,801 feet (11S 386237 4040491).

But for this trip, turn left (west) and descend steeply and then more gradually along willow-infested Rock Creek toward a lovely lake that's presently visible ahead as a gleaming blue disk in a large meadow. The lake itself looks almost heart-shaped on the topo and offers fair campsites with fine scenery (10,456´; 11S 385119 4039866; golden).

> **MITER BASIN**
>
> A dayhike to nearby Miter Basin is always a treat. Here's one route: On the way to Lower Rock Creek Lake, this route passes a hard-to-spot use trail on the main trail's right (north side); this use trail goes northward almost into Miter Basin. The use trail peters out just below the basin; work your way up Class 2 terrain into the basin proper and its unforgettable scenery. The use trail's start is just east of a large campsite that's east of Lower Rock Creek Lake's meadow.

DAY 3 (Lower Rock Creek Lake to Guyot Creek, 4.8 miles): *(Recap: Trip 81, Day 3.)* Continue generally west and downstream, fording Rock Creek, and meet the PCT again. Go ahead (west) on the PCT to another ford of Rock Creek near an overused camping area.

On the north side of the ford, pass east of an equestrian camping area and begin the climb northwest and then north to Guyot Pass. The PCT levels briefly as it reaches its ford of Guyot Creek, where there are campsites (10,373´; 11S 379725 4040980).

DAY 4 (Guyot Creek to JMT Junction, 4.7 miles): Return to the PCT. There's no reliable water between Guyot Creek and lower Crabtree Meadow. The PCT begins another steep ascent culminating at Guyot Pass (10,921´; 11S 379139 4042257). From the saddle, the trail descends moderately to the large, sandy basin of Guyot Flat and then traverses the forest east of the flat.

Beyond Guyot Flat, the trail undulates through moderate forest, bobbing over a pair of sandy ridges, before dropping steeply on very rocky switchbacks into the Whitney Creek drainage. The descent into this drainage affords views eastward to Mt. Whitney. As the route levels, it passes good campsites and then fords Whitney Creek to a junction. The PCT branches left here, while this trip turns right (east) along Whitney Creek's west bank on a lateral to the JMT/High Sierra Trail.

A half mile of easy climbing ends at upper Crabtree Meadow. Continuing northeast beside Whitney Creek, the trail ascends gradually, fords the creek, and climbs to yet another ford. Just before the ford, find a junction with a spur right (northeast) to Crabtree Ranger Station. Across the ford, arrive at a junction with the JMT/High Sierra Trail near good campsites on a rise above the creek (10,646′; 11S 379225 4047359; golden).

DAY 5 (JMT Junction to Tyndall Frog Ponds, 9 miles): Regain the JMT/High Sierra Trail and head west on it and into a foxtail-pine forest. On an overcast day, this foxtail forest, with its dead snags, fallen trees, and lack of ground cover, has an eerie, gloomy, otherworldly quality. The trail switchbacks up (views of Mt. Hitchcock, Mt. Pickering, Mt. Chamberlain, and the flanks of Mt. Whitney) to a junction where this trip rejoins the PCT while also staying on the JMT and High Sierra Trail.

Turn right (north) on what is now the combined PCT/JMT/High Sierra Trail. From the ridge, the route descends gently on a sandy trail through a moderate cover of lodgepole and foxtail to a ford (10,636′) of an unnamed creek. Beginning here the trail skirts what is called Sandy Meadow on the topo map. Small meadowy sections of trail lie beside several little streams not shown on the topo map. In season, look for senecio and monkeyflower.

Beyond, the trail ascends a moderate slope to the saddle marked 10,964′ on the topo. From this saddle, the route descends gently on a sandy trail around the west shoulder of Mt. Young. Leveling off, the trail winds among some massive boulders that make up a lateral moraine, and then leads down a rocky hillside from which there are fine views of Mt. Ericsson, Tawny Point, Junction Peak, the flank of Mt. Tyndall, Mt. Versteeg, Mt. Williamson, and, farthest right, Mt. Barnard.

After fording a tributary of Wallace Creek, the descent becomes gentle again, through moderate forest cover. Beyond the next ford, the descent steepens, and the trail switchbacks a quarter mile down to Wallace Creek (campsites). Just past the ford (very difficult in early season), the High Sierra Trail and the PCT/JMT, which have been conjoined for many miles, diverge. The High Sierra Trail turns left (west) toward Giant Forest and the PCT/JMT continues ahead (north) toward Yosemite and Canada. Nearby is an unsigned use trail east up Wallace Creek (the route to Wallace and Wales lakes). A campsite here or at Wright Creek plus a couple of layover days will allow exploration of nearby Wright Lakes as well as Wallace and Wales lakes.

This trip takes the PCT/JMT north for another 0.8 mile to the ford of Wright Creek (difficult in early season; campsites east of the trail). Several short but taxing ascents separated by level stretches take hikers onto Bighorn Plateau, where the panoramic view begins with Red Spur in the southwest and sweeps north along the Great Western Divide, then east along the Kings-Kern Divide to Junction Peak. In addition, you can see, to the southeast, Mt. Whitney, Mt. Young, and Mt. Russell. A small lake west of the trail presents great photographic possibilities in the morning.

From here, a gradual descent on a rocky trail through a sparse foxtail cover leads to good campsites (11,049′; 11S 376142 4055256) where the trail crosses the outlet of Tyndall Frog Ponds, 0.1 mile east; the ponds offer good swimming in mid- and late season. More campsites—fair ones—are located a half mile farther north just across Tyndall Creek.

DAY 6 (Tyndall Frog Ponds to Milestone Basin, 5.8 miles): Return to the PCT/JMT and continue descending toward Tyndall Creek. At a junction with a little-used trail down Tyndall Creek (the "John Dean Cutoff"), go ahead (roughly north) to meet a junction with the trail over Shepherd Pass. (Note that the topo shows these two junctions in the opposite order; the topo is wrong.) At the Shepherd Pass Trail junction, go left (north) on the PCT/JMT to ford Tyndall Creek (difficult in early season) and find campsites across the creek.

The PCT/JMT continues north to yet another junction, this one with a trail to Lake South America and Milestone Basin. Turn left (north-northwest) toward Milestone Basin on that trail, often called the Milestone Basin Trail; this trail presently curves west. A half mile farther on across alpine fell fields, go left (ahead, west) at the next junction, toward Milestone Basin. (A right turn northward goes to Lake South America.) Views in this upper Kern Basin are always panoramic and unforgettable.

Shortly after the last junction, cross the outlet stream of Lake 11450 (Lake 3490 on the metric *Mt. Brewer* 7.5´ topo; golden). The trail then skirts the north side of a small lake and makes a short, rocky climb to a ridge where the descent to the Kern River begins. From the ridge, enjoy closer views of Thunder Mountain, Milestone Mountain, Midway Mountain—all on the Great Western Divide—and Kern Ridge and Red Spur in the south. Past this viewpoint, the trail descends moderately through rocky and meadowy sections with a moderate cover of foxtail, lodgepole, and some whitebark pine, and arrives at a picture-book lake that is fast (geologically speaking) turning to meadow—the natural fate of all these lakes.

After climbing slightly, your route begins the last, steep descent to the Kern River, where it emerges to meet the Kern River Trail at an unnamed lake at 10,675 feet just west of the trail (about 3250 meters on the *Mt. Brewer* topo; golden and rainbow-golden hybrids).

Turn left (south) on the Kern River Trail to a junction with the unmapped, faint Milestone Basin Trail. This use trail, faint on this east side of the Kern River (more like a big creek here), is much more distinct on the west side. Turn right (west) onto that trail, ford the river (difficult in early season), and begin ascending into Milestone Basin.

On the other side of the river, the trail contours to meet Milestone Creek and then veers west up a rocky slope away from the creek. After a while, it rejoins the creek at a bench where, beside a waterfall, there is a good campsite (about 11,110´; 11S 370482 4056261). Fishing in Milestone Creek is good for rainbow. There are also higher and more Spartan campsites, including at the lakes themselves.

DAY 7 (Milestone Basin to Tyndall Creek, 5.2 miles): Retrace your steps as far as the campsites on Tyndall Creek (10,931´; 11S 375948 4056013).

ALTERNATE ROUTE

Hikers with an extra day or two may want to visit the remote lakes at the Kern River's headwaters. It's a detour of about 6.5 miles. At the junction of the Kern River Trail with the trail that goes right (east) back to Tyndall Creek, instead go ahead (north), following this route as it arcs northeast toward Lake South America, then east, and finally south to rejoin the trail east to Tyndall Creek at the junction just east of the outlet stream from Lake 11450 (Lake 3490). Note that the "trail" over Harrison Pass shown on the *Mt. Brewer* topo doesn't exist.

DAY 8 (Tyndall Creek to Anvil Camp, 7 miles): On the PCT/JMT, ford Tyndall Creek and ascend a little to the Shepherd Pass Trail junction. Turn left (northeast) onto the Shepherd Pass Trail and begin a long, steady ascent up the meadowy, vast, open, boulder-strewn upper basin of Tyndall Creek.

ASCENDING TOWARD SHEPHERD PASS

Views improve constantly as the trail gains elevation, and over-the-shoulder views of the peaks of the Great Western Divide take on new aspects as they are seen from new angles. To the north, the southern escarpment of Diamond Mesa hides an upper surface that is one of the most level areas in this region. The traveler who has read the incredible first chapter of Clarence King's *Mountaineering in the Sierra Nevada* (Bison Books) may speculate on where King and Richard Cotter crossed the Kings-Kern Divide and traversed this basin on their way to ascending Mt. Tyndall—which, in naming it, they believed to be the highest Sierra peak, until they were on top of it and saw other, higher ones nearby.

The path passes the tarn shown at 11,600 feet (3540 meters on *Mt. Williamson* topo) and approaches the lake just below and west of Shepherd Pass (12,002´; 3661 meters on *Mt.*

Williamson). This lake has several chilly, windy campsites and is often half frozen even in midsummer. At Shepherd Pass (12,050′), views of the Great Western Divide spread out behind you; the great Owens Valley is 8000 feet below.

The trail down the first 500 feet of Class 3 talus may be rough; it's infrequently maintained. Often this north-facing slope is covered by a snowfield well into summer, so that hikers descend a ladder of snow pockets rather than unstable talus. When the steepest part of the descent ends, the trail continues through a jumble of huge boulders. Just below treeline, the trail reaches the Pothole, an infamous 500-foot drop-and-gain, and passes an abandoned trail going northwest to Junction Pass (a part of the JMT until Forester Pass was completed).

In another mile, after descending over rough, rocky trail, cross Shepherd Creek for the first time. Presently, in welcome foxtail forest cover, reach good campsites at Anvil Camp (10,000′; 11S 381487 4061493) on either side of the creek. No wood fires are permitted.

DAY 9 (Anvil Camp to Symmes Creek Trailhead, 7.5 miles): Leaving Anvil Camp, descend on good trail through talus. Abruptly, the foxtails end and the path begins a long series of gentle switchbacks through eastside terrain—mountain mahogany and sage, plants of dry slopes—which brings it to Mahogany Flat (9000′ on *Mt. Whitney*; 2800 meters on the *Mt. Williamson*). There are several campsites here, and water if you leave the trail and descend to the creek.

Continuing the switchbacking descent, cross the only year-round creek between Mahogany Flat and Symmes Creek and then pass the burned stubs that were once a mountain mahogany "forest" of very large shrubs. A final stream crossing at 8700 feet (often dry by midsummer) marks the beginning of a discouraging 500-foot ascent. The first steep section of climbing carries you to a small ridge; there is a dry campsite with views that make up for the absence of water. Shepherd Creek has carved a steep canyon to the south, capped by towering Mt. Williamson, the only 14,000-foot peak in the Sierra not on the crestline.

The trail then traverses from Shepherd Creek's canyon into Symmes Creek's watershed by crossing two small ridges, continuing to ascend over slopes so steep they seem to exceed the angle of repose. Frequent rockslides take out sections of this trail. Reach a final welcome but waterless saddle (9200′) with ample campsites set in the trees. From this saddle, the trail descends moderately steeply through western white pine and red fir on switchback after switchback 2240 feet to Symmes Creek, the first water since Shepherd Creek.

Ford Symmes Creek four times as the steep canyon narrows—easy in a dry year or in late summer, but sure to wet feet and threaten footing most of the rest of the time. Between crossings, the trail is overgrown by alders, willows, creamberry bushes, and cottonwoods. A scant quarter mile after the last crossing, the stock trail leaves to the left, and hikers go right (east) to continue another half mile to the Symmes Creek Trailhead (6424′; 11S 385588 4065119).

83 Rocky Basin Lakes

Trip Data: 11S 381814 4034184;
27 miles; 4/1 days

Topos: *Cirque Peak, Johnson Peak*

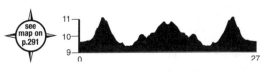

Highlights: The fine angling enjoyed at
the Rocky Basin Lakes makes them a top choice for intermediate hikers who want good recreation and a varied route. Side trips offer further adventure as well as spectacular scenery.

HEADS UP! *Wood fires are not allowed at the Rocky Basin Lakes.*

DAY 1 (Cottonwood Pass Trailhead to Stokes Stringer Campsites, 4 miles): The trail heads west, skirting Horseshoe Meadow's north edge, and, in 150 yards, it enters Golden Trout Wilderness. At the head of Horseshoe Meadow, the trail makes two quick stream crossings and climbs gradually to a small meadow. About a dozen switchbacks lead to Cottonwood Pass (11,100′). Views eastward include the Inyo and Panamint ranges, and to the west the more Sierra-like Great Western Divide.

A few feet west of the pass, you cross the famous PCT, and, from this junction, go ahead (southwest) to descend sagebrush-covered slopes southwest for a half mile to the several fair campsites to the right of the trail above Stokes Stringer.

ALTERNATE DAY 1 DESTINATIONS
Those longing for lakeside campsites can follow Trip 81 to Chicken Spring Lake, adding about a half mile to this trip's Day 1 and again to Day 2. Or, to make Day 2 shorter, continue descending Stokes Stringer to poor campsites around the junction with the Rocky Basin Lakes Trail, as described in Day 2.

DAY 2 (Stokes Stringer Campsites to Rocky Basin Lakes, 9.5 miles): About 20 steep switchbacks are required to get down to a ford of Stokes Stringer. After this, the trail zigzags down a more gentle slope to the eastern precincts of Big Whitney Meadow. Most of the tiny creeks meandering through this enormous grazeland are as unhealthy as they look; purify the water, as usual. After fording Stokes Stringer again, the trail crosses a forested ridge and descends to a muddy ford or two of an unnamed creek. The trail tops another little rise before arriving at a jump-across ford of upper Golden Trout Creek (last reliable water before Rocky Basin Lakes).

Now the sandy path enters forest cover and reaches the Siberian Pass Trail junction. Go ahead (southwest) and stroll 300 yards to a junction from where the Rocky Basin Lakes Trail departs ahead (southwest and west). Take the Rocky Basin Lakes Trail as it begins a moderate ascent through open-to-moderate stands of pine trees. This ascent makes many easy switchbacks on its southwestward traverse of the moraine just west of Big Whitney Meadow and then descends on more switchbacks to a junction and turns right (north) onto the Barigan Stringer Trail.

The ascent of Barigan Stringer, an outlet of the Rocky Basin Lakes, is gentle and then moderate, over increasingly rocky underfooting. The foxtail and lodgepole pine forest cover lining either side of this ravine is a favorite habitat for a great variety of birdlife, including long-eared owl, Steller jay, robin, chickadee, junco, calliope hummingbird, and Clark nutcracker.

Hikers may see a sign at a ford of Barigan Stringer that indicates FOOT TRAIL northwest and HORSE TRAIL west. The indistinct, unmapped foot trail offers a shorter but steeper scramble over a rocky, foxtail-clad ridge above Barigan Stringer, past a wedge-shaped lakelet, to the largest lake. The distinct, longer horse trail, shown on the topo map, winds

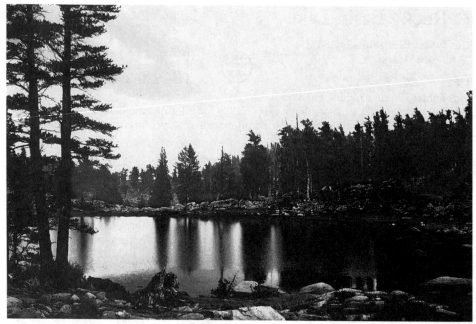

One of the Rocky Basin Lakes

over a ridge and emerges at the east end of the westernmost Rocky Basin lake. From there, it rounds the middle lakes and descends to the west side of the largest lake (10,777´; 11S 381814 4034184). There are more secluded campsites on the northeast side of the lake. Fishing is good for rainbow. The north and west walls of this cirque basin are heavily fractured granite and are a haven for marmots. Nearby Johnson Lake and the Boreal Plateau with Funston Lake offer adventurous cross-country goals.

DAYS 3–4 (Rocky Basin Lakes to Cottonwood Pass Trailhead, 13.5 miles): Retrace your steps.

Blackrock Trailhead

8971´; 11S 385863 4004218

DESTINATION/ UTM COORDINATES	TRIP TYPE	BEST SEASON	PACE (HIKING/ LAYOVER DAYS)	TOTAL MILEAGE
84 Redrock Meadows 11S 385332 4015214	Semiloop	Mid to late	3/1 Moderate	20

Information and Permits: This trailhead is in Inyo National Forest: 351 Pacu Lane, Suite 200, Bishop, CA 93514, 760-873-2400, www.fs.fed.us/r5/inyo/. Permits are required for overnight stays and are available at Inyo National Forest ranger stations in Lone Pine, Bishop, Mammoth Lakes, and Mono Basin Scenic Area Visitors Center. Permits are also available at the information station along Blackrock Road on the way to the trailhead. There are no quotas at this time.

Driving Directions: From Hwy. 395 south of Olancha and north of the junction with Hwy. 178, turn west on the signed County Road 152 to Kennedy Meadows. Drive this paved, sometimes narrow road up into the southern Sierra 23.5 miles to its intersection with Beach Meadows Road (Forest Road 21S02). Turn left (northwest) onto paved Beach Meadows Road and pass a general store. Continue 16.4 more miles to the intersection of Beach Meadows Road and paved Blackrock Road; turn right (north) and in 0.2 mile pass Blackrock Information Station (administered by Sequoia National Forest) on the right (information and permits when open; pit toilets). Continue 7.8 more paved miles to Blackrock Trailhead, with parking for hikers and equestrians, a one-overnight campground, a pit toilet, and water.

84 Redrock Meadows

Trip Data: 11S 385332 4015214; 20 miles; 3/1 days

Topos: *Casa Vieja Meadows, Kern Peak*

Highlights: Great variations characterize this

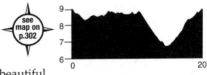

semiloop: Lovely meadows and streams lead to beautiful Redrock Meadows beneath the copper-colored monolith called Indian Head. From there, the descent of Redrock Creek leads through tragic fire devastation to the remote oasis of Jordan Hot Springs.

DAY 1 (Blackrock Trailhead to Redrock Meadows, 9.5 miles): Under a moderate canopy of red firs, head north from the roadend gate, passing signs and a hikers' sign-in box (please sign in here). Almost immediately, meet a dusty trail merging from the right from the equestrian parking; this trip continues ahead (north) on the merged, sandy trail, gradually climbing past the occasional fire-scorched tree.

The path shortly enters Golden Trout Wilderness at Blackrock Gap and begins a gradual-to-moderate descent toward Casa Vieja Meadows. Soon, a large meadow appears on the right (east) through the trees, and the trail presently crosses the meadow's seasonal creek, a tributary of Ninemile Creek, on a little bridge. With the creek now on the left (west), the trail continues downward near the creek as the fir and lodgepole forest closes in.

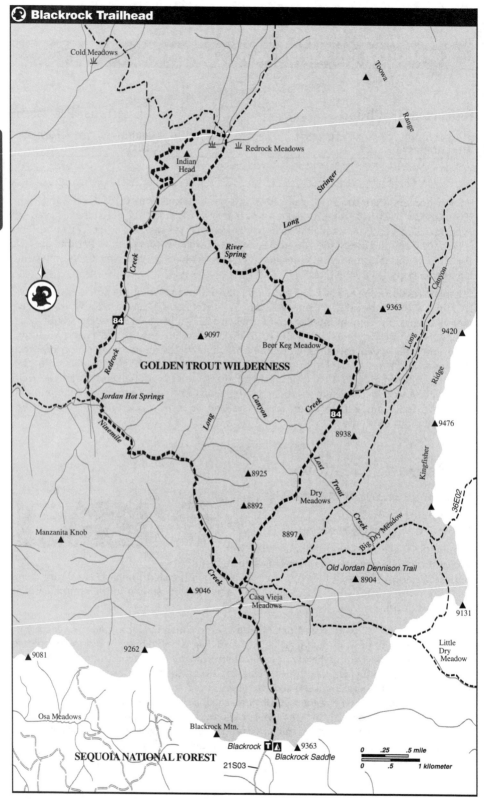

KENNEDY MDWS

Cold Meadows

Toowa

Range

Redrock Meadows

Indian
Head

Stringer

Long

River
Spring

Creek

84

▲9363

Long

Canyon

▲9420

GOLDEN TROUT WILDERNESS

▲9097

Beer Keg Meadow

Redrock

Jordan Hot Springs

Long

Canyon

Creek

84

8938▲

Long

Ridge

▲9476

Ninemile

▲8925

Lost

Trout

Kingfisher

36E02

▲8892

Dry
Meadows

Creek

Manzanita Knob
▲

8897▲

Big Dry Meadow

Old Jordan Dennison Trail

▲8904

Creek

▲9046

Casa Vieja
Meadows

▲9131

Little
Dry
Meadow

▲9081

9262▲

Osa Meadows

Blackrock Mtn.
▲

SEQUOIA NATIONAL FOREST

Blackrock T ▲
Blackrock Saddle

21S03

▲9363

| 0 | .25 | .5 mile |
| 0 | .5 | 1 kilometer |

At 1.5 miles, huge Casa Vieja Meadows opens up on the right (north) as the route steps over one and then another of Ninemile Creek's tributaries before bearing west to skirt the meadow, which is partly fenced. It's not long before the trail bends north through cowpies to an old corral and two more tumbledown buildings to a good view of the meadow, its weathered buildings, its grazing cattle, and its excellent seasonal flowers (if the cattle haven't eaten them). There are possible campsites on the granite sand under lodgepoles here and on the other side of the next tributary that the route shortly fords. "Intersecting trails" shown on the 7.5′ topo aren't apparent on the ground here.

At 2 miles, still on the edge of Casa Vieja Meadows, the trail drops to Ninemile Creek proper at a stock ford; look for a crude log bridge just downstream. The loop part of this trip begins on the other side of the stock ford at a junction signed for Jordan Hot Springs with trails left (northwest) to Jordan Hot Springs and right (northeast) to Redrock Meadows (8300′; 11S 385457 4007078 (field); mislabeled "Redrocks Meadows" on the 7.5′ topo).

Take the right fork and, in 125 yards, pass another trail sign (8334′; 11S 385636 4007164 (field)): ahead (north) toward Redrock Meadows and right (northeast) toward Monache Meadows. Go ahead on this sandy trail as it traces a dwindling, north-trending arm of Casa Vieja Meadows. From here, it's an enjoyable, varied, and gradual-to-moderate walk to Redrock Meadows. Along the way, the route undulates over low, forested ridges, through spectacular meadows, and across mostly small creeks. Campsites near the route are plentiful when water permits, so it's easy to break this long day by camping along this 7.5-mile stretch.

Beyond Casa Vieja Meadows, the trail winds between gravelly knolls and then crosses a tributary of Lost Trout Creek on a rickety bridge. Soon, the path crosses a low, bouldery ridge and climbs past a sign pointing destinations along it: Redrock Meadows, Casa Vieja Meadows, and (not on this trip) Long Canyon. Keep a lookout for apparent trail forks from here to Redrock Meadows: Typically, they're just alternate routes that split and soon rejoin (e.g., horses take one fork, hikers the other); sometimes, one's a use trail to a campsite.

Soon, the route wanders across the meadow of Lost Trout Creek, fording and then bridging it. It's not long before the track crosses the next ridge, at first through chunks of white quartz. The trail descends to a junction on the south bank of Long Canyon Creek (8475′; 11S 387389 4010327 (field)): right (east-northeast, upstream) to Long Canyon; left (briefly northeast, then north-northeast) to ford the creek (may be difficult in early season).

Go left across the creek and continue toward Redrock Meadows, tracing a tributary of Long Canyon Creek northward before winding over another ridge and curving through

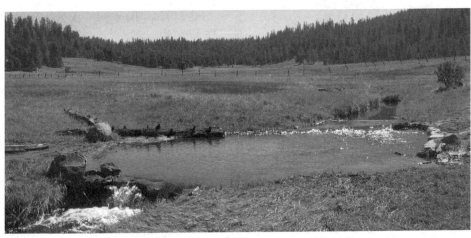

Kathy Morey

Stock crossing in Casa Vieja Meadow

and then above Beer Keg Meadow and its Long Canyon Creek tributary. Ahead lie more low ridges, another tributary, and then the drainage of Long Stringer (itself a tributary of Long Canyon Creek). Meadows along this stretch can be especially lush and flowery.

Traverse yet another ridge before descending to the forested nook from which River Spring emerges, its strong flow nourishing a downstream meadow. On the far side of the next little ridge, another "trail junction" shown on the topo again doesn't seem to exist anymore. However, the view across the hillside meadow reveals a fairly distinct line between the McNally "Incident's" devastation (extending down Redrock Creek's canyon) and the lightly forested area above. It's a sobering glimpse of things to come.

McNALLY "INCIDENT"

From July 21 to August 29, 2002, a wildfire that began near the Kern River raged, eventually burning 150,670 acres—one of the largest Sierra fires in history. A long drought had left forests ready to burst into flame; in the Sierra, most forest managers had already declared open fires forbidden, even in established campgrounds. Flouting this posted regulation, a mother built a campfire to cook dinner for her kids; the fire got out of control....You'll see the devastation while descending Redrock Creek. There, the fire burned so hot that it sterilized the soil, consuming tree seeds that might have reforested the region more quickly. For now, only scrubby vegetation has taken hold. Fire regulations: They're not just advisories. Follow them religiously!

It's not long before the trail curves around Redrock Meadows' west side, fording a fork of Redrock Creek with a wonderful view over the meadow toward the formation called Indian Head.

INDIAN HEAD

This formation gets its name from its color, which reminded early European-American visitors of a penny's color. Back then, the penny was stamped with a Native American's profile—the famous and now prized "Indian Head" penny, produced from 1859 to 1909. Perhaps some visitors even imagined they could make out a profile in the formation.

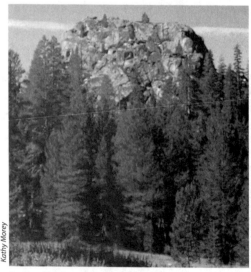

Kathy Morey

Indian Head over Redrock Meadows

The next sandy rise (good campsites) has a trail junction positioned between an old corral downhill and a ruined cabin uphill: The right fork goes northeast toward Templeton Meadows, while the left goes deeper into Redrock Meadows and (eventually) to Cold Meadows and the Kern River. Go left, ford a tributary, and find another junction where the right fork goes northwest to Cold Meadows; this trip takes the left fork as it curves west over a sandy flat with abundant campsites (8660´; 11S 385373 4014711) on the northeast edge of Redrock Meadows. This is the last good opportunity to camp before Jordan Hot Springs. Just northeast of this flat is a large, year-round tributary.

DAY 2 (Redrock Meadows to Jordan Hot Springs, 5.2 miles): Much of this day consists of the sunstruck, 2300-foot descent to Jordan Hot Springs—easier as a descent than an ascent.

Heading east-northeast, ford the tributary (may be difficult in early season; in late season, it's the last reliable chance for water before the first ford of Redrock Creek, 2 miles ahead). Follow the track westward through dense forest before tracing it across the meadow's northwest arm. It's so faint here that there's a sign to point it out. On the other side, ascend some 200 feet to a saddle behind Indian Head (reportedly Class 3 from here by the easiest route).

Begin the 2300-foot descent of Redrock Creek on a series of long, sometimes steep switchbacks under sparse, partly scorched forest. Be alert at the switchback turns; from some of which use trails extend misleadingly. Near the end of the last, very long switchback leg, pass below a clump of aspens as you near the creek. Follow the track as it veers sharply left toward the creek and drops very steeply to the first ford (if you're doing this trip in reverse, this is the last reliable chance for water before Redrock Meadows).

On the other side, by some large boulders, ignore a use trail that climbs steeply away from the creek; instead, curve right and downstream with the main trail as it continues its descent. The trail clings to the creek as far as the next ford, which comes up soon.

The trail climbs away from the creek now and soon wanders through some very meadowy spots as it intersects several springs. Enjoy these last bits of shade, for soon the path enters the burnt, sterilized zone, where lifeless, blackened sticks, soon to join the already ample deadfall, make camping impossible because it is too dangerous. Shortly, the path passes above a beautiful waterfall that's worth an admiring pause as the route continues downstream from it.

In this area, not only are all the burned trees dead, but new trees—seedlings—are, so far, completely absent. Clumps of manzanita and buckthorn sprout here and there, sometimes threatening to engulf the track, which can be sizzling hot on a sunny day. The trail presently rises high above the creek and strays westward away from it, occasionally through foamy patches of delicate white gayophytum—for now, a rare touch of beauty in the midst of so much destruction.

Near Jordan Hot Springs, ford a tributary and then angle southeast to cross Redrock Creek for the last time. (A junction shown on the topo between the tributary and the main creek doesn't exist.) Descending gradually southeast, the trail crosses some runoff channels and enters live forest as it skims the soggy meadow to the southwest on Ninemile Creek's north bank.

At a junction below Point 9097T, the right fork goes west into the meadow, where it disappears briefly, and down Ninemile Creek toward the Kern River. There are some poor campsites around here; better ones lie across the creek. Your route goes ahead (southeast) on the left fork, crosses Ninemile Creek on a bridge of two flattened logs, and reaches the vicinity of Jordan Hot Springs.

JORDAN HOT SPRINGS RESORT

For many years before the establishment of Golden Trout Wilderness, concessionaires operated a very rustic hot springs resort here on a Forest Service lease. While the lodgings consisted of dirt-floored wooden shacks with iron cots (you brought your own sleeping bag), the main lodge building housed a restaurant widely known for its wonderful views and delicious, hearty meals. Rickety bathhouses on the edge of Ninemile Creek sheltered shallow tubs where visitors could relax in the springs' warm waters. By the time the lease last expired, the resort was within the wilderness, and there was no provision for renewing the lease. Consistent with wilderness-management policies, the resort ceased operation in 1990 when the lease expired. The Forest Service has since removed all but a few of its buildings, keeping only those deemed historically significant (look for their bright metal roofs up on the hillside).

The trail, temporarily heading away from the creek, reaches an incense-cedar forested flat with a decaying cabin and packer campsite. The McNally Fire spared this immediate area and its meadows, so look for good campsites around here (6545´; 11S 383106 4010127). The footprints of a few of the old bathhouse tubs, filled with algae-scummed water, still exist downstream on this south bank of Ninemile Creek; follow use trails to find them—on cool mornings, look for steam rising from them. There's reportedly fishing for golden trout in the creek.

DAY 3 (Jordan Hot Springs to Blackrock Trailhead, 5.3 miles): Today's leg consists of the 2400-foot climb back to the trailhead; much of the climb is well-shaded by forest that large-ly escaped the McNally Fire. The climb between Jordan Hot Springs and Casa Vieja Meadows is the steeper part.

Leaving the vicinity of the old resort behind, you'll encounter a junction with a signed spur to a public pasture; continue left (southeast) on the main trail. Soon, the trail begins its climb of Ninemile Creek's narrow canyon to Casa Vieja Meadows. Through a forest of fir, pine, and incense-cedar that's partly burned, the track drops to the next ford of Ninemile Creek (may be difficult in early season). Resume the moderate ascent under shade, crossing a couple of tributaries that support hillside meadows.

Presently, the route fords Ninemile Creek again (difficult in early season). In about 0.8 more mile, in a thicket of red osier dogwood, the trail fords one of Ninemile Creek's major tributaries, Long Canyon Creek, which you first crossed on Day 1. This ford may also be difficult in early season. Continuing, the path crosses more but smaller tributaries, and the number of charred trees diminishes to almost none.

The next ford may be troublesome in early season and leads to a couple of switchbacks that carry the trail high above Ninemile Creek for a while and over more tributaries. The showy, seasonal flower gardens along this stretch include lupine, groundsel, meadow rue, ranger's button, leopard lily, potentilla, lavender asters, skyrocket, bitter cherry, currant, fireweed, madia, and gayophytum.

Close the loop part of this trip on the west edge of Casa Vieja Meadows at the junction from which, on Day 1, you headed northwest toward Redrock Meadows. Turn right (south), find the crude log bridge over Ninemile Creek just downstream of the stock ford, and retrace your steps to the trailhead from here.

INDEX

ABOUT THE AUTHORS

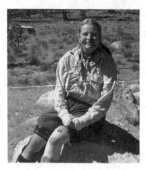

Kathy Morey

The backpacking bug hit Kathy Morey hard in the 1970s and hasn't let go yet. In 1990 she abandoned an aerospace career to write for Wilderness Press, authoring four hiking guides on Hawaii, *Hot Showers, Soft Beds, and Dayhikes in the Sierra,* and *Guide to the John Muir Trail.* She was a co-author of several previous editions of *Sierra North* and *Sierra South.* For the 8th edition of *Sierra South,* Kathy served as lead author. Kathy lives in Mammoth Lakes, California.

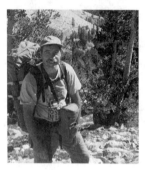

Mike White

Mike White was born and raised in Oregon and learned to hike in the Cascades. In the early 1990s, he began writing about the outdoors full time, and he has since written or contributed to almost a dozen Wilderness Press books, including *Afoot & Afield Reno-Tahoe, Kings Canyon National Park, Sequoia National Park,* and *Top Trails Lake Tahoe.* He also has written for *Sunset* and *Backpacker* magazines and the *Reno Gazette-Journal.* Mike lives in Reno and teaches backpacking and snowshoeing at Truckee Meadows Community College.

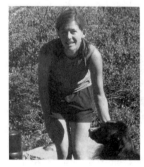

Stacy Corless

Stacy Corless is a writer and hiker based in Mammoth Lakes, California. She helped update the ninth edition of *Sierra North.*

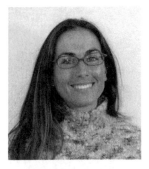

Analise Elliot

Analise Elliot is an avid hiker, surfer, bird-watcher, and backpacker. She holds a bachelor's degree in forestry from the University of California, Berkeley, and she has worked as a naturalist, environmental educator, and outdoor education program director along the California coast and Sierra Nevada. She currently directs a nature and environmental studies program at a school in Mill Valley, California. She is also the author of *Hiking & Backpacking Big Sur*.

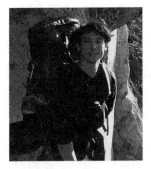

Chris Tirrell

The Sierra Nevada has always had a strong influence on Chris Tirrell, and he can often be found climbing up or riding his snowboard down a peak in the backcountry. He lives in Berkeley, California, and this is the first book he has contributed to for Wilderness Press.

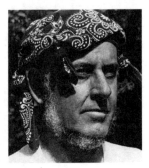

Thomas Winnett

Thomas Winnett founded Wilderness Press in 1967 with the publishing of *Sierra North*, his first guidebook. During his more than 30 years as publisher, he also wrote numerous books on how to backpack and where to hike in the wild areas of the western United States. He is now retired and lives with his wife, Lu, in Berkeley, California.

Books to the Sierra Nevada from Wilderness Press

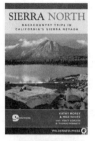

Sierra North

This completely revised and updated classic—the companion to *Sierra South*—showcases new trips and old favorites. With trips organized around major highway sections, using this guide is easier than ever.
ISBN 978-0-89997-396-8

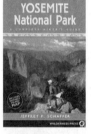

Yosemite National Park

Called the "Cadillac" of Yosemite books by the National Park Service. It details 83 trips, from dayhikes to extended backpacks and includes a foldout 4-color topographic map of the entire park.
ISBN 0-89997-383-3

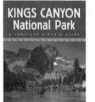

Kings Canyon National Park

An information-packed guide to the peaks and gorges of the majestic apex of the Sierra Nevada. Includes detailed maps, comprehensive trail descriptions, and enlightening background chapters.
ISBN 978-0-89997-335-7

Sequoia National Park

A comprehensive hiker's guide to 62 trips in the national park, plus information on campgrounds, outfitters, and facilities in the park and its surrounding areas.
ISBN 0-89997-327-2

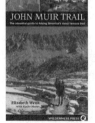

John Muir Trail

The best guide to the legendary trail that runs from Yosemite Valley to Mt. Whitney. Written for both northbound and southbound hikers and includes updated 2-color maps from Tom Harrison.
ISBN 978-0-89997-436-1

For ordering information, contact your local bookseller or Wilderness Press www.wildernesspress.com